MANAGEMENT OF END-STAGE HEART DISEASE

MANAGEMENT OF END-STAGE HEART DISEASE

Editors

Eric A. Rose, M.D.
*Valentine Mott/Johnson and Johnson
Professor and Chairman
Department of Surgery
Columbia University College
of Physicians and Surgeons;
Surgeon-in-Chief
Columbia-Presbyterian Medical Center
New York, New York*

Lynne Warner Stevenson, M.D.
*Director, Heart Failure and
Cardiomyopathy Program
Cardiovascular Division
Department of Medicine
Brigham and Women's Hospital;
Associate Professor of Medicine
Harvard Medical School
Boston, Massachusetts*

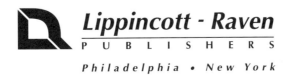

Lippincott - Raven
PUBLISHERS
Philadelphia • New York

Acquisitions Editor: Ruth W. Weinberg
Developmental Editor: Ellen DiFrancesco
Manufacturing Manager: Dennis Teston
Production Manager: Robert Pancotti
Production Editor: Loretta Cummings
Cover Designer: Marsha Cohen
Indexer: Dorothy Hoffman
Compositor: Lippincott–Raven Desktop Division
Printer: Maple Press

Printed in the United States of America

9 8 7 6 5 4 3 2 1

Library of Congress Cataloging-in-Publication Data
Management of end-stage heart disease / editors, Eric A. Rose, Lynne Warner Stevenson.
     p. cm.
    Includes bibliographical references and index.
    ISBN 0-316-75697-0
    1. Heart failure—Surgery. 2. Heart failure—Treatment. I. Rose, Eric A.
II. Stevenson, Lynne Warner.
    [DNLM: 1. Heart Diseases—surgery. 2. Cardiac Surgical Procedures. 3. Heart-Assist Devices.
    4. Heart Transplantation. 5. Heart Diseases—drug therapy. WG 169 M266 1998]
    RD598.M25 1998
    617.4'12--dc21
    DNLM/DLC
    for Library of Congress   98-15838
                                  CIP

To all the patients and their families,
who play the leading roles upon the end stage of heart failure

Contents

SECTION I: DEFINING THE PROBLEM

Lynne Warner Stevenson

SECTION II: MEDICAL THERAPY FOR CONGESTIVE HEART FAILURE

Lynne Warner Stevenson

Contributing Authors

René J. Alvarez, Jr., M.D. *Assistant Professor of Medicine, Department of Medicine, Division of Cardiology, University of Pittsburgh Medical Center, 200 Lothrop Street, S-560 Scaife Hall, Pittsburgh, Pennsylvania 15213*

Michael Argenziano, M.D. *Fellow in Cardiothoracic Surgery, Division of Cardiothoracic Surgery, Columbia University College of Physicians and Surgeons, 630 West 168th Street, New York, New York 10032*

John H. Artrip, M.D. *Research Fellow, Cardiac Transplantation, Department of Surgery, Columbia University College of Physicians and Surgeons, 177 Fort Washington Avenue, 7-435, New York, New York 10032*

Steven F. Bolling, B.S., M.D. *Professor of Surgery, Department of Surgery, Section of Thoracic Surgery, University of Michigan Hospitals, 1500 East Medical Center Drive, 2120D Taubman Center, Box 0344, Ann Arbor, Michigan 48109-0344*

Maria Rosa Costanzo, M.D. *The John H. and Margaret V. Krehbiel Professor of Cardiology, Department of Medicine, Rush-Presbyterian–St. Luke's Medical Center, 1725 West Harrison, Room 439, Chicago, Illinois 60612*

Roger W. Evans, Ph.D. *Section of Health Services Evaluation, Mayo Clinic, 200 First Street, Southwest, Rochester, Minnesota 55905*

Arthur M. Feldman, M.D., Ph.D. *Harry S. Tack Professor of Medicine, Department of Medicine, Division of Cardiology, University of Pittsburgh Medical Center, 200 Lothrop Street, S-572 Scaife Hall, Pittsburgh, Pennsylvania 15213*

Gary S. Francis, M.D. *Director, Coronary Intensive Care Unit, Department of Cardiology, Cleveland Clinic Foundation, 9500 Euclid Avenue, Cleveland, Ohio 44195*

O. Howard Frazier, M.D. *Professor of Surgery, Department of Surgery, University of Texas Medical School, 6431 Fannin, Houston, Texas 77030*

Victor Gil, M.D. *Cardiomyopathy and Transplant Center, Temple University Hospital, 3401 North Broad Street, Parkinson Pavilion, Suite 900, Philadelphia, Pennsylvania 19140-5103*

Daniel J. Goldstein, M.D. *Fellow in Cardiothoracic Surgery, Division of Cardiothoracic Surgery, Columbia University College of Physicians and Surgeons, 630 West 168th Street, New York, New York 10032*

Silviu Itescu, M.D. *Assistant Professor, Division of Surgical Sciences, Department of Surgery, Columbia University College of Physicians and Surgeons, Director, Transplant Immunology, Department of Surgery, Columbia-Presbyterian Medical Center, 622 West 168th Street, New York, New York 10032*

Vigneshwar Kasirajan, M.D. *Resident, Department of Cardiovascular Surgery, Cleveland Clinic Foundation, 9500 Euclid Avenue, Cleveland, Ohio 44195*

John A. Kern, M.D. *Assistant Professor of Surgery, Department of Surgery, Division of Thoracic and Cardiovascular Surgery, University of Virginia Health System, Jefferson Park Avenue, Charlottesville, Virginia 22908*

Irving L. Kron, M.D. *William H. Muller Jr. Professor of Surgery, Department of Surgery—TCV, University of Virginia Health System, Lee Street, Room 275, Charlottesville, Virginia 22908*

Robert T. V. Kung, Ph.D. *Senior Vice President of Research and Development, ABIOMED, Inc., 24 Cherry Hill Drive, Danvers, Massachusetts 01923*

George J. Magovern, Sr., M.D. *Department of Thoracic Surgery, Allegheny University Hospitals-Allegheny General, 320 East North Avenue, Pittsburgh, Pennsylvania 15212-4772*

George J. Magovern, Jr., M.D. *Professor of Surgery, Department of Thoracic Surgery, Division of Cardiothoracic Surgery, Allegheny University Hospitals-Allegheny General, 320 East North Avenue, Pittsburgh, Pennsylvania 15212-4772*

James A. Magovern, M.D. *Department of Thoracic Surgery, Division of Cardiothoracic Surgery, Allegheny University Hospitals-Allegheny General, 320 East North Avenue, Pittsburgh, Pennsylvania 15212-4772*

Donna M. Mancini, M.D. *Associate Professor of Medicine, Department of Medicine, Columbia University College of Physicians and Surgeons, 622 West 168th Street, New York, New York 10032*

Patrick M. McCarthy, M.D. *Surgical Director, Kaufman Center for Heart Failure, Departments of Thoracic and Cardiovascular Surgery, Cleveland Clinic Foundation, 9500 Euclid Avenue, F-25, Cleveland, Ohio 44195*

Robert E. Michler, M.D. *Karl P. Klassen Professor of Surgery; Chief, Division of Cardiothoracic Surgery, Ohio State University Medical Center, N825 Doan Hall, 410 West Tenth Avenue, Columbus, Ohio 43210*

Lynda L. Mickleborough, M.D., F.R.C.S.(C) *Professor of Surgery, Department of Surgery, University of Toronto, The Toronto Hospital, 200 Elizabeth Street, Toronto, Ontario M5G 2C4, Canada*

Oktavijan P. Minanov, M.D. *Resident in Surgery, Department of Surgery, University of North Carolina, 102 Elmwood Circle, Chapel Hill, North Carolina 27514*

John B. O'Connell, M.D. *Professor and Chair, Department of Internal Medicine, Wayne State University/Detroit Medical Center, Harper Hospital, 3990 John R, 5 Webber Green, Detroit, Michigan 48201*

Mehmet C. Oz, M.D. *Assistant Professor, Department of Surgery, Columbia University College of Physicians and Surgeons, 177 Fort Washington Avenue, New York, New York 10032*

Francis D. Pagani, M.D., Ph.D. *Assistant Professor of Surgery and Director of the Heart Transplant Program, Section of Thoracic Surgery, University of Michigan Hospitals, 1500 East Medical Center Drive, Ann Arbor, Michigan 48109-0344*

Ileana L. Piña, M.D. *Professor of Medicine, Cardiomyopathy and Transplant Center, Temple University Hospital, 3401 North Broad Street, Parkinson Pavilion, Suite 900, Philadelphia, Pennsylvania 19140-5103*

Mark A. Robbins, M.D. *Fellow in Cardiology, Department of Cardiology, Cleveland Clinic Foundation, 9500 Euclid Avenue, Cleveland, Ohio 44195*

Eric A. Rose, M.D. *Valentine Mott/Johnson and Johnson Professor and Chairman, Department of Surgery, Columbia University College of Physicians and Surgeons; Surgeon-in-Chief, Columbia-Presbyterian Medical Center, 622 West 168th Street, New York, New York 10032*

Leslie A. Saxon, M.D. *Associate Professor, Department of Cardiac Electrophysiology, University of California, San Francisco/Moffitt Hospital, 500 Parnassus Avenue, Box 1354, San Francisco, California 94143-1354*

Kathleen A. Simpson, B.S.   *Division of Cardiothoracic Surgery, Allegheny University Hospitals-Allegheny General, 320 East North Avenue, Pittsburgh, Pennsylvania 15212-4772*

Nicholas G. Smedira, M.D.   *Departments of Thoracic and Cardiovascular Surgery, Cleveland Clinic Foundation, 9500 Euclid Avenue, F-25, Cleveland, Ohio 44195*

Randall C. Starling, M.D., M.P.H.   *Associate Professor of Medicine, Department of Cardiology, Cleveland Clinic Foundation, 9500 Euclid Avenue, Cleveland, Ohio 44195*

Lynne Warner Stevenson, M.D.   *Director, Heart Failure and Cardiomyopathy Program, Cardiovascular Division, Department of Medicine, Brigham and Women's Hospital, 75 Francis Street, Boston, Massachusetts 02115; and Associate Professor of Medicine, Harvard Medical School, 25 Shattuck Street, Boston, Massachusetts 02115*

William G. Stevenson, M.D.   *Associate Professor of Medicine, Harvard Medical School, Department of Medicine, Co-director, Cardiac Arrhythmia Service and Clinical Electrophysiology Laboratory, Cardiovascular Division, Brigham and Women's Hospital, 75 Francis Street, Boston, Massachusetts 02115*

Michael O. Sweeney, M.D.   *Cardiovascular Division, Brigham and Women's Hospital, 75 Francis Street, Boston, Massachusetts 02115*

Clifford H. Van Meter, Jr., M.D.   *Chief, Division of Cardiothoracic Surgery and Transplantation, Ochsner Foundation Hospital, 1514 Jefferson Highway, New Orleans, Louisiana 70121*

James B. Young, M.D.   *Head, Section of Heart Failure and Cardiac Transplant Medicine; Medical Director, Kaufman Center for Heart Failure, Cleveland Clinic Foundation, 9500 Euclid Avenue, Desk F-25, Cleveland, Ohio 44195*

Ross R. Zimmer, M.D.   *Cardiomyopathy and Transplant Center, Temple University Hospital, 3401 North Broad Street, Parkinson Pavilion, Suite 900, Philadelphia, Pennsylvania 19140-5103*

Preface

Morbidity and mortality of end-stage heart disease continue to increase despite the remarkable proliferation of effective, preventive, and therapeutic approaches to virtually all forms of heart disease. Congestive heart failure is implicated in more than 2 million hospitalizations per year in the United States, with an annual incidence of 400,000 patients with new onset of heart failure symptoms. Despite expenditures of more than $35 billion per year on the management of heart failure patients, the five-year survival of patients approximates only 50%, a prognosis worse than that of new onset HIV infection.

The enormity of the epidemiologic problem which heart failure represents has evoked broad interest in this epidemic problem (evidenced by the range of expertise of the authors), including special interest in epidemiology, economics, bioengineering, and immunology. One of the most exciting aspects of current clinical development in this field is the energy generated by the fusion of the medical and surgical teams. For patients with end-stage heart failure, it is now clear that a multi-disciplinary team approach including cardiologists, primary care physicians, surgeons, nurses, physical therapists, and social service providers is optimal. Numerous options can be used individually and, more often, in combination in order to prolong and enhance the quality of life of afflicted patients.

This book was written to provide an overview of the nature and magnitude of the problem of end-stage heart disease and a comprehensive review of established and investigational therapies in all relevant disciplines that deal with the problem. It is intended to serve as both an extensive profile of this field for the generalist and a summary reference for the wide array of specialist professionals who now participate in the clinical management and research of end-stage heart disease. In light of the increasing sophistication of patients and their families, this book may also help them understand the benefits and limitations of the increasing number of complex treatment options that they might choose.

The range of expertise of the authors is remarkable testament to the broad interest in this epidemic problem. Authors' special interests range from epidemiology and economics to cardiology to bioengineering, cardiac surgery, and immunology.

The text is comprised of five sections. In Section I, the problem of end-stage heart disease is defined with regard to epidemiology, economics, and meaningful benchmarks for the assessment of therapeutic approaches. Section II focuses on medical therapies, including approaches to identify specifically correctable factors and the strategies by which drug therapy may be designed for individual patients. These approaches include the limited role of positive inotropic agents, the use of various agents to counteract neurohormonal derangements associated with heart failure, and antiarrhythmics. Section II also explores the measurement of exercise capacity and its prognostic significance in heart failure, concluding with a chapter directed at defining circumstances in which heart failure should be judged to be refractory to medical management.

The last three sections of the book are devoted to surgical management. Section III explores conventional reparative surgical options, including coronary artery bypass grafting, ventricular aneurysmectomy and ablative procedures for dysrhythmias, and valvular cardiac surgery. Cardiac replacement therapies are surveyed in Section IV, focusing first on cardiac alotransplantation, the current benchmark replacement technique. Investigational approaches, including cross-species transplantation and the wide range of mechanical circulatory assistance devices currently under investigation, are systematically reviewed.

Novel strategies directed at enhancement of myocardial function are explored in Section V. These include dynamic cardiomyoplasty using skeletal muscle, transplantation of myocytes into scar, and the Batista cardiac reduction operation.

The text concludes with a speculative look at future management of patients with end-stage heart disease. While the vision offered almost certainly will prove inaccurate, the pace of change and innovation in the management of heart failure has been truly remarkable. This book illustrates the breadth and depth of that change, leaving little doubt that important new developments await us.

Eric A. Rose, M.D.
Lynne Warner Stevenson, M.D.

Acknowledgments

My thanks to Ellise, Sydney, Zachary, and Gabriel, for supporting all my distractions, and to Beth Eifert, for making the surgical section really happen.

Eric A. Rose, M.D.

My gratitude always to Bill, who restores the rhythm and energy for my patients and myself, and to Susanne, for cheerfully bringing together the medical section.

Lynne Warner Stevenson, M.D.

SECTION I

Defining the Problem

Management of End-Stage Heart Disease, edited by Eric A. Rose and Lynne Warner Stevenson. Lippincott–Raven Publishers, Philadelphia ©1998.

CHAPTER 1

Economic Impact of Heart Failure

Mark A. Robbins and John B. O'Connell

Cardiovascular disease, the leading cause of mortality in the United States, accounts for 40% of annual deaths. Although important reductions in mortality of cardiovascular disease have occurred since the mid-1960s, a concurrent decrease in mortality and admissions to the hospital for patients with heart failure (HF) has not been realized. HF is the leading reason for hospital admission in patients older than 65 years of age, who account for more than 80% of the total number of patients with HF. More than 3.5 million people in the United States have HF, and this number is expected to reach 5.7 million by the year 2030.

The increasing prevalence of HF is multifactorial. Paradoxically, one contributing factor is the improvement in the management of acute coronary syndromes. Strategies such as the use of thrombolytic agents and angioplasty have decreased fatality and improved the long-term survival associated with acute myocardial infarction. Although the acute syndrome may be successfully palliated, residual, often progressive chronic coronary syndromes with cumulative myocyte loss and adverse remodeling may result. Another factor is the degree by which the U.S. population is aging. It is estimated that the population aged 85 years or older is expected to more than triple between 1980 and 2030, and will be nearly sevenfold larger by 2050 (Figure 1). Data from the Framingham Study indicate that the incidence of HF doubles with each decade of life, reaching an extraordinary 31% in men and 28% in women between the ages of 85 and 94 years (Figure 2). Hence, the number of patients with HF will continue to increase unless effective management strategies are developed and implemented.

The economic burden of HF is considerable. Each year, at least 35% of all patients with HF are admitted to the hospital. Development of a service line strategy for the management of HF is critical to effectively reduce cost. This approach includes the administration of medications with proven efficacy and cost effectiveness, the use of a multidisciplinary programmatic infrastructure to prevent early readmission and promote careful follow-up, the development of programs to ensure timely and cost-effective cardiac transplantation, and the reallocation of spending from the in-patient arena to the out-patient setting to alleviate the most costly component of HF treatment (i.e., in-patient care).

EXPENDITURES

In 1993, health care spending in the United States accounted for a larger share of the gross domestic product (13.6%) than in any other major industrialized country. Canada and Switzerland followed the United States at 10.2% and 10%, respectively. The cost attributed to HF consumes a disproportionate percentage of the total health care dollar. This cost is accounted for by hospital care, out-patient care, medications, laboratory tests, procedures, and transplantation. In addition, a societal cost not reflected by health care data is incurred by loss from the work force.

In 1993, 875,000 hospital discharges with the primary diagnosis of congestive HF, coded 428.0 according to the International Classification of Diseases, 9th Revision (ICD-9), were reported by the National Center for Health Statistics (NCHS). These discharges included 394,000 men (45%) and 481,000 women (55%). Patients 65 years of age or older accounted for 681,000 (78%) of these admissions. The average length of stay for each hospitalization was 7.5 days. That year, the Health Care Financing Administration (HCFA) data (diagnosis-related group [DRG] 127) were similar but

M. A. Robbins: Department of Cardiology, Cleveland Clinic Foundation, Cleveland, Ohio 44195

J. B. O'Connell: Department of Internal Medicine, Wayne State University/Detroit Medical Center, Harper Hospital, Michigan 48201

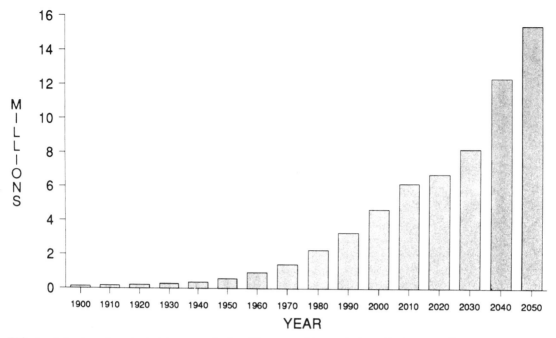

FIG. 1. Actual and projected increase in the 85+-year-old population: 1900–2050. (From U.S. Department of Health and Human Services. *Aging America: trends and projections—1991 edition.* Washington, DC: U.S. Department of Health and Human Services, 1991, with permission.)

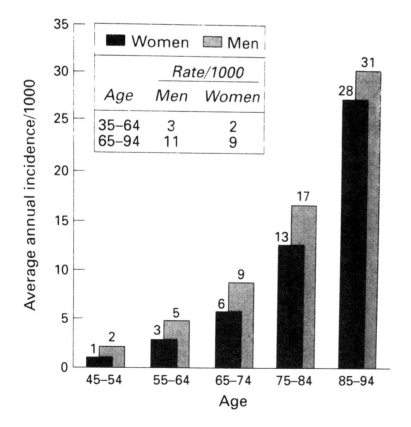

FIG. 2. Incidence of heart failure by age and sex from Framingham. (From Kannel WB, Ho K, Thom T. Changing epidemiological features of cardiac failure. *Br Heart J* 1994;72[Suppl 2]:53, with permission.)

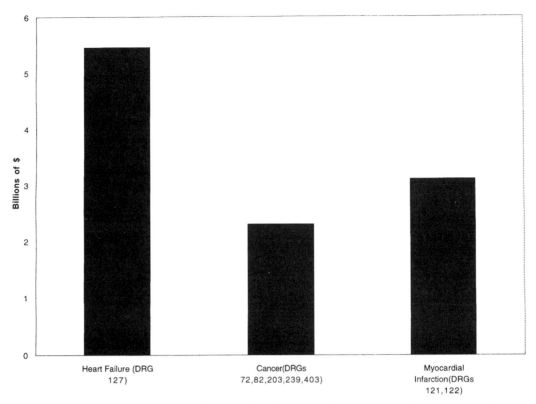

FIG. 3. Health Care Financing Administration (HCFA) expenditure on heart failure compared with that for cancer and myocardial infarction, according to Medicare in 1991. (From O'Connell JB, Bristow MR. Economic impact of heart failure in the United States: time for a different approach. *J Heart Lung Transplant* 1994;13:(Suppl 4)107, with permission.)

also included readmission rates and average charge per admission for patients older than age 65 years on Medicare. The HCFA reported 572,040 total admissions: 375,000 first admissions and 197,000 (34.1%) readmissions. The average length of stay was 7.0 days at an average charge of $8,935 per admission, totaling $5.11 billion. In 1991, Medicare expenditures for HF exceeded those for the combination of all types of cancer ($2.24 billion) and myocardial infarction ($3.18 billion; Figure 3). The charges to Medicare for readmissions in 1993 accounted for $1.75 billion or 30% of the in-patient cost. However, the average payment that Medicare assumed that year was only $4,368 per admission, or 48% of the total charge. Therefore, the $2 billion nonreimbursed charge was in all likelihood cost shifted to reduce the loss created by Medicare's reimbursement policies. Extrapolation of the HCFA expenditures to the 875,000 admissions reported by the NCHS provide the estimate that charges for in-patient care for the primary diagnosis of HF were approximately $7.7 billion in 1993.

The Department of Veterans Affairs (DVA) reported that 10,855 patients were admitted to their hospitals in 1995 with the primary diagnosis of congestive HF (DRG 127). The average length of stay was 8.57 days at an aver-

age DRG payment per stay of $3,345. The total expenditure for the treatment of HF in the DVA hospitals was approximately $36 million.

Calculations that include both the primary and secondary diagnoses of HF better estimate the total economic impact of HF admissions. In 1991, 2,280,445 hospital discharges from nonfederal hospitals were coded with primary or secondary diagnoses of HF (ICD-9 428.0, 428.1, and 428.9). The average length of stay was 7.7 days at an average charge of $10,148 per discharge, totaling $23.1 billion for in-patient care or 8.6% of the total nonfederal hospital health care costs. In 1991, 3,458,000 patients with HF were cared for in 11,396,000 ambulatory visits (3.3/patient). The average out-patient charge per year was estimated at $4,238 per patient, bringing the total out-patient expenditure to $14.7 billion (3.6% of the total out-patient health care cost). Transplantation added an estimated $270 million. By these calculations, the total health care cost attributed to HF in 1991 was an astonishing $38.1 billion, representing 5.4% of the estimated $700 billion total health care expenditure.

The extraordinary cost of HF is not confined to the United States. In the United Kingdom, it was estimated that the treatment of HF cost $326 million ($511 million) in 1990/1991, representing 1.1% of the total National

Health Service expenditure and 8.7% of the expenditure on diseases of the circulatory system. In-patient stay accounted for 65% of the United Kingdom's total cost for the treatment of congestive HF. In New Zealand, the total direct cost of HF management approximates 1.4% of the total health care expenditure.

These economic figures are discouraging. Given the fact that the expenditure dedicated to the treatment of HF can only be expected to escalate in the future, it is imperative that more cost-effective management evolve.

COST-EFFECTIVE MEDICAL THERAPY

Interest since the late 1980s has focused on developing effective medications for the management of HF. Clinical research has targeted management of potentially fatal arrhythmias and prevention of sudden death, alteration of deleterious neurohormonal responses, and the development of inotropic agents.

Angiotensin converting enzyme (ACE) inhibitors are unequivocally proven to be effective treatment for HF. These agents decrease mortality and prevent the progression of HF in both symptomatic and asymptomatic patients with left ventricular systolic dysfunction. An important aspect of treatment with ACE inhibitors is the beneficial effect on cost because of a decrease in the number of hospitalizations, nonfatal myocardial infarctions, and revascularizations compared with patients not receiving an ACE inhibitor. In the Survival and Ventricular Enlargement (SAVE) trial, captopril reduced hospital admissions from 4.9 to 3.9/100 patient years, whereas myocardial infarctions, percutaneous transluminal coronary angioplasty, and coronary bypass grafting were reduced by 21%, 27%, and 19%, respectively. The Studies of Left Ventricular Dysfunction (SOLVD) investigators calculated that 350 hospitalizations were prevented for every 1,000 patients treated by the addition of enalapril to the medical regimen.

The proof of efficacy is unequivocal, and all patients with left ventricular dysfunction should be treated with ACE inhibitors unless contraindicated. Unfortunately, clinical reality does not reflect this recommendation. In a 1991 survey, general practitioners/family physicians perceived that they prescribed ACE inhibitors only to 30% of their patients with HF; general internists to 40%; and, surprisingly, cardiologists only to 50%. Less than 20% of initial prescriptions for HF included ACE inhibitors, with cardiologists prescribing these agents more frequently than other physicians. Similar data revealed that in 1990, 1991, and 1992, patients with symptomatic HF received ACE inhibitors only 27%, 29%, and 31% of the time, respectively. More recent data suggest that this number finally approaches 50% (Figure 4).

By conservative application of the NCHS data, at least 437,500 patients not receiving ACE inhibitors were hospitalized for HF in 1993. With an estimated 90% tolerability,

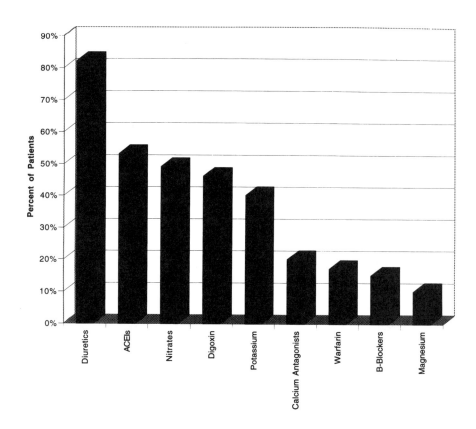

FIG. 4. Current practice in the pharmacologic treatment of heart failure.

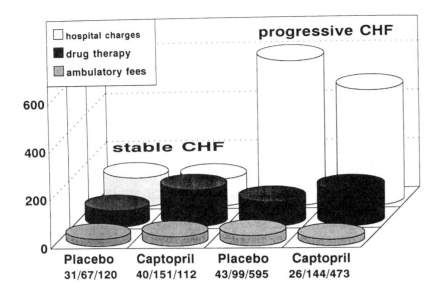

FIG. 5. Savings associated with the use of captopril for heart failure. (From Kebler FX. Socioeconomic aspects of ACE inhibitors in the secondary prevention in cardiovascular disease. *Am J Hypertens* 1994;7(Suppl 9):112–116, with permission.)

393,750 patients should have been receiving this beneficial medication. Extrapolating from the SOLVD cost-saving data and subtracting the $540 cost per year of enalapril, a net savings of over $1 billion or 12.9% of total expenditures on HF could have been realized as a result of 137,812 fewer hospitalizations. Cost savings by appropriate use of ACE inhibitors is not limited to the United States. When the SOLVD data were applied to the Canadian HF population, an average savings per patient of $1,645 was predicted, with a total savings of $100 million. Administration of captopril in the Munich Mild Heart Failure Trial resulted in profound savings, largely due to decreased hospitalization compared with the placebo (Figure 5).

The SOLVD investigators also ascertained the effect of enalapril on mortality, incidence of HF, and rate of hospitalization in patients with asymptomatic left ventricular dysfunction (ALVD; i.e., ejection fraction < 35% and no evidence of HF). The reduction in risk for development of HF, first admissions for HF, and multiple hospitalizations as a consequence of HF in the enalapril group were 37%, 36%, and 44%, respectively, compared with placebo.

These results have major implications for cost-saving strategies, given that two surveys using echocardiography as a screening tool have reported the incidence of ALVD to be between 1.2% and 4.5% of the general population. Unfortunately, the use of echocardiography to screen the general population for ALVD is probably not practical from the economic perspective. Therefore, until the development of more cost-effective technologies, symptoms and serendipity will continue to guide the diagnosis of left ventricular dysfunction.

The medical and financial benefit provided by ACE inhibitors mandates further inquiry regarding the insufficient application of this therapy in medical practice. Although cardiologists are more likely to initiate therapy with ACE inhibitors, in 1990, only 17% of patients with HF were actually treated by a cardiologist. The remaining 83% were cared for by general internists (43%), family practitioners (29%), and other providers (11%; Figure 6). If this division of care is to continue, novel strategies must be implemented to ensure appropriate management of patients with HF.

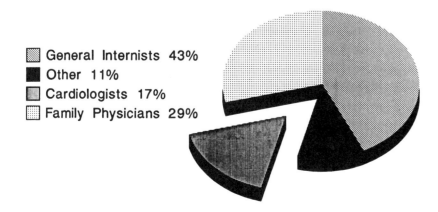

■ General Internists 43%
■ Other 11%
■ Cardiologists 17%
■ Family Physicians 29%

FIG. 6. Physicians responsible for the care of heart failure. (From O'Connell JB, Bristow MR. Economic impact of heart failure in the United States: time for a different approach. *J Heart Lung Transplant* 1994;13:(Suppl)107–112, with permission.)

When ACE inhibitors are contraindicated, the combination of hydralazine and isosorbide dinitrate should be considered. The second Vasodilator Heart Failure Trial (V-HeFT II) revealed that reduction in mortality was superior with enalapril in patients with less severe heart failure symptoms (New York Heart Association Class I and II). However, the combination of hydralazine and isosorbide dinitrate produced a significant improvement in exercise performance and left ventricular function. The hospital (DVA) admission rate for each group was nearly identical (18.9% in the enalapril group and 18.4% in the hydralazine/isosorbide dinitrate group). Hence, the cost savings described with ACE inhibitor use could in theory be extended to hydralazine/isosorbide dinitrate.

The use of digoxin for chronic HF and normal sinus rhythm remains a controversial issue. Although survival benefit is still debated, the controversies regarding symptomatic benefit have been put to rest by two clinical trials. The Prospective Randomized Study of Ventricular Failure and Efficacy of Digoxin (PROVED) and Randomized Assessment of Digoxin and Inhibitors of Angiotensin-Converting Enzyme (RADIANCE) demonstrated that withdrawal of digoxin on an ACE inhibitor background was associated with an increased risk of intensified medical therapy, HF-related emergency room visits, and hospital admission. Continuing digoxin in men with HF could prevent up to 185,000 clinic visits, 27,000 emergency room visits, and 137,000 hospital admissions,

resulting in a net savings of $406 million based on these data. Preliminary data from the Digoxin Investigators Group (DIG) trial confirm the reduction of hospitalization for men, although no benefit was demonstrated for women, a difference that may reflect differences in optimal dosing.

TRANSPLANTATION

The relatively low cost of transplantation compared with the overall expense of caring for patients with HF should not camouflage its rising cost and the complex patient base from which it draws. The cost of transplantation in some institutions has more than doubled since 1988, reaching an average of $150,000 in the first year posttransplantation. Although the volume has changed little since the early 1990s, the number of transplantations performed is consistently losing ground to the growing number of patients on transplant waiting lists. In the United States, there are at least 40% more patients on the waiting list (>3,600) on any given day than are transplanted each year (~2,500). The problems of donor shortage are consistent for all transplantations; yet, it is useful to compare the cost effectiveness of cardiac transplantation with transplantations of other organs that are more widely accepted as routine care. The cost–benefit ratio, as measured by cost per year of life saved, for heart transplantation in patients 55 years of age or younger with a

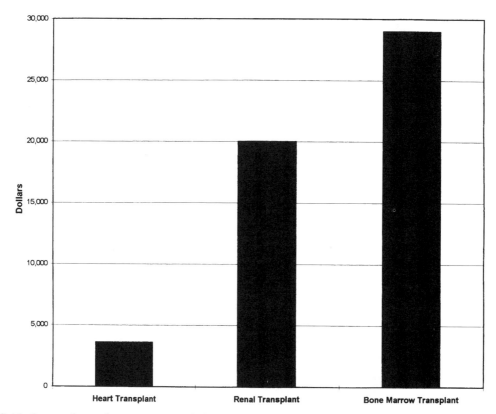

FIG. 7. Comparison of cost per year of life saved for heart, renal, and bone marrow transplantation.

favorable outcome is superior to that of both renal and bone marrow transplantation (Figure 7).

The cost of transplantation can be divided into three phases: (a) pretransplantation (i.e., HF management, evaluation, and monitoring); (b) transplantation (i.e., organ acquisition, the initial hospitalization, and physician fees); and (c) posttransplantation (i.e., immunosuppressive therapy, rejection episodes, and other complications). The largest component of the increasing costs of transplantation appears to be the increasing pretransplantation lengths of stay in the intensive care unit and regular hospital beds. Because of the critical donor organ shortage and the fact that posttransplantation survival is nearly equivalent regardless of the severity of preoperative illness, the sickest patients retain highest priority, resulting in longer pretransplantation and posttransplantation hospital stays. However, this practice of transplanting the sickest patients becomes a vicious cycle of increasing costs as the less sick become sicker while awaiting a donor. Transplantation of the less sick seems a simple and logical solution based solely on economics. However, the unequivocal survival benefit in the more seriously ill overrides consideration for an economically based organ allocation scheme.

Nearly 80% of posttransplantation patients are rehabilitated to the extent that they are able to function in the job market, yet only 45% of these patients actually do. Economic and social factors play a major role because a much higher rate of posttransplantation employment is noted in countries with a national health care plan. Some employers are unwilling to endure the economic burden of transplant recipient employees who are fully rehabilitated and return to work. Perhaps recent legislation requiring health insurance coverage for preexistent conditions may remove some of the barriers to financial rehabilitation.

New approaches and alternatives to cardiac replacement that may reduce cost and enhance access include permanently implantable left ventricular assist devices, implantable defibrillators, and xenografts. Technologically advanced portable left ventricular assist devices are beginning to reduce the number of hospital days before transplantation, which should translate into cost savings. The need for transplantation of patients solely for prevention of sudden death may be reduced by the use of implantable defibrillators with pacing capabilities. Xenografts, although still experimental, could offload the current glut of candidates waiting for transplantation, avoiding the long pretransplantation hospital stay and the inevitable costly physiologic deterioration. These new modalities may prove to be a double-edged sword. Although improved survival and early cost savings are forthcoming, the associated expense of the growing number of postreplacement patients may counterbalance the benefit. It is more expensive to be alive with a chronic illness than dead!

NEW STRATEGIES FOR THE TREATMENT OF HEART FAILURE

Hospitalizations in the United Kingdom and United States account for at least two thirds of the cost for care of patients with HF. An inordinate number of these hospitalizations represent readmission within 30 to 60 days of discharge. Therefore, hospital admissions become an easy target for cost-saving measures. A focused approach to reduce the number of hospitalizations is imperative. The factors leading to initial and early follow-up admissions, including dietary indiscretion, inadequate discharge planning and follow-up, failed social support systems, inadequate medical regimen, noncompliance with appropriate medical regimen, and failure to seek medical attention promptly when symptoms recur, must be addressed. Comorbid factors associated with an increased risk of hospitalization, such as coronary artery disease or uncontrolled hypertension, must be aggressively managed.

In the current system, office-based practices are frequently inadequate for the needs of the HF patient. In many instances, the emergency department becomes the only alternative for care, and it has been estimated that 90% of patients who present with HF are admitted to the hospital. Hospitalizations are increased and lengthened by patients' inability to recognize the early signs of HF, often because of lack of education. On the other hand, quality managers or payers encourage early discharge, which limits the time needed to modify those factors that prevent early readmission. Specific interventions shown to reduce the number of readmissions are telephone care follow-up, use of a multidisciplinary team, and HF clinics.

Provision of care over a telephone may reduce the requirement for clinic visits, further reducing cost without adversely affecting patient care. In one institution, this strategy accounted for a net savings of $1,656 per patient over a 2-year period in patients with chronic medical conditions because of fewer admissions, shorter stays, fewer out-patient clinic visits, and fewer intensive care unit days.

Use of a multispecialty team focused on eradicating those factors that are most associated with treatment failure and recurrent hospital admissions is another effective approach. The focus of these teams includes intense patient education, individualized dietary assessment, consultation with social services to facilitate discharge planning and care after discharge, analysis of medications by a cardiologist, and intensive follow-up after discharge through home health services and community-based case management. In one health care delivery system, this treatment strategy reduced the readmission rate by 56.2%, and was associated with an overall cost difference of $153 per patient per month. This approach may reduce the number of readmissions by 100,000, with potential cost savings of $1,836 per patient per year, which would have translated into $1 billion annual savings to Medicare if implemented before 1993. An alternative integrated approach emphasizing similar ambulatory strategies but providing home health nurses with the capability of administering intravenous diuretics and inotropes resulted in projected annual savings of $3,744 per patient in HF direct cost. When extrapolated to the Medicare database, the projected savings would have exceeded $2 billion in 1993.

HEART FAILURE CLINICS

The reports of cost savings by the implementation of a multidisciplinary system has spawned the development of HF clinics. These clinics are dedicated to the treatment of all stages of HF, including the evaluation and preparation for transplantation. To be efficient and cost effective, these programs have adopted many of the previously mentioned strategies in the care of their HF patients, including regimented initiation of medications proven to be beneficial and cost effective, frequent out-patient follow-up, appropriate use of laboratory and radiographic procedures, patient education concerning all facets of HF, and evaluation for transplantation for those refractory to medical management. Those clinics associated with academic health centers include clinical research programs to allow patient access to drugs under development.

Implementation of such a program shifts cost from the in-patient to the out-patient arena. To be cost effective, this increase in ambulatory care spending must be offset by savings stemming from reductions in hospitalizations, emergency room visits, lengths of stay when hospitalization is unavoidable, and the timely access to transplantation for patients when necessary.

In one documented example, this strategy decreased total medical expenses while reducing mortality and morbidity due to HF. At 10-month follow-up, a significant cost advantage was seen for the patients treated by the HF clinic compared with those followed per routine. The average total cost per patient followed in the HF clinic was $5,981, versus $7,438 for those cared for by their primary care physician. This savings of $1,457 per patient occurred despite increased spending in the out-patient setting. The average cost in out-patient care for HF clinic patients was $1,409 compared with $221 for those receiving routine care. This cost difference was accounted for by an average of 7.2 more clinic visits and more frequent laboratory assessment. However, this expense was more than offset by the 54% reduction in hospital and emergency room admissions. In addition to cost savings, survival was improved; mortality was 19% for those receiving routine care compared with 10% for patients enrolled in the HF clinic. Specific experience in out-patients awaiting transplantation indicates even greater savings in advanced HF, with an 80% reduction in hospitalization rates.

FUTURE DIRECTIONS

The future of health care will continue to be affected by cost containment. New strategies in health care delivery must be developed, especially for those areas that consume a disproportionate percentage of the health care dollar. A service line approach is ideal with respect to HF management. Currently, only 17% of HF patients are being cared for primarily by cardiologists. This percentage will not increase in the future with the projected number of symptomatic HF patients reaching 5.7 million by the year 2030. Therefore, it is imperative that a system be developed that will incorporate the primary care physician, who will work closely with HF clinics. Primary care physicians can potentially provide cost-effective management to most patients. A tiered system for the care of HF patients may include "specialized" primary care physicians, diagnostic regional referral centers, and the comprehensive HF treatment center.

Specialized primary care physicians should have a "special interest" in HF and receive appropriate training. These physicians would assume the "gatekeeper" role in the management of patients with HF, sequestering patients locally and providing initial evaluation and treatment. Patient care should be modeled after the Agency for Health Care Policy and Research or the American Heart Association/American College of Cardiology guidelines and include the initiation of beneficial and cost-effective medications and noninvasive measurement of left ventricular function. A multidisciplinary approach integrating a network of nurse educators, home health workers, and case managers should be used. The network's main objectives should be patient education, promotion of social support, home-based treatment including the use of intravenous diuretics or inotropes, decreased length of hospital stay, and, ultimately, a reduction in initial and recurrent hospitalizations. Implementation of emergency room observation units and hospital intermediate care could also be expected to shorten and prevent unwarranted hospitalizations. Patients who demonstrate refractory or persistent Class III or IV symptoms or require hospitalization despite conventional local therapy are considered to have "complex" or "advanced" HF that requires a more detailed evaluation, and should be referred to the second tier of the system.

Diagnostic regional referral centers may serve as a focus for the network of specialized primary care physicians for evaluation of failed therapy. These centers will have the capability of invasive assessment and intense pharmacologic treatment. After discharge from an HF hospitalization, some plans include passage through a "high-intensity" phase, where patients are followed closely by the specialized HF team until criteria of clinical stability are met, at which time the patients return to be followed primarily by their regular physician. It is important that access be available to HF experts. Ongoing education must be provided to the primary care physicians from the HF team.

The comprehensive HF treatment centers should formalize their relationship to a defined geographic area or provider network. Referrals may be received from diagnostic regional referral centers or, in a two-tiered system, from the specialized primary care provider. These centers provide cardiac transplantation and follow-up, and participation in clinical and basic research programs. It will be the responsibility of these centers to provide the ultimate in cost containment by new strategies to prevent HF or permanently halt its progression. Outcome data for the entire network should be generated and managed at this level. Once patients have been adequately evaluated, the primary goal will be to return the responsibility of care to their primary care physicians, thereby maintaining continuity. Communication within the network and electronic data sharing are key elements to network success.

Much of the infrastructure for this tiered system is in place, with many major teaching institutions serving as the comprehensive HF centers and larger community or metropolitan hospitals serving in the capacity of diagnostic regional referral centers. The duty of these existing facilities is to provide the education and initial financial support to implement the most important link in this tiered system, the specialized primary care physician. Generalists are responsible for over 70% of the care provided to HF patients. Therefore, it is of utmost importance that they be aware of advances in and the appropriate treatment of congestive HF.

In summary, all elements for cost-effective care of the patient with HF are in place. Creation of an organized infrastructure and information system will undoubtedly reduce the global economic burden of care for patients with HF.

SELECTED REFERENCES

American Heart Association. *Heart and stroke facts*. Dallas, Texas, 1993.

Beyond four walls: cost-effective management of chronic congestive heart failure. The Advisory Board Company, 1994.

Clinical Quality Control Investigators. Mortality risk and patterns of practice in 4606 acute care patients with congestive heart failure. *Arch Intern Med* 1996;156:1669–1673.

Eggers PW, Kucken LE. Cost issues in transplantation. *Surg Clin North Am* 1994;74:1259.

Fonarow GC, Stevenson LW, Walden JA, et al. Impact of a comprehensive heart failure management program on rehospitalization and functional status for patients with advanced heart failure. *J Am Coll Cardiol* 1997 (*in press*).

Graves EJ. *Advance Data 1993 Summary: National Hospital Discharge Survey*. U.S. Department of Health and Human Services, Center for Disease Control and Prevention, National Center for Health Statistics. 264: May 1995, 1–12.

Health Care Financing Administration. *Hospitalization data*. 1993.

Hosenpud JD, Novick RJ, Bennett LE, et al. The registry of the International Society for Heart and Lung Transplantation: thirteenth official report—1996. *J Heart Lung Transplant* 1996;15:655.

Kannel WB, Ho K, Thom T. Changing epidemiological features of cardiac failure. *Br Heart J* 1994;72[Suppl 2]:53.

O'Connell JB, Bristow MR. Economic impact of heart failure in the United States: time for a different approach. *J Heart Lung Transplant* 1994;13: S-107.

Rajfer SI. Perspective of the pharmaceutical industry on the development of new drugs for heart failure. *J Am Coll Cardiol* 1993;22[Suppl A]:198A.

Reemtsma K, Berland G, Merrill J, et al. Evaluation of surgical procedures: changing patterns of patient selection and costs in heart transplantation. *J Thorac Cardiovasc Surg* 1992;104:1308.

Rich MW, Beckham V, Wittenberg C, et al. A multidisciplinary intervention to prevent the readmission of elderly patients with congestive heart failure. *N Engl J Med* 1995;333:1190.

Stevenson LW, Hamilton MA, Tillisch IH, et al. Decreasing survival benefit from cardiac transplantation for outpatients as the waiting list lengthens. *J Am Coll Cardiol* 1991;18:919.

Tengs TO, Adams ME, Pliskin JS, et al. Five hundred life saving interventions and their cost-effectiveness. *Risk Anal* 1995;15:369.

U.S. Department of Health and Human Services. *Aging America: trends and projections—1991 edition*. Washington, DC: U.S. Department of Health and Human Services, 1991.

Veterans Affairs Hospital. *KLFMENU HCFA simulation model: fiscal year, 1995*.

Management of End-Stage Heart Disease, edited by Eric A. Rose and Lynne Warner Stevenson. Lippincott–Raven Publishers, Philadelphia ©1998.

CHAPTER 2

Cardiac Replacement: Estimation of Need, Demand, and Supply

Roger W. Evans

The epidemiology of heart failure has not been systematically studied in relationship to cardiac replacement *per se*. Although cardiovascular epidemiology is an established discipline, no epidemiologist has focused his or her research on the various aspects of transplant evaluation and candidacy. This may be due to the fact that cardiac replacement has yet to be recognized as a major public health issue. This is surprising, because transplantation is often used to underscore the importance of the dilemma health care policy makers face in making decisions about resource allocation and rationing.

Despite their relevance, rigorous epidemiologic methods are *not* essential to frame some of the most critical issues that face people interested in cardiac replacement. The problem is so large that even crude analyses readily provide a meaningful basis for further analysis. In this regard, periodic efforts, based on mortality data, have been made to estimate the *need* for heart transplantation.

The need for cardiac replacement is hardly a pedestrian issue. Heart disease remains the leading cause of death in the United States, with an age-adjusted mortality rate of 144.3 per 100,000 population. Ischemic heart disease accounts for 95.7 of these deaths. Overall, heart disease is responsible for nearly 9.0 million life years lost, defined as the number of years a person would have lived in the absence of death. In turn, these premature deaths have an annual mortality cost, defined as the value of lifetime earnings lost by people who die prematurely, of $38.7 million, or $108,278 per person.

As the foregoing data suggest, the need for cardiac replacement is a critical national health care policy issue. This was apparent during the conduct of the National Heart Transplantation Study (NHTS). Today, as in the past, the future of cardiac replacement, including mechanical substitutes and xenotransplantation, can be anticipated only relative to estimates of need.

At the completion of the NHTS, it was estimated that, given prevailing patient selection criteria, fewer than 15,000 people died each year of conditions amenable to heart transplantation. However, even at the time the Health Care Financing Administration was busy crafting its policy with respect to Medicare reimbursement, it was apparent that the criteria for patient selection were becoming increasingly liberal. In anticipation of this, the NHTS final report projected that the annual need for some form of cardiac replacement could exceed 96,000 people.

Today, it is even more apparent that cadaveric donor heart supply will be inadequate to meet *demand*, let alone *need*. Realistically speaking, the need for cardiac replacement will be met only if a viable long-term mechanical device is perfected, or xenotransplantation becomes a clinical reality.

It is the intent of this chapter to put the foregoing issues into proper perspective. Unfortunately, when it comes to need, demand, and supply, misconceptions abound. However, clinical activities, research, and public health policy must be informed by credible analyses, despite the limited scope and sometimes questionable quality of the data on which they are based.

THE CONCEPTS OF NEED, DEMAND, AND SUPPLY

Figure 1 puts the concepts of *need* and *demand* into perspective. As shown, we can differentiate among the concepts of unrecognized need, unmet demand, met demand, unmet need, total demand, and total need. Each of these concepts is defined in Table 1; however, as is

Section of Health Services Evaluation, Mayo Clinic, Rochester, Minnesota 55905

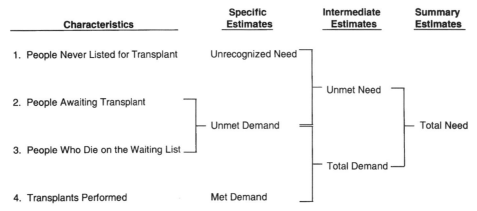

Characteristics	Specific Estimates	Intermediate Estimates	Summary Estimates
1. People Never Listed for Transplant	Unrecognized Need	Unmet Need	Total Need
2. People Awaiting Transplant	Unmet Demand		
3. People Who Die on the Waiting List		Total Demand	
4. Transplants Performed	Met Demand		

FIG. 1. The concepts of need and demand in organ transplantation. (From Roger W. Evans, Ph.D., Mayo Clinic, Rochester, Minnesota.)

TABLE 1. *Definitions of concepts*

- **Unrecognized need**—the number of suitable people never placed on the transplant waiting list
- **Unmet demand**—the number of people awaiting transplantation plus the number of people who die while on the waiting list
- **Met demand**—the number of transplantations performed
- **Unmet need**—the number of suitable people never placed on the transplant waiting list plus the number of people awaiting transplantation plus the number of people who die while on the waiting list
- **Total demand**—the number of people awaiting transplantation plus the number of people who die while on the waiting list plus the number of transplantations performed
- **Total need**—the number of people never listed for transplantation plus the number of people awaiting transplantation plus the number of people who die on the waiting list plus the number of transplantations performed.

apparent from Figure 1, unmet demand factors into our calculation of the estimate of total need twice. Thus, in calculating total need, we must exclude one estimate of unmet demand to avoid double counting.

With the rare exception of an occasional living donor heart being transplanted, cadaveric donors remain the primary source of hearts. Since 1988, between 1 and 12 living donor hearts have been transplanted each year. There are also times when a procured heart is discarded or used for research. In this regard, relevant data are summarized in Figure 2 for the period 1988 to 1994.

It is also worthwhile to distinguish between the *actual* and the *potential* supply of donor hearts. Not every suitable heart is procured because the relatives may be unwilling to consent to organ donation. As shown in Figure 3, Life-Source of Minneapolis, Minnesota, reports that for 35% of potential donors, relatives deny consent. In addition, other reasons contribute to failed procurement attempts for

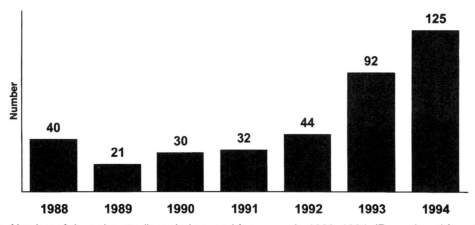

FIG. 2. Number of donor hearts discarded or used for research, 1988–1994. (Reproduced from United Network for Organ Sharing. *1995 Annual Report of the U.S. Scientific Registry of Organ Transplant Recipients and the Organ Procurement and Transplantation Network. Transplant data: 1988–1994.* Richmond, VA: United Network for Organ Sharing, 1996:262, with permission.)

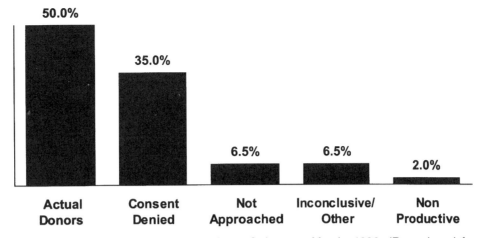

FIG. 3. What happened to potential organ donors? January–March, 1996. (Reproduced from Life-Source, Minneapolis, MN, 1996, with permission.)

another 15% of donors. Thus, only 50% of potential donor families actually consent to organ donation.

NEED AND DEMAND ESTIMATES

The *need* for heart transplantation is based on current indications. These have evolved over time. Table 2 contains a complete listing of the primary indications for *adults*. Table 3 supplements this list with the primary

indications for *pediatric* heart transplantation. Based on deaths due to these indications, Figure 4 summarizes the total need for cardiac replacement in the United States. These estimates are based on deaths wherein the *primary* cause is a suitable indication for heart transplantation. Of

TABLE 2. *Diagnoses at death for which cardiac transplantation could have been indicated[a]*

ICD-9 code	Description
164.1	Malignant neoplasm of the heart
394.0	Mitral valve stenosis
394.1	Rheumatic mitral insufficiency
394.2	Mitral stenosis with insufficiency
394.9	Other and unspecified mitral valve disease
395.0	Rheumatic aortic stenosis
395.1	Rheumatic aortic insufficiency
395.2	Rheumatic aortic stenosis with insufficiency
395.9	Other and unspecified rheumatic aortic diseases
396	Diseases of mitral and aortic valves
398.0	Rheumatic myocarditis
398.9	Other and unspecified rheumatic heart diseases
414.0	Coronary atherosclerosis
414.1	Aneurysm of the heart
414.8	Other specified forms of chronic ischemic heart disease
424.1	Aortic valve disorders
425.0	Endomyocardial fibrosis
425.4	Other primary cardiomyopathies
428.0	Congestive heart failure
428.1	Left heart failure
428.9	Heart failure, unspecified
429.0	Myocarditis, unspecified
429.1	Myocardial degeneration
429.3	Cardiomegaly

[a]Each condition must be listed as the *primary* cause of death.

TABLE 3. *Indications for pediatric heart transplantation[a]*

ICD-9 code	Description
425.0	Endomyocardial fibrosis
425.3	Endocardial fibroelastosis
745.0	Common truncus
745.1	Transposition of great vessels
745.10	Complete transposition of great vessels
745.11	Double outlet right ventricle
745.12	Corrected transposition of great vessels
745.19	Other
745.2	Tetralogy of Fallot
745.3	Common ventricle
745.4	Ventricular septal defect
745.5	Ostium secundum type atrial septal defect
745.6	Endocardial cushion defect
745.60	Endocardial cushion defect, unspecified type
745.61	Ostium primum defect
745.69	Other
745.7	Cor bioculare
745.8	Other
745.9	Unspecified defect of septal closure
746.01	Atresia, congenital
746.02	Stenosis, congenital
746.09	Other
746.1	Tricuspid atresia and stenosis, congenital
746.2	Ebstein's anomaly
746.6	Congenital mitral insufficiency
746.7	Hypoplastic left heart syndrome
746.84	Obstructive anomalies of heart, not elsewhere classified
746.85	Coronary artery anomaly
746.86	Congenital heart block
746.87	Malposition of heart and cardiac apex
746.89	Other
746.9	Unspecified anomaly of heart

[a]Each condition must be listed as the *primary* cause of death.

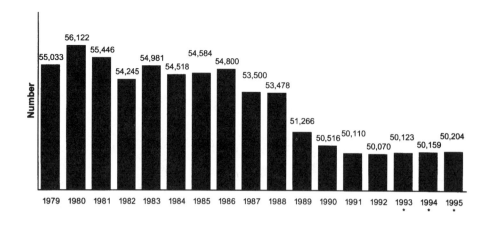

* Projected.

FIG. 4. The total need for heart transplantation, 1979–1995.

course, the people so identified may have had comorbidities or complications that could have excluded them from further consideration for cardiac transplantation. Moreover, some of these people could have died under circumstances in which heart transplantation would never have been a serious consideration from a temporal perspective (e.g., out-of-hospital cardiac arrest). Thus, there will always be some uncertainty associated with the estimates presented in Figure 4.

Figure 5 provides a slightly different perspective on the data presented in Figure 4. Clearly, as the size and composition of the U.S. population changes each year, it makes sense to evaluate the need for heart transplantation based on the number of cases per million population (PMP). As shown in Figure 5, the need for heart transplantation has declined from 244.5 PMP in 1979 to 190.6 PMP in 1995.

As is apparent from Figure 6, the *unmet need* for heart transplantation has dropped considerably over the aforementioned period and has now stabilized. In 1995, it is estimated that 47,843 people died who could have potentially benefited from a heart transplant, compared with 51,802 in 1988.

For various reasons, not every person who could potentially benefit from a heart transplant is placed on the waiting list, thereby becoming a demand consideration. Nonetheless, as shown in Figure 7, the *unrecognized need* for heart transplantation continues to decline. This conclusion is consistent with the data presented in Figures 8 and 9. Since 1986, the year-end waiting list for heart transplantation has increased from 282 to 3,468 people in 1995. Unfortunately, the number of patient deaths on the waiting list has also increased since 1988, but, since 1991, has been somewhat stable between 724 and 780 deaths annually.

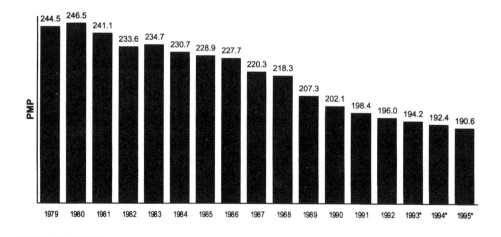

* Projected.

FIG. 5. The total need for heart transplantation per million population (PMP), 1979–1995.

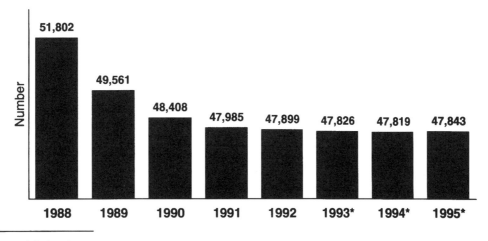

* Projected.

FIG. 6. The unmet need for heart transplantation, 1988–1995.

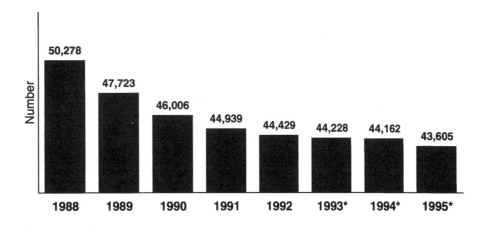

* Projected.

FIG. 7. The unrecognized need for heart transplantation, 1988–1995.

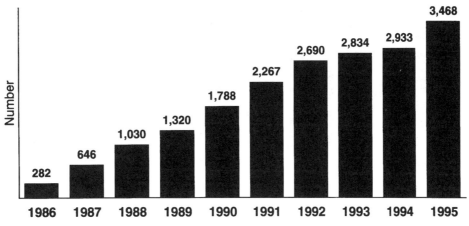

FIG. 8. The waiting list for heart transplantation, 1986–1995.

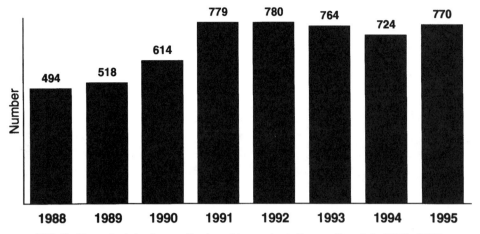

FIG. 9. Reported deaths on the heart transplantation waiting list, 1988–1995.

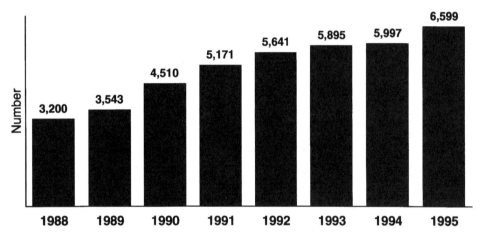

FIG. 10. The total demand for heart transplantation, 1988–1995.

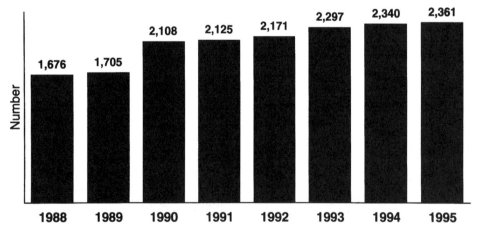

FIG. 11. The met demand for heart transplantation, 1988–1995.

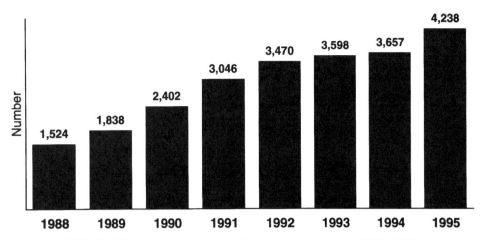

FIG. 12. The unmet demand for heart transplantation, 1988–1995.

As defined in Table 1, the *total demand* for heart transplantation over the course of 1 year is equal to the number of people awaiting transplantation at year end, plus the number of people who die while on the waiting list, plus the number of transplantations performed during the course of the year. In this regard, the relevant data are summarized in Figure 10. As indicated, since 1988 the total demand for heart transplantation has more than doubled. Meanwhile, the *met demand* for heart transplantation (i.e., the number of transplantations performed) has become relatively stable, as shown in Figure 11. Not surprisingly, therefore, the *unmet demand* for heart transplantation has continued to *increase* each year since 1988 (Figure 12).

DONOR SUPPLY ESTIMATES

Donor supply remains an intractable problem and greatly limits our ability to meet both the need and the demand for heart transplantation. Although studies continue to show that *potential* donor organ supply is greater than the number of organs procured, we have made little headway in our efforts to address the problem of a shortage in the face of plenty.

Figure 13 provides annual estimates of the number of potential organ donors available each year in the United States for the period 1988 to 1995. In 1995, approximately 11,500 donors should have been available; however, as shown in Figure 14, there were only 5,361 organ donors. Thus, as is apparent from Figure 15, since 1988, *actual* donor organs have been procured from between only 38% and 47% of *potential* donors, results remarkably consistent with the data presented in Figure 3.

Unfortunately, not every suitable potential donor is a source of a transplantable heart. Figure 16 summarizes the relevant data for the period 1988 to 1995. As shown, in 1995, it is estimated that 8,749 *potential* donor hearts were available in the United States, but only 2,506 were *actually* procured (Figure 17). Thus, as is apparent from Figure 18, actual donor hearts are procured from between 22% and 29% of potential donors.

The foregoing data can be readily placed in perspective. Figure 19 summarizes the relationships among

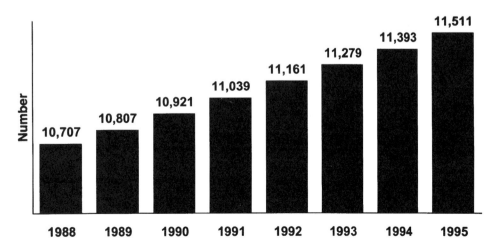

FIG. 13. Estimated number of potential cadaveric organ donors by year, 1988–1995.

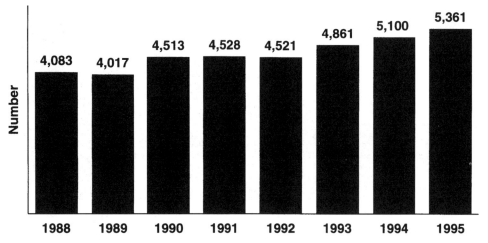

FIG. 14. Estimated number of cadaveric organ donors by year, 1988–1995.

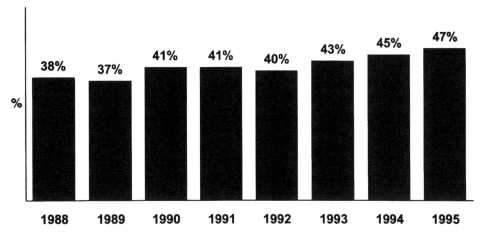

FIG. 15. Percentage of potential cadaveric donors from which actual organs were procured, 1988–1995.

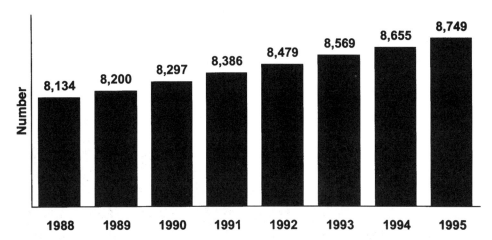

FIG. 16. Estimated number of potential cadaveric donor hearts available by year, 1988–1995.

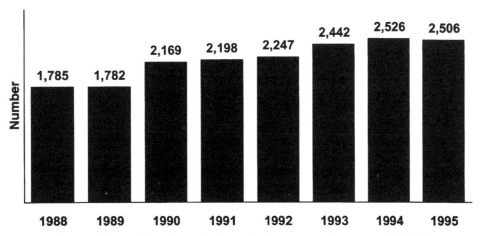

FIG. 17. Estimated number of cadaveric donor hearts by year, 1988–1995.

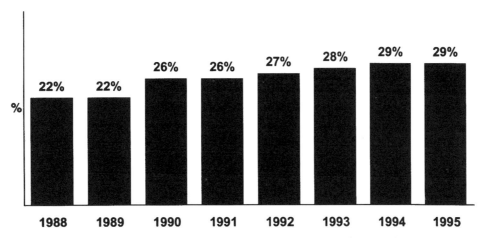

FIG. 18. Percentage of potential cadaveric donors from which actual donor hearts were procured, 1988–1995.

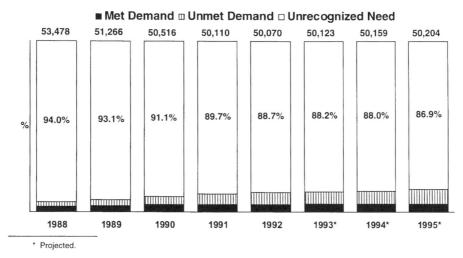

FIG. 19. The relationships among unrecognized need, unmet demand, and met demand, 1988–1995.

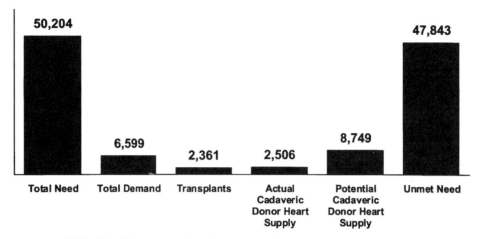

FIG. 20. Heart transplantation: need, demand, and supply, 1995.

unrecognized need, unmet demand, and the number of transplantations performed (i.e., met demand). As shown, since 1988, the unrecognized need for heart transplantation has decreased from 94% to 86.9% of the total. However, both the met and unmet demand for heart transplantation continue to increase.

Figure 20 puts all of the data for 1995 into perspective. As shown, over 50,000 people could have potentially benefited from a heart transplant. Of the 2,506 donor hearts that were procured, only 2,361 (94%) were actually transplanted. Finally, what is most noteworthy is the remarkable discrepancy between potential cadaveric donor heart supply and the total need for heart transplantation. Even if a donor heart was procured from every potential donor, over 40,000 people who could have benefited from heart transplantation would have died in 1995.

DISCUSSION

Considerable progress has been made in the management of heart failure. However, more work is required. The demand for heart transplantation has more than doubled since 1988, and the number of deaths on the waiting list has increased by 56%. Nonetheless, our ability to meet both need and demand is tempered by donor organ supply, over which physicians and surgeons have little control. More donors translates into fewer deaths and, potentially, better outcomes because surgeons have a better opportunity to time the transplant procedure optimally. Thus, any decline in the waiting list must be viewed as an important victory for transplant cardiologists. In the absence of their efforts, the death rate on the waiting list could be much higher than it is already.

Since the mid-1980s, there has been a remarkable decline in deaths due to cardiovascular disease. Many factors have contributed to this decline, including changes in lifestyle and improved treatment modalities.

Unfortunately, compared with lifestyle changes, the net benefits associated with heart transplantation are rather unimpressive. From a public health perspective, we have probably accomplished as much, if not more, through changes in the way we live than we have achieved through clinical interventions *per se*. Behavior modification can yield substantial benefits in the long term, even if it can do little in the near term.

As the data presented here indicate, some form of long-term cardiac replacement, whether it be xenotransplantation or a viable mechanical circulatory support system, could go a long way to ameliorate the considerable health care burden associated with cardiovascular disease. However, such options are likely to prove expensive, both in terms of development and application. The economics of cardiac replacement are now constrained by donor organ supply. By removing this constraint, we make way for a very different economic, social, ethical, and legal reality.

In the past, we have adopted a very conservative approach to need estimation. In 1984, we anticipated the possibility of, but did not realistically project, where we are today. For example, although we were certain that patient selection criteria would become increasingly liberal, we did not base our health care policy recommendations on the same data we would today. Realistically, the data suggest that the *actual* need for cardiac replacement has increased by nearly 350%. Meanwhile, actual donor supply has probably changed very little. The increase in the number of heart donors is most likely attributable to more liberal donor selection criteria. In other words, we have simply changed the definition of what constitutes a suitable heart donor.

Projecting the future of cardiac replacement will remain speculative at best, although there is considerable merit in pursuing further studies concerning the epidemiology of heart failure. The results of these analyses, coupled with a better understanding of current drug therapy, would greatly enhance the knowledge base on which we derive future projections. However, advances in mechanical assist and permanent replacement technology are likely to have a more significant near-term impact than xenotransplantation. Even optimistic projections concerning xenotransplantation would place its availability in the next decade. Although there has been some intriguing initial work, none of it could yet be classified as promising. It is simply too early to anticipate what implications it could have for long-term cardiac replacement. Therefore, through the foreseeable future, those who are skeptical about xenotransplantation will continue to outnumber those who see a brighter future in animals than machines.

ACKNOWLEDGMENT

The author thanks Ms. Leisa Leisen for her expert secretarial assistance.

SELECTED REFERENCES

Alexander JW, Vaughn WK. The use of "marginal" donors for organ transplantation: the influence of age on outcome. *Transplantation* 1991;51: 135–141.

Alexander JW, Vaughn WK, Carey MA. The use of marginal donors for organ transplantation: the older and younger donors. *Transplant Proc* 1991;23:905–909.

Ashton RC Jr, Goldstein DJ, Rose EA, et al. Duration of left ventricular assist device support affects transplant survival. *J Heart Lung Transplant* 1996;15:1151–1157.

Bart KJ, Macon EJ, Whittier FC, et al. Cadaveric kidneys for transplantation: a paradox of shortage in the face of plenty. *Transplant Proc* 1981;31:379–382.

Bennett LE, Glascock RF, Breen TJ, et al. Organ donation in the United States: 1988 through 1992. In: Terasaki PI, Cecka JM, eds. *Clinical transplants, 1993*. Los Angeles: UCLA Tissue Typing Laboratory, 1994:85–93.

Bowling A. Health care rationing: the public's debate. *Br Med J* 1996;312: 670–674.

Chapman LE, Folks TM, Salomon DR, et al. Xenotransplantation and xenogeneic infections. *N Engl J Med* 1995;333:1498–1501.

Cohn JN. The management of chronic heart failure. *N Engl J Med* 1996; 335:490–498.

Committee on Evaluation and Management of Heart Failure. Guidelines for the evaluation and management of heart failure: report of the American College of Cardiology/American Heart Association Task Force on Practice Guidelines. *Circulation* 1995;92:2764–2784.

Committee on Xenograft Transplantation. *Xenotransplantation: science, ethics, and public policy*. Washington, DC: National Academy Press, 1996.

Copeland JG, Pavie A, Dureau D, et al. Bridge to transplantation with the CardioWest total artificial heart: the international experience 1993 to 1995. *J Heart Lung Transplant* 1996;15:94–99.

Dec GW. Idiopathic dilated cardiomyopathy. *N Engl J Med* 1994;331: 1564–1575.

Dyer O. Nontransplanted organs can be used for research. *Br Med J* 1996; 312:1631.

Edwards EB, Breen TJ, Guo T, et al. The UNOS OPTN waiting list: 1988 through November 30, 1992. In: Terasaki PI, Cecka JM, eds. *Clinical transplants, 1992*. Los Angeles: UCLA Tissue Typing Laboratory, 1993:61–75.

Edwards EB, Guo T, Breen TJ, et al. The UNOS OPTN waiting list: 1988 to 1993. In: Terasaki PI, Cecka JM, eds. *Clinical transplants, 1993*. Los Angeles: UCLA Tissue Typing Laboratory, 1994:71–83.

Ellison MD, Breen TJ, Glascock RF, et al. Organ donation in the United States: 1988 through 1991. In: Terasaki PI, Cecka JM, eds. *Clinical transplants, 1992*. Los Angeles: UCLA Tissue Typing Laboratory, 1993:119–128.

Evans RW. The actual and potential supply of organ donors in the United States. In: Terasaki PI, ed. *Clinical transplants, 1990*. Los Angeles: UCLA Tissue Typing Laboratory, 1990:329–341.

Evans RW. Organ transplantation and the inevitable debate as to what constitutes a basic health care benefit. In: Terasaki P, Cecka M, eds. *Clinical transplants, 1993*. Los Angeles: UCLA Tissue Typing Laboratory, 1994: 359–391.

Evans RW. Socioeconomic aspects of heart transplantation. *Curr Opin Cardiol* 1995;10:169–179.

Evans RW. The demand for transplantation in the United States. In: Terasaki PI, ed. *Clinical transplants, 1990*. Los Angeles: UCLA Tissue Typing Laboratory, 1990:319–325.

Evans RW. Need, demand, and supply in organ transplantation. *Transplant Proc* 1992;24:2152–2154.

Evans RW. Social, economic, and insurance issues in heart transplantation. In: O'Connell JB, Kaye MP, eds. *Intrathoracic transplantation 2000*. Austin, TX: RG Landes Co., 1993:1–17.

Evans RW. Heart transplants and priorities [Letter]. *Lancet* 1984;1: 852–853.

Evans RW. The economics of heart transplantation. *Circulation* 1987;75: 63–76.

Evans RW. Invited commentary on "The potential contribution of cardiac replacement to the control of cardiovascular diseases." *Arch Surg* 1990; 125:1151.

Evans RW, Manninen DL, Garrison LP, Maier A. Donor availability as the primary determinant of the future of heart transplantation. *JAMA* 1986;255:1892–1898.

Evans RW, Manninen DL, Gersh BJ, et al. The need for and supply of donor hearts for transplantation. *J Heart Transplant* 1984;4:57–62.

Evans RW, Manninen DL, Overcast JD, et al., eds. *The National Heart Transplantation Study: final report, volumes 1–5*. Seattle, WA: Battelle Human Affairs Research Centers, 1984.

Evans RW, Orians CE, Ascher NL. The potential supply of organ donors: an assessment of the efficiency of organ procurement efforts in the United States. *JAMA* 1992;267:239–246.

Evans RW, Orians CE, Ascher NL. Estimates of organ-specific donor availability for the United States. *Transplant Proc* 1993;25:1541–1542.

Faltin DL, Jeannet M, Suter PM. The decrease in organ donations from 1985 to 1990 caused by increasing medical contraindications and refusals by relatives. *Transplantation* 1992;54:85–88.

Farrar DJ, Hill JD. Recovery of major organ function in patients awaiting heart transplantation with Thoratec ventricular assist device. *J Heart Lung Transplant* 1994;13:1125–1132.

Frazier OH, Duncan JM, Radovancevic B, et al. Successful bridge to heart transplantation with a new left ventricular assist device. *J Heart Lung Transplant* 1992;11:530–537.

Garrison LP Jr, Evans RW. The economic impact of heart transplantation on the Medicare program, 1985–1989. In: Baumgartner WG, Reitz BA, eds. *Heart and heart–lung transplantation*. Baltimore: Williams & Wilkins, 1989:41–50.

Ham C. Health care rationing. *Br Med J* 1995;310:1483–1484.

Heginbotham C. Health care priority setting: a survey of doctors, managers, and the general public. In: Smith R, ed. *Rationing in action*. London: BMJ Publishing Group, 1993:141–156.

Hogness JR, VanAntwerp M, eds. *The artificial heart: prototype, policies, and patients*. Washington, DC: National Academy Press, 1991.

Jacquet L, Dion R, Niorhomme P, et al. Successful bridge to retransplantation with the wearable Novacor left ventricular assist system. *J Heart Lung Transplant* 1996;15:620–622.

Kaiser J. IOM backs cautious experimentation. *Science* 1996;273:305–306.

Kaiser J. Xenograft guidelines clearing last hurdles. *Science* 1996;271:585.

Kondro W. Canadians float artificial heart on stock exchange. *Lancet* 1996;348:1441.

Kottke TE, Pesch DG, Frye RL, et al. The potential contribution of cardiac replacement to the control of cardiovascular diseases: a population-based estimate. *Arch Surg* 1990;125:1148–1151.

Lin SS, Platt JL. Immunologic barriers to xenotransplantation. *J Heart Lung Transplant* 1996;15:547–555.

Marwick C. British, American reports on xenotransplantation. *JAMA* 1996; 276:589–590.

Maynard A. Rationing health care. *Br Med J* 1996;313:1499.

Mehta SM, Aufiero TX, Pae WE Jr, et al. Combined registry for the clinical use of mechanical ventricular assist pumps and the total artificial heart in conjunction with heart transplantation: sixth official report—1994. *J Heart Lung Transplant* 1995;14:585–593.

Murphy FA. The public health risk of animal organ and tissue transplantation into humans. *Science* 1996;273:746–747.

Myllykangas M, Ryynanen O-P, Kinnunen J, Takala J. Comparison of doctors', nurses', politicians' and public attitudes to health care priorities. *Health Serv Res Policy* 1996;1:212–216.

Nathan HM, Jarrell BE, Broznik B, et al. Estimation and characterization of the potential renal organ donor pool in Pennsylvania: report of the Pennsylvania Statewide Donor Study. *Transplantation* 1991;51:142–149.

National Center for Health Statistics. *Health, United States, 1995.* Hyattsville, MD: Public Health Service, 1996.

Nowak R. Xenotransplants set to resume. *Science* 1994;266:1148–1151.

Nuffield Council on Bioethics. *Animal-to-human transplants: the ethics of xenotransplantation.* London: Nuffield Council on Bioethics, 1996.

O'Connell JB. Immunosuppression for dilated cardiomyopathy. *N Engl J Med* 1989;321:1119–1121.

O'Connell JB, Bourge RC, Castanzo-Nordin MR, et al. Cardiac transplantation: recipient selection, donor procurement, and medical follow-up. A statement for health professionals from the Committee on Cardiac Transplantation of the Council on Clinical Cardiology, American Heart Association. *Circulation* 1992;86:1061–1079.

Packer M, Bristow MR, Cohn JN, et al. The effect of carvedilol on morbidity and mortality in patients with chronic heart failure. *N Engl J Med* 1996;334:1349–1355.

Packer M, Carver JR, Rodeheffer RJ, et al. Effect of oral milrinone on mortality in severe chronic heart failure: the PROMISE Study Research Group. *N Engl J Med* 1991;325:1468–1475.

Pennington G, McBride L, Miller LW, Swartz MT. Eleven years' experience with the Pierce–Donachy ventricular assist device. *J Heart Lung Transplant* 1994;13:803–810.

Ratner LE, Kraus E, Magnuson T, Bender JS. Transplantation of kidneys from expanded criteria donors. *Surgery* 1996;119:372–377.

Roper WL. Medicare coverage criteria for Medicare coverage of heart transplants; proposed notice. *Federal Register* 1986;51:37164–37170.

Roper WL. Medicare program: criteria for Medicare coverage of heart transplants. *Federal Register* 1987;52:10935–10951.

Shelton DL. Physicians hold key to boosting organ donation, awareness. *American Medical News* 1996;39(17):7.

Shirley S, Cutler J, Heymann C, Hart M. Narrowing the organ donation gap: hospital development methods that maximize hospital donation potential. *J Heart Lung Transplant* 1994;13:817–823.

Shuldiner AR. Transgenic animals. *N Engl J Med* 1996;334:653–655.

Smith R, ed. *Rationing in action.* London: BMJ Publishing Group, 1993.

Stevenson LW, Warner SL, Steimle AE, et al. The impending crisis awaiting cardiac transplantation: modeling a solution based on selection. *Circulation* 1994;89:450–457.

United Network for Organ Sharing. *1995 Annual report of the U.S. Scientific Registry of Organ Transplant Recipients and the Organ Procurement and Transplantation Network. Transplant data: 1988–1994.* Richmond, VA: United Network for Organ Sharing, 1996.

U.S. Bureau of the Census. *Statistical abstract of the United States: 1995.* 115th ed. Washington, DC: U.S. Bureau of the Census, 1996.

U.S. Department of Health and Human Services. *Healthy people 2000: national health promotion and disease prevention objectives.* DHHS Publication No. (PHS) 91-50212. Washington, DC: U.S. Government Printing Office, 1991.

Wight C, Cohen B. Shortage of organs for transplantation. *Br Med J* 1996;312:989–990.

Management of End-Stage Heart Disease, edited by Eric A. Rose and Lynne Warner Stevenson. Lippincott–Raven Publishers, Philadelphia ©1998.

CHAPTER 3

End-points for Evaluation of Therapies

Ileana L. Piña, Ross R. Zimmer, and Victor Gil

The population with heart failure continues to increase. Many of these patients will either present with end-stage disease, or the disease will develop in them over time. As we continue to search for the "ideal" therapeutic approach that will be applicable to all New York Heart Association (NYHA) classifications, data regarding the success of therapy in this special group remain scant. The management of the end-stage population is often driven by the experience of the clinicians caring for them and ranges from aggressive, hemodynamic-driven therapy to cautious increments in medications based on clinical signs and symptoms. Similarly, the use of intravenous inotropic support falls into a wide range of applications from none, to out-patient intermittent programs, to home continuous therapy. Because mortality remains high, other end-points need to be sought in the management of this unique group of patients in a resource-efficient manner. Other end-points should include functional capacity, quality of life, and frequency of hospitalizations (Table 1). This chapter explores end-points of therapy as they pertain specifically to the patient group with moderate to severe heart failure.

MORTALITY

The 4-year mortality rate reported from the Framingham study for patients who were diagnosed with heart failure was 52% for men and 34% for women. From the 12-year cumulative experience at Duke University, the 1- and 5-year mortality rates for Class II and III were similar, whereas that of Class IV was 66% and 82% at 1 and 5 years, respectively (Figure 1). Another population studied between 1979 and 1981 with moderate to severe heart failure had a 1-year mortality rate of 34%, 59% at 2 years, and 76% at 3 years.

Improvement in survival is an obvious and desirable end-point for any patient with heart failure. Unfortunately, large, multicenter therapeutic trials that have been published to date have included only small numbers of Class IV patients, as shown in Table 2. Nonetheless, the therapies proven for less severe heart failure are ultimately applied to the patients with more severe disease as well. One transplantation center has reported an improvement in survival of the most severely ill group of patients with heart failure when analyzing mortality data for the periods 1986 to 1988, 1989 to 1990, and 1991 to 1993, in spite of a longer waiting time for transplantation and a relatively stable number of transplantations performed. This improvement could be attributed to the application of proven therapeutic interventions, such as the increased use of angiotensin-converting enzyme (ACE) inhibitors and general improvements in medical management using a comprehensive treatment plan. This study, however, did not include a randomized, prospective trial of therapy.

Vasodilators and Angiotensin-Converting Enzyme Inhibitors

The Cooperative North Scandinavian Enalapril Survival Study (CONSENSUS) was the first trial prospectively to evaluate mortality in the NYHA Class IV patient group. The study group consisted of 253 patients randomly assigned to placebo or enalapril. The follow-up was short, at a mean of 188 days, and the study was stopped 20 months after the first patient was enrolled. The 1-year mortality rate was reduced by 31%, and by the end of the study, the reduction in deaths was 27% in the enalapril-treated group.

A comprehensive review of ACE inhibitor trials was undertaken by Garg and Yusuf. Only prospective, randomized trials that had a placebo group, lasted at least 8 weeks,

Cardiomyopathy and Transplant Center, Temple University Hospital, Philadelphia, Pennsylvania 19140-5103

TABLE 1. *End-points in the evaluation of therapies for heart failure*

Mortality
Symptoms
Hospitalizations
Quality of life
Functional capacity
Hemodynamics

and had determined that mortality by an intention to treat were included in the analysis. Of 3,870 patients in the ACE inhibitor group and 3,235 in the placebo group, 253 (6.5%) and 213 (6.6%) patients were enrolled with Class IV symptoms, respectively. Twenty-eight percent of the patients in the ACE inhibitor group and 45.1% in the placebo group died, with an odds ratio of 0.55 in favor of the ACE inhibitor group. This odds ratio is significantly different from that of the Class III patients, which was 0.76 in favor of the ACE inhibitors and where 16.5% of the group on ACE inhibitors died versus 23.8% in the placebo group. Analysis of hospitalizations is discussed later.

Adrenergic Blocking Agents

Beta-adrenergic blocking agents have shown promise by improving symptoms, functional capacity, and ventricular function in patients with heart failure secondary to either dilated cardiomyopathy or coronary artery disease. Fisher and coworkers prospectively randomized 50 patients with heart failure due to coronary artery disease, 60% of whom were Class III and IV, to metoprolol or placebo. Patients were treated on a background of digoxin, diuretics, and vasodilators. The patients on metoprolol exhibited a decrease in hospital admissions, an improvement in functional class, and an increase in ejection frac-

tion and functional capacity. Although encouraging, the number of patients in this study and others has been small. More recently, one of four parallel carvedilol trials that was specifically addressing the end-stage population was stopped prematurely because of beneficial effects of the drug in the other trials. Therefore, only 32 Class IV patients were enrolled, with a short follow-up period and with four deaths occurring during the study period. Therefore, with one of the more promising new agents, carvedilol, the amount of data on the end-stage patient again falls short. Two ongoing trials plan to enroll a greater number of Class IV patients. The Beta Blocker Evaluation Survival Trial (BEST trial) is a large, randomized, prospective, placebo-controlled study of bucindolol in a large group of patients with Class III and IV chronic heart failure on a background of digoxin, diuretics, and ACE inhibitors. Similarly, the Prospective Randomized Amlodipine in Survival Evaluation (PRAISE) II trial will study the effects of amlodipine in a population of Class III and IV patients with dilated, nonischemic cardiomyopathy. The first PRAISE trial is briefly discussed later.

Amiodarone

Amiodarone is frequently used for arrhythmia management in patients with heart failure. The GESICA trial (Grupo de Estudio de la Sobrevida en la Insuficiencia Cardiaca en Argentina) enrolled 516 patients, 79% of whom were Class III and IV, and prospectively randomized them to 300 mg of maintenance amiodarone or to control in a nonblinded fashion. The study did not include placebo in the control group. The risk reduction of deaths in the amiodarone group was 28% ($p = 0.024$), with 26% risk reduction in Class IV and 24% in Class III. The Veterans Affairs Survival Trial of Antiarrhythmic Therapy in Congestive Heart Failure failed to demonstrate a reduc-

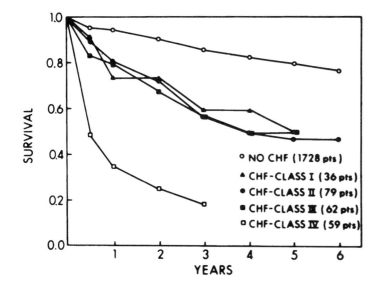

FIG. 1. Survival probabilities in 236 patients with congestive heart failure (CHF) and coronary artery disease according to the NYHA classification and compared with 1,728 patients without a history of CHF. (From Califf RM, Bounous P, Harrell FE, et al. The prognosis in the presence of coronary artery disease. In: Braunwald E, ed. *Congestive heart failure: current research and clinical applications*. New York: Grune & Stratton, 1982:31–40.)

TABLE 2. *Number and percentage of New York Heart Association Class III and Class IV patients enrolled in major heart failure studies (all studies have had at least 8 weeks of follow-up and had mortality as an end-point)*

Trial	Total no. of patients	No. and percentage of class III patients	No. and percentage of class IV patients
Vasodilator Heart Failure Trial (V-HeFT-II)	804	345 (42.9%)	28 (0.35%)
Studies of Left Ventricular Dysfunction (SOLVD) Treatment Trial	2,569	784 (31%)	43 (1.6%)
Cooperative North Scandinavian Enalapril Survival Study (CONSENSUS)	253	0	253 (100%)
Metoprolol in Dilated Cardiomyopathy (MDC) Trial Study Group	383	186 (49%)	15 (4%)
Carvedilol Study	1,094	480 (44%)	32 (3.0%)
Grupo de Estudio de la Sobrevida en la Insuficiencia Cardiaca en Argentina (GESICA)[a]	516	250 (48%)	158 (31%)
Congestive Heart Failure Survival Trial of Anti-arrhythmic Therapy (CHF STAT)	674	278 (29%)[b]	
Total	5,619[c]	2,045 (36%)[c]	807 (14%)[c]

[a]No placebo group.
[b]Represents a grouping of Class III and IV.
[c]Does not include the CHF STAT.

tion in mortality, with a trend toward reduction in mortality in the nonischemic group.

Although the results of both trials appear contradictory, there may be reasons for the discrepancy. First, there was a greater severity of heart failure in the GESICA group, with 79% of Class III and IV patients versus 41% in the Veterans Affairs trial. The Veterans Affairs trial, on the other hand, included a greater proportion of ischemic cardiomyopathy patients (71%) compared with the GESICA trial (40%). Whether the cause of the heart failure or its severity will have an impact on the long-term outcome of patients on amiodarone therapy still needs to be determined.

Digoxin

Although used by clinicians for many decades, digoxin has remained controversial in its applicability to different functional classifications of heart failure. As in other drug categories mentioned in this chapter, the data on the benefits of digoxin for patients with Class IV heart failure remain few. The effects of digoxin alone on mortality have been difficult to assess from the large, randomized trials in which digoxin has been standard background therapy. To answer this important question, the Digitalis Investigator Group (DIG) trial was designed. Although 7,788 were enrolled, most were Class II and III. In the total population, there was no difference in mortality between the group receiving digoxin therapy and the placebo group. A subgroup analysis, however, showed significant benefit of digoxin for the combined end-point of overall mortality and hospitalizations, which was greater in those with worse symptoms, larger hearts, and lower ejection fractions.

Calcium Channel Blockers

Calcium channel blockers have in general been avoided in patients with advanced heart failure because of their negative inotropic effects. The third generation of dihydropyridine compounds, of which amlodipine and felodipine are examples, has received renewed interest after the PRAISE I and Veterans Administration Vasodilator in Heart Failure Trial (V-HeFT)-III trials. Neither agent appeared to worsen heart failure symptoms. Felodipine had a neutral effect on survival, whereas amlodipine had a neutral overall effect on survival but a slight advantage in survival for the nonischemic heart failure group. This finding has prompted a second trial, PRAISE II, to evaluate survival in dilated cardiomyopathy in patients with Class III and IV chronic heart failure. A third calcium channel blocker, mibefradil, which selectively affects T channels, is being studied in patients with Class III and IV heart failure in a mortality study called the Mortality Assessment in Congestive Heart Failure Trial (MACH-1).

HOSPITALIZATIONS

Hospitalizations have also been used as end-points for therapies in patients with heart failure. Hospitalizations could also easily be listed among factors contributing to quality of life. Because patients with end-stage disease are often rehospitalized at a high health care cost, this end-point is a reasonable one to examine further. The same problem encountered with the randomized trials exists in the search for hospitalizations as an end-point, given the small percentage of Class IV patients in trials. The rate of readmission has varied widely among studies, depending on the age of the population being studied and whether the study is prospective or retrospective. Vinson and colleagues prospectively followed a population of elderly patients with heart failure, 49% of whom were Class III and 12% Class IV, to determine the rate of readmission. The NYHA Class did not distinguish those being readmitted from those not requiring readmission. Of interest, patients who had more than four prior admissions were more likely to be readmitted. Gooding et al. found a 36% hospital readmission rate for patients 65 years of age or older admitted with heart failure to a large city hospital.

Therapeutic Strategies

The V-HeFT-I trial did not demonstrate any significant differences in hospitalizations among groups in spite of an improvement in survival in patients randomized to the hydralazine–isosorbide dinitrate combination compared with placebo. Similarly, the second trial, V-HeFT-II, also failed to demonstrate differences in rate of hospitalization in spite of a better survival in the enalapril-treated group. The predictors of hospitalization for heart failure overall were similar in both studies and included peak $\dot{V}O_2$, left ventricular ejection fraction, plasma norepinephrine, increased cardiothoracic ratio, and coronary artery disease. Time to first hospitalization after randomization was shorter for patients with peak $\dot{V}O_2$ less than 10 mL/kg/minute compared with the group with peak $\dot{V}O_2$ greater than 15 mL/kg/minute. The factors predicting hospitalizations are not surprising because they are indirect measurements of more advanced disease as well as prognostic indicators.

Although demonstrating improved survival with enalapril, the CONSENSUS study of Class IV patients did not address the question of hospitalizations in this moderately to severely ill group of patients. The Studies of Left Ventricular Dysfunction (SOLVD) had a primary end-point of mortality, but repeated hospitalizations constituted a major secondary end-point. Patient recruitment exceeded 2,500, 90% of whom were in Class II and III heart failure. At the end of follow-up, 971 hospitalizations had occurred in the placebo group and 683 in the enalapril-treated group (Table 3). Repeated hospitalizations were also less frequent in the enalapril group. The combined end-point of total mortality and hospitalization was also favorable for the enalapril-treated group, with 616 patients of 1,285 and 737 of 1,284 in the enalapril and the placebo groups, respectively, either hospitalized or dying during the follow-up period. In the summary trials of ACE inhibitors by Garg and Yusuf, of a total of 3,810 patients in the group who received an ACE inhibitor, 253 were Class IV, and of 3,178 in the control group, 213 were Class IV. For the combined end-point of mortality and hospitalization, the odds ratio in favor of ACE inhibitors for Class IV was 0.69, similar to Class II (0.68) and Class III (0.58). In the GESICA trial, subgroup analyses by NYHA class showed a 37% risk reduc-

TABLE 3. *Frequency of hospitalization for heart failure in the Studies of Left Ventricular Dysfunction (SOLVD) treatment arm*

Variable	Placebo		Enalapril	
	No.	%	No.	%
Vital status/hospitalizations				
Alive				
0[a]	548	42.7	672	52.3
1	123	9.6	95	7.4
2	48	3.7	31	2.4
3	27	2.1	15	1.2
>4	28	2.2	20	1.6
Death				
0	266	20.7	281	21.9
1	113	8.8	80	6.2
2	70	5.4	38	3.0
3	32	2.5	25	1.9
>4	29	2.2	28	2.2
Patients hospitalized				
At least once	470	36.6	332	25.8
Twice or more	234	18.2	157	12.2
All hospitalizations	971	—	683	—
Patients dead or hospitalized	736	57.3	613	47.7

[a]Number of hospitalizations.

tion for combined death or hospitalization in favor of the amiodarone-treated group.

In patients with multiple rehospitalizations, experience continues with intravenous inotropic infusions, which range from home care with 24-hour infusions to outpatient intermittent therapy. Friedman and colleagues reported on 13 patients with frequent readmissions, using 24-hour infusion of inotropes in 11 and intermittent outpatient therapy in 2. Hospital days decreased from 447 to 334, whereas days between hospitalizations increased from 1,462 to 3,280, although there were deaths in the group. Despite many anecdotal reports of experience with chronic inotropic support, prospective controlled data are lacking for hospitalization or other end-points. Out-patient infusion treatment is considered experimental and each center decides on its use based on their own experience.

HEMODYNAMICS

Most patients with advanced heart failure possess some degree of hemodynamic abnormality. The abnormal hemodynamics may be manifest at rest or be initiated by exercise and contribute to symptoms. Hemodynamics, therefore, is a reasonable end-point to discuss. The degree of resting hemodynamic disruption may not always correlate with prognosis. The response to therapy tailored for improvement in hemodynamics and the response to exercise are both of great importance.

The patient with Class IV or end-stage heart failure referred for further treatment or transplantation would have a measurement of baseline hemodynamics followed by intravenous therapy with either nitroglycerin, nitroprusside, or inotropic agents such as dobutamine or milrinone, which, along with diuretics, are tailored to hemodynamic goals. Typical end-points of tailored therapy include a pulmonary capillary wedge pressure (PCWP) no greater than 15 mm Hg and a systemic vascular resistance (SVR) no greater than 1,200 dynes/second/cm^5 with a systolic blood pressure of 80 mm Hg or more. The aim is to attain these end-points within 1 to 2 days with concurrent upward titration of high-dose ACE inhibitors and other oral vasodilators such as nitrates and hydralazine, with hopes for a subsequent slow wean off the intravenous support. Once ambulation and other normal activities are resumed, fine tuning of the medical regimen continues, including optimization of diuretic therapy. The patient should simultaneously be receiving detailed education regarding heart failure symptoms, dietary restrictions, and an exercise program.

The degree of the initial hemodynamic abnormalities does not predict which patients will achieve the end-points of tailored therapy. It is also worth noting that there are no untoward effects in attempting to achieve a PCWP within the normal range, rather than allowing the PCWP to remain elevated to maintain a good cardiac output, as had been suggested by the experience in patients with acute myocardial infarction.

A more valuable predictor of outcome than the initial hemodynamic profile is the individual patient's response to tailored therapy. In an analysis of 152 patients with a mean ejection fraction less than 20% and end-stage heart failure referred for transplantation, application of tailored therapy resulted in a right atrial pressure and PCWP decrease of approximately 40%, an SVR decrease of 26%, and a cardiac index increase of almost 50%. After discharge, the actuarial survival rate was 73% at 3 months and 62% at 1 year (Figure 2). Univariate analysis demonstrated that baseline hemodynamics were not predictive of mortality, but that the response of filling pressure to tailored therapy was highly predictive. In multivariate analysis, the independent predictor of overall mortality was an elevated final PCWP. Those patients with a final PCWP greater than 16 mm Hg despite tailored therapy had a 1-year survival rate of only 38%, compared with 83% when the PCWP could be reduced to less than 16 mm Hg. In a parallel fashion, the patients who presented with normal filling pressures (14% of the total group) had a 95% 1-year survival rate. It is unclear whether the results of this study suggest that tailored therapy is actually beneficial for these patients for the long term, or whether the lack of response selects a high-mortality group.

The hemodynamic response to exercise is emerging as an interesting and perhaps important end-point in heart failure. Wilson and coworkers have described the varied exercise hemodynamic responses of a group of 64 sequential patients undergoing cardiac transplant evaluation, all of whom had left ventricular ejection fraction less than 33% and a peak $\dot{V}O_2$ less than 14 mL/kg/minute. Forty-two percent exhibited a reduction in cardiac output to exercise accompanied by an increase in the PCWP to greater than 20 mm Hg. In contrast, 20% of the patients had a normal cardiac output response to exercise while keeping the PCWP less than 20 mm Hg at peak exercise. It is reasonable to propose that the group with a normal exercise response may be a target for a conditioning exercise program and a follow-up evaluation. This study underscores the complexity of using strict end-points in the selection of patients with moderate to severe heart failure as candidates for transplantation. Although exercise hemodynamics could be cumbersome, the process may allow better selection of a group of patients who fall at the borderline of ventricular function and functional capacity indices.

It is important to recognize that hemodynamic response as an end-point of therapy does not always translate into a favorable outcome. The type of therapy

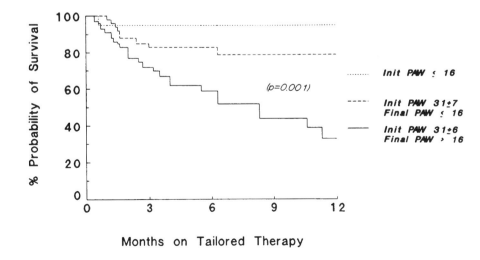

(p=0.001)

.... Init PAW ≤ 16

- - - - Init PAW 31±7
Final PAW ≤ 16

——— Init PAW 31±6
Final PAW > 16

FIG. 2. Relation between survival and pulmonary artery wedge (PAW) pressure at baseline and on tailored therapy in 152 patients discharged after referral for cardiac transplantation with ejection fractions greater than 20%. (From Stevenson LW, Tillisch JH, Hamilton MA, et al. Importance of hemodynamic response to therapy in predicting survival with ejection fraction ≤20% secondary to ischemic or nonischemic dilated cardiomyopathy. *Am J Cardiol* 1990;66:1348–1354.)

used to achieve hemodynamic goals is also important. This point became clearly evident in the oral milrinone trial (PROMISE) in which the drug initially had a favorable hemodynamic profile, only later to have a deleterious effect on survival. Paradoxically, ACE inhibitors, which have become the cornerstone of therapy in heart failure because of mortality benefits, have not consistently led to improvements in hemodynamics when used alone; nor have they consistently produced early improvements in functional capacity. The Hy-C trial enrolled 117 patients being evaluated for cardiac transplantation. Eighty percent of those patients had Class IV symptoms and were randomized to receive either captopril or hydralazine and isosorbide dinitrate. Tailored therapy goals were achieved initially with intravenous nitroprusside and diuretics and subsequently with oral therapy. Nearly 40 patients in the initial captopril group and 22 patients in the vasodilator group required a change in therapy because of a poor response or side effects. Although the hemodynamic targets were achieved with both regimens, the actuarial 1-year survival rate was 81% in the captopril/nitrate group and 51% in the hydralazine/nitrate group. In this study, as in the other discussed previously, PCWP was an independent predictor of survival.

In summary, a valuable intermediate end-point in the management of the patient with advanced heart failure is the degree to which hemodynamics, particularly filling pressures, can be optimized with a combination of diuretics, digoxin, ACE inhibitors, and vasodilators. A knowledge of the response to tailored therapy can give the clinician another early prognostic indicator in this very ill population.

FUNCTIONAL CAPACITY

Because reduction in functional capacity owing to symptoms of fatigue or dyspnea is the hallmark of end-stage heart failure, it is reasonable and clinically relevant to use exercise capacity as an end-point of any therapy. A drug that improves symptoms also should be able to demonstrate improvements in objective forms of exercise testing in a parallel fashion. In general, drugs that have improved symptoms during placebo-controlled trials in patients with heart failure have also led to objective improvements in exercise capacity. In addition, and of great importance, is the role that exercise testing, particularly determination of $\dot{V}O_{2max}$, plays in prognostic allocation. It must be borne in mind, however, that improvement in functional capacity does not always translate to improvement in survival, as was unfortunately observed with the drug flosequinan.

Vasodilators

Keeping in mind the limited number of Class IV patients enrolled in large trials, as discussed earlier, some results of these studies merit a brief review. In the V-HeFT-II trial, a subset of patients underwent functional capacity assessment by cardiopulmonary exercise testing. In spite of the ACE inhibitor, enalapril, having the survival edge, the vasodilator combination of hydralazine and isosorbide dinitrate performed better in $\dot{V}O_2$ response, albeit to a modest degree (Figure 3). Furthermore, the changes in peak $\dot{V}O_2$ were poorly correlated to changes in quality-of-life scores, except for the group whose peak $\dot{V}O_2$ improved by more than 2.5 mL/kg/minute (Figure 4).

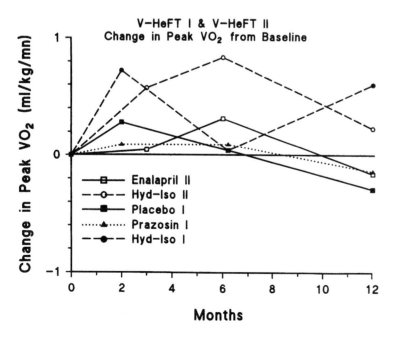

FIG. 3. Changes in peak $\dot{V}O_2$ after randomization in the first and second Vasodilator in Heart Failure Trials (V-HeFT-1 and V-HeFT-II). The vasodilator combination resulted in a modest increase in functional capacity. However, enalapril, prazosin, and placebo were not associated with any significant change.

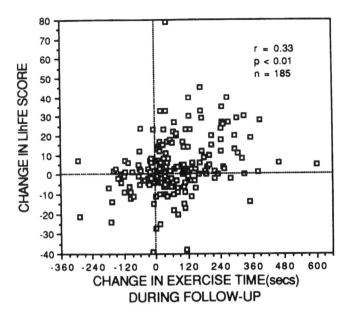

FIG. 4. Changes in peak VO_2 compared with an improvement in quality-of-life score after randomization to pimobendan or placebo. An increase in peak VO_2 to greater than 2.5 mL/kg/minute usually has been associated with an improvement in the Minnesota Living with Heart Failure Questionnaire score.

In smaller trials, nitrates alone have also been shown to improve exercise tolerance. The improvement, however, is not seen immediately but occurs with time. Flosequinan, a direct-acting vasodilator with mild inotropic effects, was also shown to improve exercise function as well as symptoms. Unfortunately, the survival data were not in favor of the drug, and thus flosequinan was removed from the market.

ACE Inhibitors

Early trials of captopril were favorable with respect to exercise tolerance. Shortly thereafter, similar observations were made with enalapril. Unfortunately, neither the SOLVD nor the CONSENSUS trial studied functional capacity with exercise testing prospectively. A subset of the SOLVD subjects underwent the 6-minute walk test, which is discussed later. ACE inhibitors also fall into the category where lack of early increase in exercise tolerance does not translate to similar late findings or lack of efficacy.

Digoxin

Using functional capacity as an end-point of therapy, the results of digoxin trials have been varied. In the milrinone–digoxin trial, the addition of digoxin improved exercise tolerance compared with the placebo or milrinone groups. By contrast, in the captopril–digoxin trial, digoxin did not affect exercise tolerance, as was the case in the digoxin–xamoterol trial. The explanation for these

discrepancies may lie in the type of patient enrolled in each of these trials and in the severity of heart failure. At least one study has shown improvement in exercise duration only in the most limited group. Therefore, digoxin therapy designed to ameliorate exercise-induced symptoms and hence improve function may be best suited to the population with end-stage disease.

Diuretics

Although diuretics are the standard mainstay of therapy in heart failure, to date there are no published large-scale trials to evaluate the effects of diuretic therapy on functional capacity. Improvement in exercise duration seems a relevant point in a patient whose volume overload or edema is relieved by any given diuretic.

Inotropes

As noted earlier, an increase in exercise duration has not always been associated with an increase in survival, as has been shown by oral milrinone, xamoterol (a beta₁ agonist), and flosequinan. Each of these drugs led to initial improvements in exercise function but eventually increased mortality.

6-Minute Walk Test

Early efficacy studies of vasodilators and ACE inhibitors attempted to demonstrate beneficial drug effects with serial testing to a maximum level. The addition of gas exchange parameters gave investigators a better assessment of a maximum effort and therefore a more reliable peak exercise end-point. Among the patient group to whom this book is dedicated, maximum exercise testing could be unrealistic. Furthermore, self-assessments of function derived from questionnaires show striking discrepancies between physician-assigned functional capacity and more objective measures of exercise tolerance.

Among exercise testing protocols, the 6-minute walk test has become more popular in recent years because of its ease of administration, inexpensive nature, and its approximation to daily tasks. Originally described in a chronic pulmonary disease population as a 12-minute walk, the test uses a 20-meter–long, level, enclosed corridor. Instructions are given to the patient to cover as much ground as possible in 6 minutes by walking continuously, if possible. Lipkin and colleagues adapted the test to the heart failure population and tested it in 26 patients with chronic heart failure. The 6-minute walk test was preferred by the patients to the maximum treadmill test. The 6-minute walk test did not discriminate between NYHA Class II and III as well as a $\dot{V}O_{2max}$ test, but was more sensitive for distinguishing changes in functional status in the patients with more advanced disease. The walk test, therefore, may be better suited for the patients with moderate to severe heart failure in whom repeated testing is used for serial monitoring. In a small group of 18 patients with heart failure, the 6-minute walk correlated better with other instruments, such as the Baseline Dyspnea Index and the Specific Activity Scale, than a cycle ergometer test. The test is therefore valid. Of interest, a substudy of the SOLVD registry reported that the 6-minute walk test was safe and simple to perform as well as an independent, strong predictor of mortality and morbidity. Among 898 patients in the SOLVD registry, those with the higher performance level had the lowest chance of death and hospitalization during the follow-up period.

The 6-minute walk has also been included by some centers as part of an overall assessment of quality of life in advanced heart failure. Dracup and associates included the 6-minute walk in a study designed to evaluate quality of life in a group of patients who had been referred to a transplantation center. Fifty-six percent of those patients were in Class IV heart failure and 37% in Class III. Although challenging for some, all the patients completed the 6-minute walk test without complications. The 6-minute walk distance correlated with NYHA classification and the self-assigned multiple of the resting metabolic oxygen requirements (MET) level in a functional status inventory, thus confirming the findings of Lipkin et al. In summary, the 6-minute walk test seems to offer an advantage over maximum treadmill/bicycle exercise testing in patients with advanced heart failure because of its ease of administration, safety, validity, and evidence of prognostic import in at least one large trial. It may particularly be useful as an adjunct measurement of quality of life when assessing the effect of medical therapy.

Peak $\dot{V}O_2$

The prognostic significance of a low peak $\dot{V}O_2$ has been more extensively studied. There is disagreement among heart failure specialists as to the timing of this test vis-à-vis medical therapy. The ability to exercise should be significantly better once adequate medical therapy is instituted. It is for this reason that many cardiac transplantation centers perform the index cardiopulmonary test for transplant evaluation only after medical therapy is optimized. Although levels from 10 to 14 mL/kg/minute have been suggested, a definitive cut-off for $\dot{V}O_2$ may not be appropriate as the only prognostic factor. This fact is underscored by some observations by Wilson and colleagues, who reported that as many as 20% of patients with a $\dot{V}O_2$ less than 14 mL/kg/minute have only mild hemodynamic impairment with exercise. Similarly, even when an improvement in $\dot{V}O_2$ is achieved as an end-point by either exercise training or medical therapy, there are no data available that support an automatic improvement in prognosis. Using this value as the sole criterion of listing or delisting for transplantation may be unwise. The total clinical picture remains the most important of all observations.

QUALITY OF LIFE

The term "quality of life" encompasses many factors, such as the ability to function in daily life, social roles, psychological well-being, and coping, among others. Wenger describes three major components that wholly define quality of life. These are functional capacity, perceptions, and symptoms and their consequences (Table 4). Functional capacity includes items such as mobility, independence, and ability to perform self-care, participate in work or recreational activities, and obtain needed rest and sleep. This category also includes intellectual function such as memory and judgment, as well as emotional status and economic status. Perceptions are colored by a patient's belief system and perspectives. Symptoms may result in repeated hospitalizations and administration of medications, with their consequent side effects. In the patient with advanced heart failure, all of these factors may play a significant role and are interrelated. The ability to work may not be an issue in this population, but certainly independence with regard to self-care and intellectual function, as well as relief of symptoms and freedom from hospitalizations, characterize quality of life for these patients.

The term "health-related" quality of life perhaps best describes the type of quality of life assessment pertinent to patients with end-stage heart disease. As Guyatt points out, other factors that affect quality of life such as the environment are far removed from the needs and concerns of a patient who is severely ill. Instruments used to assess quality of life in patients with coronary artery disease may not be applicable to patients with end-stage heart failure, for whom more basic necessities are often luxuries. Nonetheless, quality-of-life analysis has been used in clinically controlled trials of heart failure. In the SOLVD trial, quality of life was assessed by a questionnaire derived from previously validated instruments. The SOLVD study, however, was composed primarily of ambulatory Class II and III patients and included less than 3% Class IV cohorts. This large and critical trial underscores the problems with lack of verifiable instru-

TABLE 4. *Quality of life*

Functional capacity
  Ability to perform activities of daily living
  Social function
  Intellectual function
  Emotional function
  Economic status
Perceptions
  General health status
  Level of well-being
  Satisfaction with life
Symptoms and their consequences
  Of presenting illness
  As a result of therapy
  Concurrent illnesses

ments in a prospective trial of a population composed of patients with moderate to severe heart failure.

Properties Necessary for Measurements

There are four indispensable aspects of quality-of-life measurements: reliability, responsiveness, validity, and sensitivity. *Reliability* refers to the ability of an instrument to discriminate accurately among subjects tested in relation to changes in the facet being studied. *Responsiveness* is defined as the ability of an instrument to detect changes in an individual, even if the change is small. In patients who have had a stable clinical picture, the clinical instrument should reflect a stable score. Similarly, the instrument should reflect a significant change in score to parallel a significant change in a specific quality-of-life aspect. *Validity* refers to the ability of an instrument to measure what it was designed to measure. For example, an instrument to measure a patient's ability to perform daily living activities should relate to a test of exercise capacity. *Sensitivity* refers to the ability of a measurement to detect true changes or differences in quality of life.

Questionnaire Administration

For quality-of-life instruments to be successful in any clinical setting, several principles should be addressed. First, questionnaires for quality-of-life assessment should be considered of equal importance to other aspects of the study. Second, personnel who administer the instruments must be properly trained, avoiding bias. Third, monitoring mechanisms must be in place to ensure compliance with instrument administration. Self-administered instruments may prevent inherent bias and have been used in several published reports of quality of life in patients with heart failure. Wiklund and colleagues used a self-assessment instrument called the Quality of Life Questionnaire in Severe Heart Failure (QLQ-SHF) during the CONSENSUS trial and found it to be relevant and reliable. However, the investigators found methodologic problems with a trial that had a high mortality rate in the placebo group, creating an imbalance in the follow-up patient-driven objectives over time. The SOLVD investigators also used a self-administered short questionnaire in all patients in the trial and a more detailed assessment administered by a trained psychologist in a subset of patients in 5 of 23 centers. The brief questionnaire was thought to be discriminatory among patients with different degrees of severity, although there was a considerable amount of missing quality-of-life data as the study progressed.

Instruments

In general, there are two type of instruments for measurements of health-related quality of life, generic and disease specific. Generic measures are broad based and applicable to a wide array of disease entities, and can be divided into health profiles and utility instruments. The best known of the health profiles is the Sickness Impact Profile (SIP), which measures the impact of disease on physical and psychosocial behavior and other items such as sleep/rest and work. In a small group of patients with heart failure who were given the SIP and underwent a cardiopulmonary test, there was only a weak correlation between the peak oxygen uptake achieved and the score of the SIP, with considerable overlap across three levels of functional capacity. Utility instruments such as the Quality of Well-Being Scale measure symptoms, social activities, and actual patient preferences of treatment processes, including hospitalizations. These instruments many not be sensitive enough to pick up small changes in clinical status.

Disease-specific measures focus on aspects of quality of life relevant primarily to patients with a specific disease. These instruments are the most commonly used in studies of patients with heart failure. Perhaps the best known of these is the Minnesota Living with Heart Failure Questionnaire, which contains 21 items covering physical, social, psychological, and economic aspects as they directly affect the patient with heart failure symptoms. This questionnaire has been shown to be a valid representation of symptoms in patients with Class II and III heart failure, and in the SOLVD trial could distinguish between Class I and Class II to III patients. This instrument, however, has not been validated in a more impaired group of patients with heart failure. Three other instruments that have been used in patients with heart failure include the Yale Scale or Fatigue–Dyspnea Index, the Chronic Heart Failure Questionnaire (CHQ), and the QLQ-SHF.

The Yale Scale

Because patients with heart failure experience a change in quality of life directly related to symptoms of dyspnea and fatigue, Feinstein and coworkers have developed a simple instrument to assess the clinical impact of fatigue and dyspnea on the quality of life of patients with heart failure. Made up of three components, the instrument is administered by experienced personnel and uses a five-point scale. The components include the specific task that provoked dyspnea or fatigue, the effort with which the task is performed, and the patient's overall functional capacity. A rating of 0 indicates severe impairment, and 4, no impairment. The individual scores are added to give a composite score. Tested in a total of 362 patients with heart failure from two randomly assigned trials of lisinopril versus captopril and lisinopril versus placebo, the index proved to be reliable and valid, and concentrates on an area of physical distress that affects the functional aspects of quality of life.

The Chronic Heart Failure Questionnaire

This questionnaire is meant to evaluate longitudinal changes over time; its feature include (a) measures of physical and emotional health; (b) items to reflect functional areas important to patients with heart failure; (c) scores that can be analyzed statistically; (d) responsiveness to clinical changes, including small ones; (e) validity; and (f) a short enough length to be time- and cost-effective. It consists of 123 questions, 61 of which deal with physical function and 62 with emotional or social function. Table 5 lists the highest-scoring items in 88 patients with heart failure. During a randomized trial of digoxin versus placebo, the CHQ dyspnea score correlated better with global changes in shortness of breath, changes in walk test, and changes in heart failure score than the NYHA and the Specific Activity Scale (SAS) (Table 6).

Quality of Life Questionnaire in Severe Heart Failure

Wiklund et al. developed a self-administered, health-related questionnaire specifically to evaluate the population with severe heart failure. A better quality of life was defined as decreased symptoms, increased well-being, and improved capacity to function in daily living activities. The items are divided as follows:

1. Somatic, functional, and emotional disturbances: symptoms of fatigue, dyspnea, palpitations—20 items
2. Emotional and cognitive symptoms—21 items
3. Life satisfaction reflecting subjective well-being/happiness—10 items
4. Self-care activities and light to moderate exertion in ambulation/mobility/physical activity—24 items
5. Social/recreational activity—15 items

A subset of this questionnaire was used during the CONSENSUS trial. The authors found methodologic problems in such a trial that had parallel groups comparing enalapril to placebo where mortality was expected to be high in the placebo-treated group. The high mortality created an imbalance in follow-up of patient-measured objectives such as symptoms and psychological stress. The value of this type of questionnaire for individual patients not enrolled in a mortality trial has not been assessed.

In summary, questionnaires assessing quality of life in severe heart failure should be short and standardized, and address the very specific areas that relate to the severity of the disease. To date, such an ideal instrument for this specific population is lacking.

Measured Quality of Life in Advanced Heart Failure

Quality of life in patients with advanced heart failure was studied by Dracup and colleagues in a group of 134 patients who were being evaluated for possible cardiac transplantation. Using a set of instruments that included the 6-minute walk, NYHA classification, and the Heart Failure Functional Status Inventory, among others, they

---

TABLE 5. *Areas of dysfunction as reported by 88 patients with heart failure*

Dyspnea	Difficulty in concentrating
Hurrying	Emotional
Walking upstairs	Anxiety
Going for a walk	Restlessness
Carrying, such as groceries	Depression
Being angry or upset	Discouraged
Bending	Down in the dumps
Walking uphill	Inadequate
Fatigue	A burden on others
Worn out	Embarrassment
Low in energy	Need to rest frequently because of fatigue or
Generally tired	tiredness
Sluggish	Aching, tired legs
Exhausted	Need to rest frequently because of shortness of
Not having enough energy to get through the day	breath
Sleep disturbance	Frustration
Trouble getting to sleep	Frustrated
Waking up during the night	Impatient
Not getting a good night's sleep	Mastery
Social	A feeling of fear or panic when you could not get your
Doing your usual social activities	breath
Cognitive	Feeling out of control of your breathing problems
Forgetfulness	

Adapted from Guyatt GH, Nogradi S, Halcrow S, et al. Development and testing of a new measure of health status for clinical trials in heart failure. *J Gen Intern Med* 1989;4:101–107.

TABLE 6. *Correlations between Congestive Heart Failure Questionnaire (CHQ) dyspnea dimension, New York Heart Association (NYHA) functional classification, and Specific Activity (SAS) Classification[a]*

	Global rating of change in shortness of breath	Change in walk test score	Change in heart failure score
CHQ dyspnea score	0.65	0.60	0.42
NYHA functional classification	0.20	0.24	0.10
SAS classification	0.34	0.11	0.04

[a]In natural units, correlations between NYHA and SAS and other measures are negative; sign has been reversed for comparison purposes. All correlations greater than or equal to 0.20 are statistically significant at the 0.05 level.

From Guyatt GH, Nogradi S, Halcrow S, et al. Development and testing of a new measure of health status for clinical trials in heart failure. *J Gen Intern Med* 1989;4:101–107.

found no significant relation between quality of life and resting ejection fraction. There were significant correlations, however, among the 6-minute walk, the NYHA classification, and the self-reported functional status with psychosocial adjustment. Depression, hostility, and MET level of function accounted for a significant portion of the psychosocial adjustment. It is reasonable, then, to pursue improvements in depression, hostility, and functional status when assessing interventions to improve quality of life in patients with advanced heart failure.

SUMMARY

This chapter has attempted to present reasonable end-points in patients with end-stage heart failure. In this extremely ill patient population, end-points other than mortality alone need to be considered. The ability to carry out tasks associated with daily living, less frequent hospitalizations, and quality of life may be more important to the patient than quantity of life. Evaluation of the impact of therapies for this group of patients continues to present a challenge to the clinical heart failure team.

SELECTED REFERENCES

Cohn J, Johnson G, Ziesche S, et al. A comparison of enalapril with hydralazine-isosorbide dinitrate in the treatment of chronic congestive heart failure. *N Engl J Med* 1991;325:303–310.

Doval HC, Nul DR, Granceli HO, et al. Randomized trial of low-dose amiodarone in severe congestive heart failure. *Lancet* 1994;344:493–498.

Dracup K, Walden JA, Stevenson LW, Brecht ML. Quality of life in patients with advanced heart failure. *J Heart Lung Transplant* 1992;11:273–279.

Feinstein AR, Fisher MB, Pigeon JG. Changes in dyspnea–fatigue ratings as indicators of quality of life in the treatment of congestive heart failure. *Am J Cardiol* 1989;64:50–55.

Fonarow GC, Chelimsky-Fallick C, Stevenson LW, et al. Effect of direct vasodilation with hydralazine versus angiotensin-converting enzyme inhibition with captopril on mortality in advanced heart failure: the Hy-C trial. *J Am Coll Cardiol* 1992;19:842–850.

Garg R, Yusuf S. Overview of randomized trials of angiotensin-converting enzyme inhibitors on mortality and morbidity in patients with heart failure. *JAMA* 1995;273:1450–1456.

Guyatt GH. Measurement of health-related quality of life in heart failure. *J Am Coll Cardiol* 1993;22[Suppl A]:185A–191A.

Lipkin DP, Scriven AJ, Crake T, Poole-Wilson PA. Six-minute walking test for assessing exercise capacity in chronic heart failure. *Br Med J* 1986; 292:653–655.

Packer M, Bristow MR, Cohn JN, et al. The effect of carvedilol on morbidity and mortality in patients with chronic heart failure: U.S. Carvedilol Heart Failure Study Group. *N Engl J Med* 1996;334: 1349–1355.

Rector TS, Kubo SH, Cohn JN. Patients' self-assessment of their congestive heart failure: part 2. content reliability and validity of a new measure, the Minnesota Living with Heart Failure Questionnaire. *Heart Failure* 1987; 1:198–209.

Stevenson LW, Dracup KA, Tillisch JH. Efficacy of medical therapy tailored for severe congestive heart failure in patients transferred for urgent cardiac transplantation. *Am J Cardiol* 1989;63:461–464.

Stevenson LW, Tillisch JH, Hamilton MA, et al. Importance of hemodynamic response to therapy in predicting survival with ejection fraction ≤20% secondary to ischemic or nonischemic dilated cardiomyopathy. *Am J Cardiol* 1990;66:1348–1354.

Stevenson WG, Stevenson LW, Middlekauff HR, et al. Improving survival for patients with advanced heart failure: a study of 737 consecutive patients. *J Am Coll Cardiol* 1995;26:1417–1423.

Swedberg K. Effects of enalapril on mortality in severe congestive heart failure: results of the Cooperative North Scandinavian Enalapril Survival Study. *N Engl J Med* 1987;316:1429–1435.

The SOLVD Investigators. Effect of enalapril on survival in patients with reduced left ventricular ejection fractions and congestive heart failure. *N Engl J Med* 1991;325:293–302.

Singh SN, Fletcher RD, Fisher SG, et al. Amiodarone in patients with congestive heart failure and asymptomatic ventricular arrhythmias. *N Engl J Med* 1995;333:77–82.

Waagstein F, Bristow MR, Swedberg K. Beneficial effects of metoprolol in idiopathic dilated cardiomyopathy. *Lancet* 1994;342:1441–1446.

Wiklund I, Swedberg. Some methodological problems in analyzing quality of life data in severe congestive heart failure patients. *Journal of Clinical Research and Pharmacoepidemiology* 1991;5:265–273.

Medical Therapy for Congestive Heart Failure

Management of End-Stage Heart Disease, edited by Eric A. Rose and Lynne Warner Stevenson. Lippincott–Raven Publishers, Philadelphia ©1998.

CHAPTER 4

Approach to the Patient with Severe Heart Failure

Gary S. Francis

Heart failure is a complex clinical syndrome that defies simple definition. The incidence in the United States is growing, particularly in the elderly (Figure 1). The diagnosis of heart failure remains largely a clinical exercise, and requires a careful history and physical examination. Virtually any form of heart disease can lead to heart failure, and there is no single laboratory test by which it can be consistently diagnosed. Like fever or renal failure, the diagnosis of "heart failure" by itself is inadequate, and the etiologic factors should always be considered. A thorough knowledge of the natural course of the syndrome is very helpful in the management of these patients. Determining prognosis for individual patients has proven to be notoriously difficult because the syndrome is characterized by a waxing and waning of the clinical course.

These difficulties, along with the growing awareness that heart failure is an expanding problem in the aging population, have resulted in a multifaceted teamwork approach to the care of these complicated patients. Although the clinical recognition of the syndrome is relatively straightforward, the management of the patient with heart failure requires an ongoing commitment from medical and nursing personnel. The care of the patient with heart failure has largely evolved into a team effort at most major medical centers. Each physician specializing in end-stage heart failure may have a somewhat different approach to the problem. Nevertheless, a number of unifying principles have emerged over time that may be helpful for health care workers encountering this ever-growing population of patients. For some of these principles, we now have abundant "evidence-based" clinical trials to guide us (Table 1). Other nuances of management are not always based on sound evidence, but experience

can be a helpful teacher. As I have worked in a heart failure clinic since 1979 and have observed the evolution of treatment over this period, it is of some interest for me to reflect on my personal experiences with these fragile but very grateful patients and to provide a rather personal approach toward their case.

APPROACH TO THE NEW PATIENT WITH ADVANCED HEART FAILURE

The Role of Conventional Therapy

For more than 200 years, the treatment of congestive heart failure has included digitalis and bed rest. In the 1950s, diuretics were added to the regimen, and in the 1960s potent loop diuretics were included in the therapeutic armamentarium. The model for the treatment of heart failure changed perceptibly in the 1970s, when the concept of vasodilator therapy became widely embraced. Although physiologists had long appreciated that manipulation of loading conditions directly influenced left ventricular performance in the failing heart, the attractiveness of pharmacologically "unloading" the heart finally took hold when drugs such as nitroprusside and oral agents such as hydralazine and nitrates became widely available. It eventually became clear that chronic heart failure was characterized by excessive neuroendocrine activation that was not a simple epiphenomenon, but contributed importantly to the pathogenesis of the syndrome. With the introduction of angiotensin-converting enzyme (ACE) inhibitors, further dramatic strides were made in the management of patients with heart failure. Today, ACE inhibitors are the cornerstone of therapy for the management of patients with heart failure.

The era of clinical trials began with the publication of the Veterans Administration Cooperative Vasodilator–Heart Failure Trial (V-HeFT I) in 1986. Since then, there

Department of Cardiology, Cleveland Clinic Foundation, Cleveland, Ohio 44195

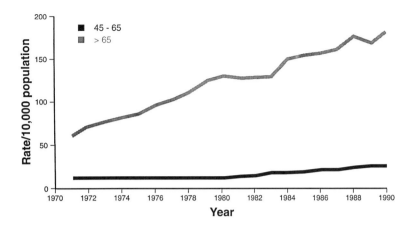

FIG. 1. Rates of admission to hospital for heart failure according to age in the United States, 1971–1990. (From Kannel WB, Ho K, Thom T. Changing epidemiological features of cardiac failure. *Br Heart J* 1984;72:S3–9, with permission.)

has been a series of clinical survival trials reporting on a myriad of therapies for the management of heart failure (see Table 1). What has emerged is a clearer picture of treatment. The combination of digitalis, diuretics, and ACE inhibitors remains the standard for conventional management of heart failure. Although the results of the Digitalis Investigator Group (DIG) trial indicate that digoxin had an overall neutral effect on the all-cause mortality of patients with heart failure, the investigators did report a highly statistically significant reduction in the number of deaths due to pump failure and a reduction in the need for hospitalization. Diuretics have remained the mainstay of therapy for patients with heart failure fluid retention, although no survival study has ever been reported. Based on the results of the Studies of Left Ventricular Dysfunction (SOLVD) treatment and prevention trials, as well as data derived from the V-HeFT II, ACE inhibitors have emerged as important therapy for patients with Class I to IV heart failure. Uncertainty remains regarding the primary use of beta-adrenergic blockers, calcium channel blockers, and amiodarone and the chronic or intermittent use of intravenous inotropic drugs, anticoagulation, and implantable cardioverter defibrillators. Some of these issues are addressed elsewhere in this chapter. Patients with a past history of systemic emboli, mitral stenosis, or atrial fibrillation are prime candidates for chronic anticoagulation. However, the routine use of chronic anticoagulation for less ill patients with chronic heart failure cannot be supported by available data.

The patient with advanced heart failure or refractory heart failure is superficially defined as one who is already being treated with digitalis, diuretics, and ACE inhibitors but fails to demonstrate an adequate clinical response. It has been our experience that many patients with so-called "refractory heart failure" are prescribed inadequate doses of ACE inhibitors. Although it is possible that small dosages of ACE inhibitors, such as 6.25 mg of captopril twice a day or 2.5 mg of enalapril per day, are effective, there simply are no data available to support such a strategy. I always try to gradually titrate the ACE inhibitor dose recommended by the large clinical trials. For captopril, the target dosage should be 50 mg three or even four times a day. For enalapril, the target dosage should be 10 mg twice a day. The usual dosage of lisinopril is 20 mg/day. There is much less information available regarding alternative ACE inhibitors.

It is likely that some physicians are reluctant to titrate the dose of ACE inhibitor to a higher level based on concerns about hypotension and renal insufficiency. Although these are realistic concerns, in many patients it is possible to gradually titrate the dose upward without causing symptomatic hypotension or meaningful renal insufficiency. Nevertheless, patients must be monitored carefully during the up-titration phase of treatment, and it is prudent to follow the response of blood pressure and renal function on a regular basis in the out-patient clinic. Low blood pressure induced by an ACE inhibitor, in the range of 85/50 mm Hg, is not necessarily an indication to withdraw the ACE inhibitor or reduce the dose, provided that the patient is having no symptoms of hypotension such as lightheadedness or severe fatigue. It must be kept in mind that blood pressure and blood flow are not synonymous, and that blood flow can be maintained despite a seemingly very low blood pressure. Likewise, patients with advanced heart failure frequently have abnormal baseline renal function, and it might be expected that the serum creatinine may rise further with the introduction of ACE inhibitor therapy. Nonetheless, although there may be a small initial increment in serum creatinine, long-term therapy is usually not associated with a progressive rise in serum creatinine or renal failure. The clinical experience with the ACE inhibitors is now vast, and there is simply no question that they have emerged as the most important form of therapy for advanced heart failure. Unless contraindicated or poorly tolerated because of symptomatic hypotension, cough, or hyperkalemia, an attempt should always be made to titrate the dose of the ACE inhibitor to the doses used in the large clinical trials (see Table 1).

The Clinic Visit and the Evaluation Process

Given the complexities involved in the diagnosis and management of patients with advanced heart failure, it is reasonable to assume that it will require at least 1 hour to see a new out-patient with advanced heart failure. Approximately half of the visit should be dedicated to extracting a thorough history and performing a complete cardiovascular examination on the patient. The other half of the visit should be focused on the patient's therapy and educating the patient about the nuances of heart failure. Particular emphasis should be placed on consideration of dietary restrictions, physical activity limitations, and prognosis. It is imperative that patients understand the nature of the "heart failure" problem, which is best explained in their terms. It is also important to have family members present in the clinic, particularly spouses, whenever possible. A large and comfortable room, adjusted for appropriate temperature, should be made available.

It has been our practice at the University of Minnesota to have a nurse first contact a new patient by phone to get a "feel" for the patient's sense of urgency and apprehension. This same nurse then meets with the patient for 5 to 10 minutes before the physician enters the examining room. This allows the nurse briefly to present the case to the physician and point out the specific concerns that need to be addressed when seeing the patient.

Every new patient requires some laboratory evaluation, in addition to the history and physical examination. It has been our practice to obtain an electrocardiogram, a chest radiograph, and a panel of serum electrolytes, a blood urea nitrogen (BUN), serum creatinine, and a complete blood count. Often these routine laboratory data are provided by the referring physician. Every new patient should have an echocardiogram to assess left ventricular size and performance characteristics, and to evaluate valvular function. We now know that as many as one third of patients referred to a center with the diagnosis of heart failure have relatively preserved ejection fraction, with presumed "diastolic" heart failure. The treatment and natural history of diastolic heart failure may be quite different from those of systolic heart failure. The echocardiogram should preferably be reviewed in detail by the physician before the patient is seen in the clinic.

Depending on the individual circumstances, it has been our practice to have nearly all patients undergo a maximal cardiopulmonary exercise test sometime during the evaluation. This is particularly true for younger patients who can still readily exercise. Using standard gas-exchange techniques, the test allows the clinician to determine both anaerobic threshold and maximum oxygen consumption ($\dot{V}O_2$). In addition, the time spent exercising by the patient on the treadmill, the response of heart rate and blood pressure to exercise, and the electrocardiographic response to exercise should be carefully noted. The reasons for dis-

continuing the test should be explored in detail. We find that exercise testing is of particular value when determining the extent of disability. In many cases, the patient's history and personal recollection of his or her disability bears little relationship to the extent of left ventricular function.

Left ventricular function at rest fails to relate to $\dot{V}O_2$. In general, when the patient's level of performance is less than 50% of that expected for body size and age, we consider the patient to be seriously impaired and a potential candidate for heart transplantation.

Perhaps one of the most contentious issues in the evaluation process concerns the need for a right-heart catheterization and coronary angiography. Since the late 1980s, it has become clear that many patients referred for management of advanced heart failure have severe underlying coronary disease, although there may be virtually no symptoms of angina pectoris or its equivalents. With experience, it has become apparent that some of these patients will have reversal of severe left ventricular dysfunction when revascularized. These findings have led many to consider coronary angiography patients presenting with advanced heart failure, even in the complete absence of symptoms due to ischemic heart disease. Some physicians choose not to perform invasive hemodynamic measurements or coronary angiography unless there is some noninvasive evidence of ischemic heart disease. If the patient is being seriously considered for heart transplantation, coronary angiography should be performed, because some of these patients will have severe coronary artery disease, which may be amenable to coronary artery bypass surgery. In such cases, coronary artery bypass surgery is clearly preferable to heart transplantation. However, depending on the age of the patient and the circumstances of the referral, whether to proceed with hemodynamic measurements and coronary angiography remains the prerogative of the physician who will be primarily responsible for the patient's care. In general, the more information the physician has, the more rationally he or she can make decisions about treatment. Therefore, I generally favor obtaining current right-heart catheterization hemodynamic data and coronary angiography in nearly every case.

Discussion of Prognosis

Once the patient has been thoroughly evaluated with a history and physical examination, laboratory data, echocardiography, and a cardiac catheterization, the physician has substantial information regarding prognosis (Table 2). Knowledge of hemodynamics is useful in knowing when a patient is truly "advanced." Still, sequential follow-up may provide the most important information. It should be explained to the patient and family that, in general, heart failure has a poor prognosis, but that treatment with ACE inhibitors has been shown to improve outcome. It is important to emphasize, however,

TABLE 1. *Randomized, controlled, multicenter survival trials in heart failure*

Acronym	Full title	Study drugs	NYHA class	Outcome	Publication
V-HeFT I	Vasodilator Heart Failure Trial I	Placebo vs. hydralazine and isosorbide dinitrate vs. placebo. Background therapy—digitalis and diuretics	II, III	Hydralazine (75 mg q.i.d.) and isosorbide dinitrate 40 mg q.i.d.) improved survival.	Published: *N Engl J Med* 1986;314: 1547–1552
CONSENSUS I	Cooperative New Scandinavian Enalapril Survival Study	Placebo vs. enalapril 10 mg b.i.d. Background therapy—digitalis, diuretics, some vasodilators	IV	Enalapril improved survival (average dose 18.4 mg/day).	Published: *N Engl J Med* 1987;316: 1429–1435
V-HeFT II	Vasodilator Heart Failure Trial II	Enalapril vs. hydralazine and isosorbide dinitrate. Background therapy—digitalis, diuretics	II, III	Enalapril 20 mg/day improved survival more than hydralazine–isosorbide dinitrate. Exercise tolerance and EF were improved more by hydralazine–isosorbide dinitrate.	Published: *N Engl J Med* 1991;325: 303–310
SOLVD–Treatment	Studies of Left Ventricular Dysfunction—Treatment	Enalapril 10 mg b.i.d. vs. placebo in patients with symptomatic heart failure. Background therapy—digitalis and diuretics	II, III	Enalapril improved survival.	Treatment trial published: *N Engl J Med* 1991;325:293–302
SOLVD–Prevention	Studies of Left Ventricular Dysfunction—Prevention	Enalapril 10 mg b.i.d. vs. placebo in asymptomatic patients with EF ≤35%	I	Enalapril delayed progression of heart failure, but did not improve survival.	Prevention trial published: *N Engl J Med* 1991;327:685–691
PROMISE	Prospective Randomized Milrinone Survival Evaluation	Milrinone 10 mg q.i.d. vs. placebo. Background therapy—digitalis, diuretics, ACE inhibitors	III, IV	Milrinone increased mortality.	Published: *N Engl J Med* 1991;325: 1468–1475.
Vesnarinone (OPC-8212)	Vesnarinone (OPC-8212)	Vesnarinone 60 mg/day and 120 mg/day vs. placebo. Background therapy—digoxin, diuretics, ACE inhibitors	III, IV	Vesnarinone 60 mg/day improved survival, whereas 160 mg/day increased mortality.	Published: *N Engl J Med* 1993;329: 149–155
VEST	Vesnarinone Survival Trial	Vesnarinone 60 or 30 mg/day vs. placebo 3500 patients, EF ≤30%	III, IV	Vesnarinone increased mortality.	Preliminary results reported
PROFILE	Prospective Randomized Flosequinan Longevity Evaluation	Flosequinan 100 mg/day vs. placebo. Background therapy—digoxin, diuretics, ACE inhibitors	III, IV	Terminated May, 1993, because of excess mortality with flosequinan.	Preliminary results reported
MDC	Metoprolol in Dilated Cardiomyopathy	Metoprolol vs. placebo; after slow titration dose of metoprolol 100–150 mg/d	II, III, IV	Trend for improved survival plus reduced need for heart transplantation in patients treated with metoprolol.	Published: *Lancet* 1993;342: 1441–1446
BEST	Beta-blocker Evaluation Survival Trial	Bucindolol 6.25 to 200 mg b.i.d. vs. placebo: EF ≤35%	III, IV	In progress.	

Trial	Description	Comparison	NYHA Class	Results	Publication
PRAISE	Prospective Randomized Amlodipine Survival Evaluation	Amlodipine (dihydropyridine) 10 mg/day vs. placebo Background therapy—digoxin, diuretics, ACE inhibitors	III, IV	No overall difference in survival vs. placebo; trend for "nonischemic" cardiomyopathy patients to have improved survival.	Published: N Engl J Med 1996;335: 1107–1114
PRAISE II	Prospective Randomized Amlodipine Survival Evaluation II	Amlodipine vs. placebo in patients with nonischemic cardiomyopathy	III, IV	In progress.	
CHF-STAT	Congestive Heart Failure Survival Trial of Anti-arrhythmic Therapy	Amiodarone vs. placebo in patients with heart failure and >10 premature ventricular contractions per hour	I, II, III, IV	No overall difference in survival vs. placebo; trend for patients with nonischemic cardiomyopathy to have improved survival and improved EF.	Published: N Engl J Med 1995;333: 77–82
GESICA	Group Study of Heart Failure in Argentina	Nonrandomized placebo-controlled trial of amiodarone (300 mg/day)	II, III, IV	Mortality and hospital admission rate reduced by low-dose amiodarone independent of complex ventricular arrhythmias.	Published: Lancet 1994;344:493–498
PRECISE/MOCHA	Prospective Randomized Evaluation of Carvedilol on Symptoms and Exercise/Multicenter Oral Carvedilol Heart Failure Assessment	Carvedilol vs. placebo	II, III, IV	Significant improvement in survival with Carvedilol.	Published: N Engl J Med 1996;334: 1349–1355
FIRST	Flolan International Randomized Survival Trial	Intravenous epoprostenol vs. conventional therapy	IV	Terminated in June, 1993 because of increased mortality and clinical deterioration in the epoprostenol	Published: Am Heart J 1997; 134:44–54
DIG	Digitalis Investigators Group	Digoxin vs. placebo in stable heart failure Background therapy—diuretics and ACE inhibitors; 7,788 patients	II, III	No overall effect on mortality; fewer hospitalizations and pump failure deaths with digitalis; trend for more arrhythmic deaths with digitalis.	Published: N Engl J Med 1997;336: 525–533
ATLAS	Assessment of Treatment with Lisinopril and Survival	Survival study of high vs. low-dose lisinopril in moderate to severe congestive heart failure	II, III, IV	Completion in 1996.	
RALES	Randomized Aldactone Evaluation Study	Placebo vs. spironolactone in patients on triple therapy with digoxin, diuretics, ACE inhibitors	II, III, IV	In progress.	
MACH-1	Mortality Assessment of Congestive Heart Failure Trial	Mibefradil vs. placebo in 2,400 patients on conventional treatment for heart failure	II–IV	Completed	Presented 1998

ACE, angiotensin-converting enzyme; EF, ejection fraction.

TABLE 2. *Prognostic factors in patients with congestive heart failure*

Prognostic Factor	Comments
Left ventricular ejection fraction	This prognostic factor is valid only if one is examining a broad range of ejection fractions. For patients referred to transplant centers, all of whom have a very low ejection fraction, it carries much less diagnostic weight.
Maximal or peak oxygen consumption	Patients with a $\dot{V}O_2 \geq 14$ ml/kg/min tend to have a somewhat better prognosis regardless of the extent of left ventricular dysfunction. Some investigators "normalize" the $\dot{V}O_2$ for body size and age. Patients who are able to exercise at 50% or more of the normal level for their body size and age may be "too well" for transplantation.
Serum sodium concentration	Patients with a low serum sodium in general have a worse prognosis, but this factor was of no prognostic value in some of the large clinical trials such as SOLVD and V-HeFT.
Syncope	Any loss of consciousness, whether cardiac related or not, implies a poor prognosis.
Plasma norepinephrine levels	These have repeatedly been demonstrated to be associated with prognosis. In general, patients with plasma norepinephrine levels in excess of 600–900 pg/mL have a much worse prognosis. As with other neurohormonal measurements, this measurement remains largely a research tool.
Atrial natriuretic peptide level	The *N*-terminal pronatriuretic factor appears to be an independent predictor of long-term prognosis, particularly after myocardial infarction.
Endothelin levels	At least two studies have now suggested that an elevated plasma endothelin level is associated with poor prognosis.
Cytokine levels	This is a very new area of research, but emerging data suggest that cytokines are important in the progression of heart failure.
New York Heart Association Functional Class	Patients in New York Heart Association Functional Class IV have been consistently demonstrated to have a very poor prognosis.
Left ventricular dimension by echocardiography	The group from University of California, Los Angeles, has suggested that the left ventricular dimension is an important predictor of prognosis.
Demonstrable improvement in left ventricular ejection	The V-HeFT II investigators found that an increase in ejection fraction of five or more fraction units during the course of the study was associated with improved prognosis.
Symptomatic or asymptomatic sustained/nonsustained ventricular tachycardia	There has been some controversy regarding the importance of ventricular arrhythmias as prognostic factors.
Signal-averaged electrocardiogram	As with ventricular arrhythmias, some data suggest that an abnormal finding on signal-averaged electrocardiography may be associated with a poor prognosis.
Duration of disease	
Clinical stability or deterioration	Ability to achieve and maintain better clinical status may be more important than status at presentation.
Etiology of disease	The etiology of the heart failure (ischemic vs. nonischemic) has been controversial with regard to its prognostic importance. Some studies have suggested that ischemic cardiomyopathy is associated with a worse prognosis than nonischemic cardiomyopathy.
Left ventricular filling pressure and its response to therapy	"Tailored therapy" has been demonstrated to optimize left ventricular filling pressure and is associated with improved short-term survival.
Heart rate	
Cardiac index	Less predictive of outcome than parameters related to intracardiac filling pressures.

SOLVD, Studies of Left Ventricular Dysfunction; V-HeFT, Vasodilator Heart Failure Trial.

that patients with very advanced heart failure still have a high 6-month mortality rate, in the range of 20% to 30%. This discussion gives the physician and nurse an opportunity to focus meticulous attention on the details of management, including the low-sodium diet, the need for daily exercise, and the nuances of drug therapy. I often take time to explain to the patient that sudden and unexpected death is a frequent and sometimes unavoidable consequence of advanced heart failure. It is my personal view that patients should have a serum potassium of at least 4.5 mEq/L to prevent lethal arrhythmias, although there are no data bearing directly on this point. A period of intensive therapy before the final evaluation process is extremely helpful. Invariably, some patients dramatically improve with intensification of their medical regimen.

It seems imprudent to tell a patient that they have only "6 months to live." In my experience, predicting short-term prognosis in such patients is hazardous, and even very experienced physicians are frequently inaccurate. Today, patients with the most advanced heart failure appear to have a 1-year survival rate of almost 68%, whereas in 1987 such patients were reported to have a 54% survival rate as part of the initial Cooperative North Scandinavian Enalapril Survival Study (CONSENSUS) trial. If one has information regarding $\dot{V}O_{2max}$, further refinement of the prognostic determination is possible. For example, patients with reasonably intact exercise tolerance and a $\dot{V}O_{2max}$ greater than 14 mL/kg/minute are considered by many cardiologists to be "too well" for heart transplantation. They have a somewhat better prognosis.

Last, it must be emphasized to the new patient that a single visit often does not provide enough information to predict how the course of events is going to unfold. Multiple studies now emphasize the importance of serial evaluation in patients after the initial referral. Often patients have not been vigorously treated by the referring physician, and the condition of the patient at the time of initial referral simply may not reflect his or her underlying capacity for compensation. It is always important to keep adjusting therapy until clinical congestion has resolved, or the patient does not tolerate higher doses of drugs.

Physicians can be more confident about prognosis once they have seen the patient sequentially over time. Should the patient improve after referral, the prognosis is much better than if the patient remains in an advanced stage of heart failure. A small number of patients have spontaneous improvement in left ventricular function, and their prognosis also is better. Even patients without major improvement in left ventricular function may clinically improve on intensification of medical therapy. Likewise, although sudden death continues to account for about half of the mortality, the absolute incidence of this devastating complication has diminished over time. This is perhaps due to the increasing use of ACE inhibitors and the avoidance of Class I antiarrhythmic agents. It is also possible that the increasing use of amiodarone has contributed to improved survival in patients with advanced heart failure, but this improvement may be restricted to those patients with nonischemic cardiomyopathy. More data are required regarding the use of amiodarone and its influence on survival in patients with advanced heart failure.

A comprehensive management program to lower the hospitalization rate for patients with advanced heart failure is possible. The group from University of California, Los Angeles, reported an 80% decrease in hospital admissions for heart failure after referral to a heart transplantation center. Patients frequently bring up the idea of heart transplantation, even when it is not very appropriate. It should always be remembered that heart transplantation is not an option for most patients. Only about 2,400 heart transplantations are performed each year, whereas more than 1 million patients are admitted to the hospital each year with worsening heart failure. Most patients are beyond the age limit for transplantation. Nevertheless, quality of life can be improved and savings can be extended to high- and low-risk patients using the heart failure team approach to intensification of medical therapy.

APPROACH TO THE PATIENT WITH CHRONIC FAILURE WHO HAS ACUTELY DECOMPENSATED

Invariably, nearly every patient with advanced heart failure has episodes of acute decompensation. Because this is a frequent complicating event, it is very helpful to have a phone system whereby patients can have easy access to nurses trained in the care and management of advanced heart failure. Even if the nurse cannot directly help the patient, the patients find it very useful to discuss their change of condition with experienced medical personnel. In most cases of acute decompensation, we advise that the patient be seen either in the clinic or the emergency room without hesitation. If the patient is reluctant to be seen at once, case management changes can sometimes be safely negotiated by phone.

It is important that physicians caring for patients with heart failure be thoroughly familiar with the factors that contribute to decompensation (Table 3). In every case, a search should be made for superimposed acute myocardial ischemia. If the patient should give any indication of worsening or progressive symptoms of coronary insufficiency, hospitalization is indicated. At the very least, a careful history, physical examination, and electrocardiogram are always indicated, with a specific search made for the electrocardiographic changes of myocardial ischemia. High blood pressure, although unusual, can occur with advanced heart failure and must be aggressively treated. Weight loss must be strongly encouraged in overweight patients.

New-onset atrial fibrillation is well known to result in decompensation of previously stable congestive heart failure. Although the literature is at variance with regard to the prognostic importance of atrial fibrillation in the setting of heart failure, there is a general consensus that the onset of new atrial fibrillation can lead to acute hemodynamic compromise. In many cases, heart rate control is all that is necessary. However, because the contribution of atrial contraction may be critical to the patient's hemodynamic stability, electrical cardioversion to normal sinus rhythm should always be considered. Therefore, it is important to carefully review the electrocardiogram of patients who present with acute decompensation of heart failure. The diagnosis of new-onset atrial fibrillation may be an indication for hospitalization, heart rate control, and elective cardioversion. Patients with atrial fibrillation of less than 48 hours' duration can be safely cardioverted

TABLE 3. *Exacerbating factors in chronic heart failure*

- Acute myocardial ischemia
- Uncorrected high blood pressure
- Obesity
- Atrial fibrillation and other arrhythmias
- Negative inotropic drugs (e.g., verapamil, nifedipine, diltiazem, beta-adrenergic blockers)
- Nonsteroidal antiinflammatory drugs
- Excessive alcohol
- Endocrine abnormalities (e.g., diabetes mellitus, hyperthyroidism, hypothyroidism)
- Drug and Na$^+$ noncompliance; lack of information given to patient about diet and medications
- Concurrent infections (e.g., pneumonia, viral illnesses)

without warfarin, but they should still be considered for long-term chronic anticoagulation therapy because recurrence of the arrhythmia is likely.

Another cause of acute decompensation is the injudicious use of drugs that are negatively inotropic. Our experience has been that the first-generation calcium channel blockers such as verapamil, nifedipine, and diltiazem all have the potential to aggravate congestive heart failure, particularly in patients with advanced stages of the disease. Often such agents are used inappropriately as primary vasodilator therapy, or may be added more appropriately to conventional therapy in an attempt to control high blood pressure or worsening angina pectoris. It has been my practice to discontinue calcium channel blockers when there is acute decompensation of heart failure. It is possible that the second-generation dihydropyridines, such as amlodipine and felodipine, may have more vasculoselective properties, and hence may be less negatively inotropic. Nevertheless, caution is still urged in the use of such drugs for patients with advanced heart failure.

Nonsteroidal antiinflammatory agents are notorious for causing additional salt and water retention in patients with advanced heart failure. Such patients are highly dependent on prostaglandin synthesis to maintain adequate renal function. Therefore, the clinician must caution patients with advanced heart failure against the use of nonsteroidal antiinflammatory agents. Consideration should be given to discontinuing them in the face of acute decompensation. Because many such agents are now available over the counter, time must be taken to explain their specific disadvantages to patients. For example, episodes of acute gouty arthritis are perhaps more safely treated with oral colchicine and intraarticular instillation of corticosteroids than by treatment with nonsteroidal antiinflammatory agents.

Patients must also be reminded that consumption of large amounts of alcohol can depress myocardial function. Although the acute hemodynamic effects of alcohol include vasodilation and an increase in heart rate, leading to an increase of cardiac output, the chronic use of alcohol can clearly lead to diminished left ventricular function in some people. Moreover, the regular use of alcohol can cause systemic hypertension, which is well known to aggravate congestive heart failure. It is perhaps prudent to discuss the use of alcohol in detail with each patient, and make it clear that abstinence, under most circumstances, is the most appropriate course of action. Patients are sometimes not familiar with the concept of alcoholic cardiomyopathy, and traditionally underreport their use of alcohol. Heavy consumption of alcohol should always be considered a possible etiologic factor in patients with decompensation of heart failure.

Superimposed systemic infections, even "simple" viral infections, can strain the compromised cardiovascular system and precipitate acute heart failure. Patients with chronic heart failure should always be vaccinated against influenza and should have a one-time vaccination against pneumonia. Despite these precautions, the onset of a surprisingly mild respiratory tract infection or gastroenteritis can sometimes lead to acute decompensation of chronic heart failure. This should always be kept in mind when trying to decipher the etiology of acute decompensation.

Endocrine abnormalities, including hypothyroidism, hyperthyroidism, and poorly controlled diabetes mellitus, can lead to acute decompensation of heart failure. Because complaints of chronic fatigue, apathy, and mild depression are common in patients with heart failure, the clinician must specifically seek out clinical laboratory evidence of hypothyroidism. Diabetes mellitus-induced severe hyperglycemia can lead to polyuria, thus complicating fluid and electrolyte balance. Relative volume depletion is a frequent cause of mild symptomatic hypotension in patients receiving ACE inhibitors, and could easily be further aggravated by diabetes mellitus-induced polyuria and dehydration.

Last, patients with little information or who are poorly educated regarding compliance with sodium restriction, prescribed medications, and daily weights are at risk for acute decompensation of chronic heart failure. In our experience, this is a common cause of acutely decompensated heart failure. A considerable amount of time and energy must be expended for patients to understand how much sodium is allowed on a daily basis. Somewhat arbitrarily, we encourage a low-sodium diet of 2 g or less per day. In my practice, I almost never restrict fluids, unless the patient is hyponatremic. Other heart failure specialists consider fluid restriction to 2 L a day to be a useful adjunct once the daily diuretic requirement exceeds 120 mg of furosemide. On the other hand, sodium must be restricted in every patient who demonstrates fluid retention. For reasons that are unclear, patients often indicate that they are gaining weight and becoming edematous without any perceived change in their diet. Almost invariably, they are ingesting excessive dietary sodium. Excessive sodium ingestion is also responsible for many cases of "diuretic resistance." At the University of Minnesota, our heart failure nurses spend a considerable amount of time explaining to the patients, their patients' spouses, and their patients' families the critical importance of sodium restriction. To the extent that they can restrict their dietary sodium, patients with advanced heart failure can be kept out of the hospital for prolonged periods of time, thereby improving their quality of life.

FLEXIBLE DIURETIC USE

It is well known to physicians that patients with insulin-dependent diabetes mellitus can usually alter their insulin dose on an "as needed" basis without necessarily having a formal clinic appointment with their physician. Likewise, patients with advanced heart failure can learn to adjust their diuretic dose as needed to control their fluid balance. For many years, we have encouraged all patients with advanced heart failure to weigh themselves daily. They should be instructed to keep a daily log of their weight. If there is an increase in weight of 3 or more pounds, or if the patient feels particularly "bloated" or congested, some can be improved by a modest up-titration of their diuretic dosage. For example, if they are taking 40 mg of furosemide a day, they should be encouraged to take 60 or 80 mg for 2 or 3 days until they are back to their baseline weight. At that point, they can go back on their usual maintenance of 40 mg of furosemide per day. For patients with a more pronounced propensity to retain salt and water, the intermittent concomitant use of a nonloop diuretic such as metolazone is most beneficial. I have encouraged patients to take 2.5 or 5 mg of metolazone 0.5 hour before their usual dose of morning furosemide. The two drugs act synergistically to augment the diuresis.

However, it is well known that metolazone can lead to severe fluid and electrolyte depletion, including loss of excessive amounts of potassium and magnesium in the urine. Therefore, the patient should be instructed on how to supplement his or her potassium chloride dose, should a substantial diuresis ensue. Importantly, the use of metolazone should usually be restricted to 2 or 3 days until the baseline weight is reestablished. The purpose of allowing the patient to participate in a flexible diuretic dosage scheme is to prevent the need for excessive visits to the emergency room and clinic, and, ultimately, hospitalization. Our experience has been that most patients are able to make a diuretic adjustment appropriately without formally engaging the help of their physician. In addition, the responsibility for adjusting diuretics often reinforces the patient's appreciation of the relationship between occasional sodium indiscretion and subsequent fluid retention. Once again, the use of nurses who are specialized in the management of advanced heart failure is particularly helpful in this regard.

Just as diuretics may need to be adjusted upward in the face of excessive salt and water retention, they may have to be adjusted downward in patients with evidence of postural hypotension or progressive renal insufficiency. The need to adjust the dosage of diuretics downward can be more subtle, and often requires direct interaction with the physician. Patients who are receiving ACE inhibitors and who are having difficulty with intermittent symptomatic hypotension frequently benefit from a reduction in diuretic dose. For example, the dose of furosemide might be adjusted from 40 to 20 mg/day. This appears to be a far more prudent strategy than reducing or temporarily withholding the ACE inhibitor. The development of a serum electrolyte "contraction alkalosis" is also sometimes a sign that overdiuresis and volume depletion are occurring, thereby indicating the need to reduce the diuretic dose.

Despite the now widespread strategy of allowing patients to adjust their diuretic schedule to their own needs, there are few or no data in direct support of this strategy. It is unlikely that any pharmaceutical company will support such a study, and nonpharmaceutical company support for such a project would be difficult to obtain in this age of diminishing resources for clinical investigation. Nevertheless, experience to date would indicate that a very flexible diuretic schedule might be able to allow patients to reduce the need for hospitalization.

CLINIC VISIT FREQUENCY

Patients with advanced heart failure, such as those requiring frequent adjustment of their medications, need to be seen in the clinic on a regular basis, perhaps as often as once a week in some cases. For patients who remain relatively stable, a visit to the clinic every 3 or 4 months is often sufficient. Nevertheless, this is a purely judgmental exercise that must be individualized and tailored to the needs of each patient.

WHEN TO HOSPITALIZE THE PATIENT

The need for hospitalization is a subjective judgment and always involves some interaction between patient and physician. At our institution, the nurses often detect that the patient is in need of hospitalization through a patient-initiated phone contact, and then discuss the case further with the supervising physician. In general, patients should be admitted to the hospital who demonstrate the problems discussed in the following sections.

Clinical or Electrocardiographic Evidence of Acute Myocardial Ischemia

Patients who complain of accelerating or worsening angina pectoris or who have a new abnormality on their electrocardiogram suggesting underlying myocardial ischemia should always be considered for admission to the hospital. Such patients are usually placed in the intensive care unit and undergo the appropriate tests to exclude acute myocardial infarction. In some cases, coronary angiography may be necessary.

Pulmonary Edema or Severe Respiratory Distress

It is seemingly self-evident that any patient who is experiencing acute pulmonary edema needs to be hospitalized in the intensive care unit. However, there are less extreme and more subtle changes that occur, such as increase in respiratory rate or progressive dyspnea, that might also sway the physician toward hospitalizing the patient. Patients who demonstrate increasing jugular venous distention; evidence of progressive fluid retention such as increasing weight gain, edema, and new onset of orthopnea; or tender hepatic congestion are candidates for hospitalization.

Oxygen Saturation Below 90 Percent (Not Due to Pulmonary Disease)

Patients who are complaining of increasing shortness of breath who have direct evidence of oxygen desaturation should be admitted to the hospital. In many cases, this is evidence for impending acute pulmonary edema.

Severe Complicating Medical Illnesses

Patients with chronic heart failure who have a serious superimposed systemic illness such as bronchial pneumonia should always be admitted to the hospital. The combination of pneumonia and congestive heart failure is frequently lethal, particularly in the elderly population.

Anasarca

Patients in whom severe peripheral edema including anasarca develops are best treated in the confines of the hospital. They frequently need intravenous loop diuretics, and in some cases a continuous intravenous loop diuretic drip along with dobutamine or nitroprusside is necessary to rid them of their severe edema and improve their hemodynamic profile.

Symptomatic Hypotension or Syncope

Patients with symptomatic hypotension or frank syncope in the setting of heart failure have an extremely poor prognosis, even if the syncope is not due to a direct cardiac cause. Mild symptomatic hypotension can sometimes be treated with down-titration of the diuretic dose. However, patients who are persistently weak or lightheaded or who demonstrate frank syncope should be given serious consideration for admission to the hospital. In some cases, lethal arrhythmias may account for the symptoms, and in other cases they may be due to overdiuresis and volume depletion. In either event, consequences can be serious, including injuries related to a fall. Hospital admission is advised.

Heart Failure Refractory to Out-patient Therapy

This is always a somewhat subjective indication for hospitalization, but nevertheless those patients who fail to improve on conventional therapy should be considered candidates for in-patient care. In general, such patients are usually admitted to the intensive care unit for invasive monitoring and treated with additional therapy including intravenous loop diuretics, metolazone, nitroprusside, dobutamine, and possibly milrinone. It is sometimes very difficult to know precisely at what point such patients

should be admitted to the hospital. This problem can be obviated, to some extent, by repeated clinic visits with the same physician over time. In my practice, I pay particular attention to the jugular venous pressure, and would take evidence of a progressively rising venous pressure as a sign of refractoriness to out-patient therapy. In many instances, such patients should be admitted to the hospital, particularly if they are increasingly dyspneic, refractory to diuretics, and unable to sleep. In milder cases, an increase in out-patient diuretic therapy may be all that is necessary.

Inadequate Social Support for Safe Out-patient Management

There is no question that some patients simply do poorly because they have little or no family or social support system at home. Elderly patients who are unable to care for themselves are likely candidates for admission, even when the heart failure may not be overtly decompensated. An experienced physician can sometimes anticipate problems when it is clear the patient has no intention of taking medications or avoiding excessive salt intake. In such cases, it may be hazardous to send the patient back home, particularly if there are medical indications that the heart failure may be worsening. Under these circumstances, I have a relatively low threshold to admit the patient for in-patient care. Arrangements for a more structured out-patient support system can often be aided by hospital social services.

IN-PATIENT MANAGEMENT OF ADVANCED HEART FAILURE

There are perhaps few more daunting challenges than the care of the patient with advanced and progressive heart failure. However, a number of guiding principles are available to physicians to help them through a series of complex therapeutic decisions. First, the cause of the acute decompensation should always be considered (see Table 3). When the precipitating cause is identifiable, such as rapid atrial fibrillation, steps should be taken rapidly to correct the problem. For example, in the case of rapid atrial fibrillation, electrical cardioversion may be appropriate, or slowing of the rate with intravenous digoxin or diltiazem may be preferred.

After a thorough history and physical examination, the clinician usually has a reasonable idea as to what the hemodynamic profile might be, although the physical examination may be misleading. The time-honored findings of acute heart failure include a third heart sound, pulmonary rales, an abnormal jugular venous pulse, and peripheral edema. The chest radiograph is often confirmatory. Unlike acute heart failure, chronic heart failure is characterized by a host of compensatory mechanisms that may reduce the accuracy of the usual physical findings. In a study of 50 patients with chronic heart failure,

Stevenson and Perloff noted that rales, edema, and elevated mean jugular venous pressure were absent in 18 of 43 patients with pulmonary capillary wedge pressures of 22 mm Hg or higher. However, a narrow pulse pressure did correlate with a low cardiac index (r = 0.82). In chronic heart failure, pulmonary rales are rarely present, even when pulmonary capillary wedge pressure is 35 mm Hg or more. The bedside examination may be completely misleading if only rales and edema are sought. However, when jugular venous pressure is obviously elevated and the patient has pulmonary rales, the clinician can be confident that filling pressures will be elevated. On the contrary, the absence of jugular venous distention, a third heart sound, or pulmonary rales does not exclude severe elevation of pulmonary capillary wedge pressure because these signs, although specific, are lacking in sensitivity. The accuracy of the physical examination for the diagnosis of suspected ascites is also questionable. Ultrasonography is recommended in questionable cases.

All patients admitted to the hospital for management of advanced heart failure should have an echocardiogram performed. The size and the performance of the heart should be carefully evaluated. As many as 40% of patients with heart failure, particularly the elderly, have systolic function preserved, thereby suggesting the diagnosis of diastolic heart failure. Evidence for valvular stenosis or valvular insufficiency should be carefully evaluated. Nearly all patients with advanced heart failure have some degree of mitral and tricuspid insufficiency. The degree of left ventricular hypertrophy should be assessed. Spherical enlargement of the heart is more likely to be associated with mitral insufficiency. Severe right heart dilatation and flagrant tricuspid regurgitation sometimes exclude the use of a left ventricular assist device.

SPECIFIC THERAPEUTIC STRATEGIES

Patients hospitalized with severe heart failure should have hemodynamic monitoring to help assess their prognosis (Figure 2) and manage their response to therapy. Once baseline hemodynamic findings have been assessed, a plan of specific therapeutic measures should be discussed with the patient and family. If urine output has been inadequate, a Foley catheter should be placed in the urinary bladder to assess accurately hourly urine volume. Baseline weight should be obtained. Nearly all patients are already receiving ACE inhibitors, digitalis, and diuretics. Baseline electrolytes, BUN, serum creatinine, hemoglobin, and white blood cell count should be obtained.

If blood pressure and renal function are adequate, although not normal, the doses of conventional therapy should be optimized. Because diuretics are sometimes not well absorbed by the edematous gut, consideration should be given to the use of intravenous loop diuretics. The loop diuretics act to inhibit chloride absorption in the thick ascending loop of Henle, thereby restricting Na+

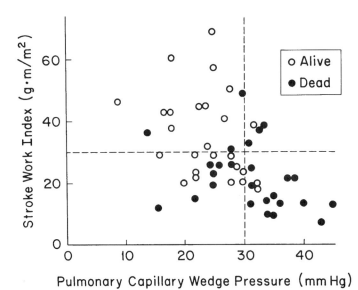

FIG. 2. Six-month mortality is related to hemodynamic measurements. Nearly all patients presenting with a pulmonary capillary pressure greater than 30 mm Hg and a stroke work index of less than 30 g·m/m² were dead 6 months after the invasive study. (From Massie BM, Ports T, Chatterjee K, et al. Long-term vasodilator therapy for heart failure: clinical response and its relationship to hemodynamic measurements. *Circulation* 1981;63:269, with permission.)

reabsorption as well. The choice and dose of loop diuretic varies substantially, but furosemide 40 to 120 mg intravenously (i.v.), bumetanide 0.5 to 2 mg i.v. as a single dose, or torsemide 20 to 40 mg i.v. may be sufficient. Combining a nonloop diuretic, such as chlorothiazide 500 mg intravenously over 5 to 15 minutes, or metolazone 2.5 to 10 mg orally, may provide pharmacologic synergy and thereby enhance the effects of the loop diuretic. The use of a continuous i.v. furosemide or bumetanide drip may sometimes be more effective than bolus administration. The continuous infusion of loop diuretics may provide a more efficient delivery of diuretic to the nephron, eliminate compensatory sodium retention ("rebound") during the diuretic-free interval, and diminish the development of tolerance. The risk of ototoxicity may also be less, but this is not proven. Severe myalgia may be more frequent with bolus diuretic injection, particularly with bumetanide, but can also occur with continuous intravenous infusion of loop diuretics. This complication may be dose related, is not associated with any laboratory abnormality, and responds to discontinuation of the diuretic. Bumetanide is sometimes given as a continuous drip at 0.5 mg/hour (12 mg/24 hours) or furosemide at 40 mg/hour to afford a continuous blood level. In patients who use large doses of loop diuretics continuously as out-patients, hypertrophy of the distal renal tubule and enhanced chloride and sodium reabsorption at this site can develop, thus diminishing the natriuretic effect over time.

Provided that hyperkalemia is not present, potassium-sparing diuretics such as spironolactone (initial dose 25 mg/day) or amiloride (5 mg/day) might also be considered. In some patients, the addition of spironolactone seems to initiate a diuresis when conventional diuretics are less effective. The choice and dose of diuretic remains somewhat arbitrary. Bumetanide is sometimes more effective when furosemide has failed, but it is considerably more expensive. We have observed excellent results with i.v. torsemide when i.v. furosemide has failed to produce an effective diuresis.

In rare cases, patients fail to respond to conventional diuretics and renal failure ensues. An attempt should be made to improve renal blood flow by increasing cardiac output and renal blood flow with dobutamine, but some patients may remain diuretic resistant. Low-dose dopamine, although long touted to improve renal blood flow, has not been any more effective in our experience than dobutamine. In some cases, large volumes of excess body water can be rapidly removed by ultrafiltration or hemodialysis. Ultrafiltration or hemodialysis can be performed while supporting blood pressure with arterial vasoconstrictors such as dopamine (5–15 mg/kg/minute). This often results in a reduction in right atrial pressure and pulmonary capillary wedge pressure with a stabilization of cardiac index. Dyspnea may be relieved and a more favorable water balance achieved. A chronic reduction in plasma norepinephrine, plasma renin activity, and plasma aldosterone may occur in patients responsive to ultrafiltration, although the procedure is strictly palliative.

CONTROL OF HEMODYNAMIC DERANGEMENT

Careful consideration should be given to control of abnormal hemodynamic findings. It must always be remembered that pump failure is a cardiac disorder, and that no therapy has ever been demonstrated to improve symptoms in the absence of improvement in hemodynamics. Therapy that stabilizes or improves hemodynamics will influence long-term survival, although there are exceptions to this rule. The immediate goal in patients with advanced heart failure is to provide freedom from pulmonary and circulatory congestion. Orthopnea is nearly always evident in patients with advanced heart failure, and can usually be relieved without compromising cardiac output.

The first goal is to reduce cardiac filling pressure, and an optimal cardiac output can nearly always be achieved at near-normal filling pressures (Figure 3). Left ventricular size is diminished, which reduces wall stress and myocardial oxygen demand. A higher stroke volume can be achieved at a lower filling pressure if there is redistribution of mitral regurgitant flow, which can at times consume more than 50% of total left ventricular ejected volume. Stroke volume can improve even as pulmonary

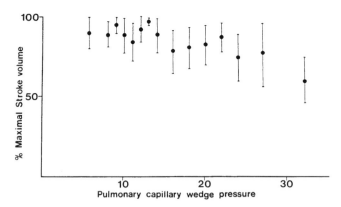

FIG. 3. Stroke volume can be maintained even as pulmonary capillary wedge pressure is reduced, suggesting that left ventricular filling pressure can be safely reduced in patients with advanced heart failure without compromising cardiac output. (From Stevenson LW. Therapy tailored for symptomatic heart failure. *Heart Failure* 1995;11:87–107, with permission.)

capillary wedge pressure is reduced to 10 mm Hg. It therefore seems reasonable to reduce left ventricular filling pressures to the 10- to 15-mm Hg range whenever possible. An occasional patient may demonstrate no improvement in stroke volume with reduction in filling pressure, usually because there is no associated mitral insufficiency to redistribute back to forward flow. Such patients are unusual in our experience, but may require a higher-than-normal left ventricular filling pressure to maintain an adequate cardiac output.

Despite its popularity, there is no rationale for "targeting" a specific reduction in systemic vascular resistance other than as a means to decrease filling pressure. The primary goal is to reduce filling pressure while maintaining or improving cardiac output. Systemic vascular resistance is a contrived index, not a true measurement.

Although experience with agents that directly increase cardiac output has proven that they are detrimental as long-term therapy, it is important nevertheless to achieve a cardiac index greater than 2.0 L/minute/m². On the other hand, it seems far more important to relieve circulatory congestion than to increase the cardiac index toward some fixed target. It is not clear that a cardiac index of 3.0 L/minute/m² is preferable to the cardiac index of 2.5 L/minute/m². The limitations of drugs that have been designed directly to stimulate contractility and cardiac output are now well known to physicians caring for patients with advanced heart failure. Myocyte dysfunction and arrhythmias often limit the use of such drugs, at least on a chronic basis. Even acutely, there may be some detrimental effects of severely driving the inotropic state of the failing myocardium.

It is rarely necessary to perform hemodynamic monitoring to diagnose heart failure, unless there is severe concomitant intrinsic pulmonary disease or sepsis present. For most patients, the history and physical examination are sufficient to establish the baseline hemodynamic profile, which can vary widely in patients referred for treatment of advanced heart failure (Figure 4).

The utility of invasive hemodynamic monitoring is primarily to facilitate treatment and safely maximize the use of potent drug therapy. Once conventional therapy has been optimized and the patient is sufficiently oxygenated and diuresed, the need for quick-acting and powerful vasodilator therapy is often still evident. In such cases, nitroprusside is perhaps the treatment of choice. Unlike dobutamine or milrinone, it is energetically neutral and does not increase myocardial oxygen consumption. Nitroprusside simultaneously reduces afterload and preload, thereby improving myocardial performance and relieving circulatory congestion. The use of nitroprusside is primarily limited by its tendency to lower blood pressure. However, the expected increment in cardiac output with nitroprusside is usually enough to maintain an adequate blood pressure. It has been my practice to begin with 5 to 15 μg/minute of nitroprusside and increase the dose as necessary to optimize loading conditions. In general, when doses in excess of 400 μg/minute are necessary, the patient is likely "refractory" to nitroprusside. Such patients, in our experience, are often acidotic and have substantial renal insufficiency. In such cases, in view of the potential for thiocyanate toxicity, it is perhaps prudent to abandon the use of nitroprusside and use dobutamine or milrinone. The combination of dobutamine and nitroprusside is frequently used in our intensive care unit to manage patients with severely compromised left ventricular function. In general, 48 to 72 hours of nitroprusside, alone or in combination with dobutamine or milrinone, is usually sufficient to demonstrate improvement in hemodynamics. Diuretics reduce left ventricular filling pressure, but do not usually improve myocardial performance. Nitroprusside, milrinone, and dobutamine reduce left ven-

tricular filling pressure and increase stroke volume. Dopamine improves stroke volume, but has a more variable effect on left ventricular filling pressure (Figure 5).

The first goal of therapy is always relief of symptoms. However, it is important to achieve specific hemodynamic goals, such as reducing the pulmonary capillary wedge pressure to no greater than 15 mm Hg and the right atrial pressure to no greater than 8 mm Hg, and maintaining a systolic blood pressure of at least 80 mm Hg. These hemodynamic goals should be sustained for at least 48 hours. All patients are treated with concomitant oral agents such as ACE inhibitors and nitrates. Patients who are unable to maintain optimal filling pressures on withdrawal of nitroprusside or dobutamine occasionally benefit from the addition of hydralazine. The usual starting dose of hydralazine is 10 to 25 mg three or four times a day, which is gradually titrated up to a dose of 100 mg four times a day. Diuretics and digoxin should be continued unless they are specifically contraindicated. If suitable hemodynamic goals cannot be achieved or if patients continue to be symptomatic, a short-acting ACE inhibitor such as captopril can be given four times a day in combination with nitrates such as isosorbide dinitrate, which is usually dosed three times a day. Occasionally patients with severe heart failure, low baseline blood pressure, and low serum sodium may not tolerate any dose of ACE inhibitors without symptomatic hypotension. Such patients can often be treated with hydralazine and nitrates.

It is distinctly unusual for the combination of ACE inhibitor therapy, long-acting nitrates, and hydralazine to remain ineffective, and in nearly all cases, nitroprusside and dobutamine can be safely withdrawn. Invasive monitoring can usually be withdrawn after 72 hours of intravenous support, and the patient can then be safely placed on the ward. Stability of fluid balance without clinical evidence of congestion or symptomatic hypotension

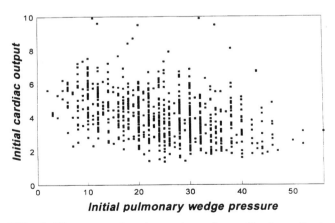

FIG. 4. The presenting hemodynamic profile in patients referred for management of advanced heart failure can vary widely. These data represent 700 patients referred for cardiac transplantation (average left ventricular ejection fraction, 22%). (From Stevenson LW. Therapy tailored for symptomatic heart failure. *Heart Failure* 1995;11:87–107, with permission.)

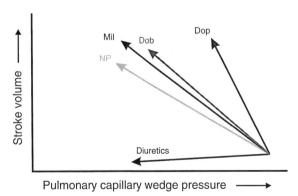

FIG. 5. Diuretics reduce pulmonary capillary wedge pressure but fail to improve myocardial performance. Dobutamine (Dob), milrinone (Mil), and nitroprusside (NP) dramatically improve stroke volume and simultaneously reduce left ventricular filling pressure. Dopamine also improves stroke volume, but has a less consistent effect on left ventricular filling pressure.

should prompt comfortable ambulation. Patients who remain stable without evidence of renal dysfunction, angina pectoris, symptomatic arrhythmias, or recurrent heart failure can usually be safely discharged after a total of 4 to 7 days in the hospital. Clearly, such patients are fragile and must be followed carefully by the therapy team. Most important, the patient must understand the medications, the need for sodium restriction, the necessity of daily weight monitoring, and the need to adjust his or her own diuretics. In rare instances, dobutamine cannot be withdrawn because of persistent pump dysfunction and hypotension. These patients are sometimes placed on chronic low-dose dobutamine, 1 to 3 µg/kg/minute, using a continuous-infusion pump to deliver the drug through a Hickman catheter. Such patients are often considered urgent candidates for heart transplantation (status I). A small minority of patients with advanced heart failure are truly dependent on intravenous inotropic therapy.

ADJUNCTIVE THERAPY

In selected patients, consideration should be given to the use of warfarin, amiodarone, and beta-adrenergic blocking agents. Patients with underlying coronary disease should be treated with daily aspirin. At present, beta-adrenergic blockers and calcium channel blockers should not be considered first-line therapy. However, studies are underway to further evaluate the role of these agents and to determine whether they have selective beneficial properties in patients with severe heart failure.

SUMMARY

It has become clear that despite the presence of advanced and refractory heart failure, most patients can be helped without surgical intervention. Admission to the hospital and expert care by a team of specialists highly experienced in the treatment of severe heart failure is crucial to management success. Nurses, physicians, and surgeons trained in the management of advanced heart failure work as a team to make decisions about both short-term and long-term management of these desperately ill patients. There is no simple treatment algorithm that applies to every patient with advanced heart failure. Drug therapy is constantly changing and being reevaluated, and new surgical techniques and transplantation strategies are continuously emerging. It is unrealistic to expect that physicians who care for such patients only on an occasional basis will be familiar with all of the latest treatment and management strategies. Therefore, it is perhaps best that the patients with truly advanced heart failure be

referred to a center where a team of experts is available to manage the patients through this critical time frame.

Although clinical trials have allowed for the emergence of drugs such as ACE inhibitors that improve survival, this improvement is usually measured only in months rather than in years. More than a million patients are admitted to the hospital each year in the United States for treatment of advanced heart failure. Yet, the number of heart transplantations has remained relatively static at about 2,400 cases per year. Therefore, most patients will not undergo heart transplantation for various reasons, and will require long-term medical support by the heart failure management team. As heart failure continues to extract an enormous emotional and economic toll on life, we can expect that considerable attention will continue to be directed to the development of new therapies and new therapeutic strategies for the management of this condition.

SELECTED REFERENCES

ACC/AHA Task Force. Guidelines for the evaluation and management of heart failure. *J Am Coll Cardiol* 1995;26:1376–1398.

Baker DW, Wright RF. Management of heart failure: IV. Anticoagulation for patients with heart failure due to left ventricular dysfunction. *JAMA* 1994;272:1614–1618.

Cattau EL, Benjamin SB, Knuff TE, Castell DO. The accuracy of the physical examination in the diagnosis of suspected ascites. *JAMA* 1982;247:1164–1166.

Francis GS. Determinants of prognosis in patients with heart failure. *J Heart Lung Transplant* 1994;13:[Suppl]113–S116.

Francis GS. Vasodilators and inotropic agents in the treatment of congestive heart failure. *Semin Nephrol* 1994;14:464–478.

Francis GS, Archer SL. Diagnosis and management of acute congestive heart failure in the intensive care unit. *Journal of Intensive Care Medicine* 1989;4:84–92.

Konstam M, Dracup K, Baker D, et al. Heart failure: management of patients with left-ventricular systolic dysfunction. In: *Quick reference guide for clinicians no. 11.* AHCPR Publication no. 94-0613. Rockville, MD: Agency for Health Care Policy and Research, Public Health Service, U.S. Department of Health and Human Services, June, 1994.

Kukin ML. Understanding refractory heart failure: pathophysiology and management. *Cardiovasc Rev Reports* 1993;27–47.

Rickenbacher PR, Trindade PT, Haywood GA, et al. Transplant candidates with severe left ventricular dysfunction managed with medical treatment: characteristics and survival. *J Am Coll Cardiol* 1996;27:1192–1197.

Stevenson LW. Managing "refractory" heart failure. *Choices in Cardiology* 1993;7:324–327.

Stevenson LW. Therapy tailored for symptomatic heart failure. *Heart Failure* 1995;87–107.

Stevenson LW, Perloff JK. The limited reliability of physical signs for estimating hemodynamics in chronic heart failure. *JAMA* 1989;261:884–888.

Stevenson LW, Tillisch JH, Hamilton M, et al. Importance of hemodynamic response to therapy in predicting survival with ejection fraction ≤20% secondary to ischemic or nonischemic dilated cardiomyopathy. *Am J Cardiol* 1990;66:1348–1354.

Stevenson WG, Stevenson LW, Middlekauff HR, et al. Improving survival for patients with advanced heart failure: a study of 737 consecutive patients. *J Am Coll Cardiol* 1995;26:1417–1423.

Management of End-Stage Heart Disease, edited
by Eric A. Rose and Lynne Warner Stevenson.
Lippincott–Raven Publishers, Philadelphia ©1998.

CHAPTER 5

Positive Inotropic Agents in the Treatment of Heart Failure

René J. Alvarez, Jr., and Arthur M. Feldman

Congestive heart failure (CHF) due to dilated cardiomyopathy (idiopathic or ischemic) is a major public health concern in the United States and the world. It is difficult to accurately calculate the incidence and prevalence of heart failure due to dilated cardiomyopathy, but it is estimated that approximately 4 million Americans carry this diagnosis and that about 400,000 new cases are diagnosed on an annual basis. CHF, therefore, is a major cause of morbidity and mortality in the United States.

Heart failure is a syndrome that results in an inability of the cardiac output to adequately meet the body's demands for blood flow. Patients with heart failure have left ventricular (LV) dysfunction (systolic, diastolic, or both), resulting in exercise intolerance, ventricular dysrhythmias, and shortened life expectancy.

The most common abnormality in patients with CHF is systolic dysfunction. It is this mechanical problem that ultimately leads to the observed symptoms, including shortness of breath, exercise intolerance, orthopnea, fatigue, and edema. Furthermore, activation of compensatory mechanisms, including the renin–angiotensin system and other neurohormonal pathways, further compromises the already failing heart and is implicated in the progression of the disease.

It can be extrapolated from the underlying pathophysiology of systolic dysfunction that pharmacologic interventions (inotropic agents) could be targeted at improving the contractile or inotropic state of the myocardium. This intervention then should result in improved symptoms, exercise tolerance, and longevity of patients. Intuitively, these interventions would be beneficial not only by improving the inotropic state of the myocardium, but by ultimately favorably altering the neurohormonal,

cytokine-mediated, and molecular events that lead to progressive dilatation and systolic dysfunction.

Unfortunately, the clinical application of inotropic agents has been hampered by the observed potential deleterious side effects associated with these drugs. These agents have been shown to exert a deleterious effect on the myocardium by inducing arrhythmias, impairing the diastolic properties of the myocardium, adversely altering metabolism and cellular energetics, and contributing to the progression of the disease. These adverse effects have been seen in clinical trials of inotropic agents and have been associated with increased mortality. However, inotropic agents still remain a mainstay of acute treatment in patients with symptomatic heart failure and of chronic therapy in those patients with end-stage heart failure who are being bridged to cardiac transplantation. This dichotomy of clinical outcomes and benefits is confusing and frustrating. Understanding the underlying cellular, molecular, and mechanistic differences among inotropic agents may allow investigators to identify factors that contribute to adverse outcomes, and may allow risk stratification of patients who could benefit from a particular class of inotropic drug.

It has been over two centuries since Withering described the clinical, therapeutic, and toxic side effects of the common foxglove plant, *Digitalis purpurea.* Since that classic report, the cardiac glycosides have been used extensively in the treatment of patients with CHF. Despite the extensive experience with this class of inotropic agent, controversy exists about its mechanism of action and role in the treatment of patients with heart failure. The role of other inotropic agents has not been as long lived as that of the cardiac glycosides. In fact, there are only three other inotropic agents that have gained U.S. Food and Drug Administration approval in the management of patients with heart failure. These agents are for

Department of Medicine, Division of Cardiology, University of Pittsburgh Medical Center, Pittsburgh, Pennsylvania 15213 parenteral use only and have been associated with adverse outcomes when used chronically. In this chapter, we discuss the pharmacology and therapeutic uses of inotropic agents approved in the management of patients with CHF. We also discuss agents that are promising but not yet approved for use. Where possible, we attempt to review the cellular and molecular events that characterize the specific drug or class of inotropic agent. Finally, we review the results of recent, large clinical trials and discuss the potential role that these agents may have in the future treatment strategies of patients with CHF.

CLASSIFICATION AND MECHANISM OF ACTION OF INOTROPIC AGENTS

Clinical heart failure due to systolic dysfunction results from a loss of myocardial contractile elements, or a generalized process that depresses myocardial contractile function. Therefore, it is reasonable to assume that agents that enhance the contractile function of the myocardium would translate into clinical benefit from

alleviation of symptoms and perhaps by favorably affecting the survival of patients. Inotropic agents are not all the same, and over the past several years we have gained insights into their modes of actions and their clinical usefulness. What is clear is that the process of excitation–contraction coupling is complex, and inotropic agents can exert their effects at various points within this cascade of events. Figure 1 summarizes schematically the various processes that have been reported to be important in excitation–contraction coupling in myocytes. Figure 2 clearly illustrates not only that different agents can exert their effects in very different manners, but that different clinical responses might be expected depending on the mechanism used. Furthermore, by virtue of the methodology used to discover these agents, they may often have unrecognized cellular effects.

Therefore, it has become clear that if inotropic agents are to continue to have a role in the management of patients with CHF, it is necessary to understand the mechanism of action of these agents at the cellular and

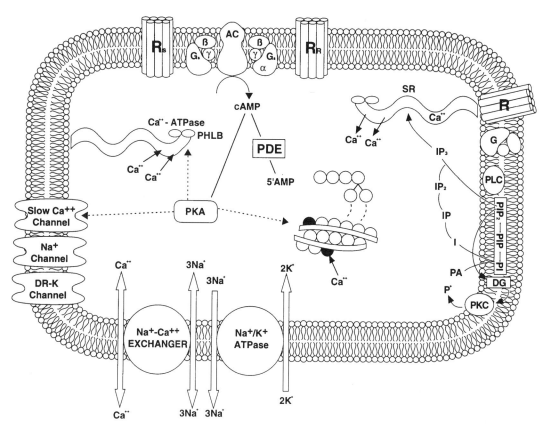

FIG. 1. Biochemical pathways important in regulation of cardiac contractility. AC, adenylyl cyclase; ATP, adenosine triphosphate; cAMP, cyclic adenosine monophosphate; DG, diacylglycerol; DR, delayed rectifier; G, guanine nucleotide-binding regulatory proteins that may stimulate (αG_s) or inhibit (αG_i) adenylyl cyclase; I, inositol; IP, inositol phosphate; IP_2, inositol diphosphate; IP_3, inositol triphosphate; PDE, phosphodiesterase; PHLB, phospholamban; PI, phosphotidylinositol; PIP, phosphotidylinositol 4 phosphate; PIP_2, phosphotidylinositol 4,5-biphosphate; PKA, protein kinase A; PKC, protein kinase C; PLC, phospholipase C; R, sarcolemmal receptor; R_i, inhibitory receptor; R_s, stimulatory receptor; SR, sarcoplasmic reticulum; Tn, troponin. (Adapted from Feldman AM. Classification of positive inotropic agents. *J Am Coll Cardiol* 1993;22:1223–1227, with permission.)

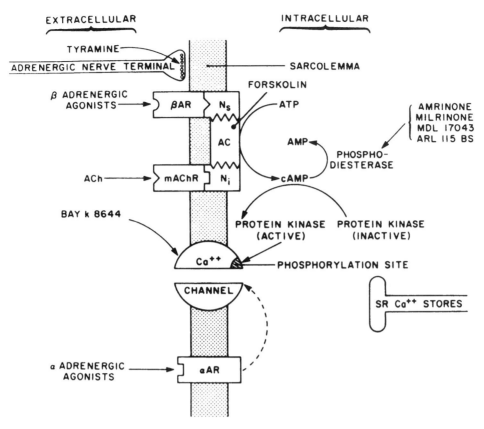

FIG. 2. Diagram illustrating the sites of action of several positive inotropic agents. Circulating catecholamines, catecholamines released from adrenergic nerve terminals, and exogenous sympathomimetic drugs act on beta-adrenergic and alpha-adrenergic receptors (β-AR and α-AR, respectively). Stimulation of beta-adrenergic receptors causes activation of adenylate cyclase (AC), resulting in increased cyclic adenosine monophosphate (cAMP) production, which in turn causes an increase in calcium influx through slow calcium channels, presumably due to the activation of protein kinases that phosphorylate the slow calcium channel. The mechanism by which stimulation of alpha-adrenergic receptors causes an increase in myocardial contractility is not fully understood, but it may also involve an action on the slow calcium channel. Tyramine acts on adrenergic nerve terminals to release catecholamines, which then act on adrenergic receptors. Calcium channel agonists (e.g., the drug Bay k 8644) act directly on the calcium channel to increase calcium influx. Intracellular cAMP is degraded by phosphodiesterases, and inhibition of cardiac phosphodiesterases therefore results in an increase in intracellular cAMP levels. Several of the newer positive inotropic agents appear to act largely by this mechanism. cAMP can also be increased independently of beta-adrenergic receptors by direct stimulation of adenylate cyclase with forskolin. N_s, guanine nucleotide stimulatory subunit; ACh, acetylcholine; mAChR, muscarinic ACh receptor; N_i, guanine nucleotide inhibitory subunit; SR, sarcoplasmic reticulum. (Adapted from Colucci WS, Wright RF, Braunwald E. New positive inotropic agents in the treatment of congestive heart failure. *N Engl J Med* 1986;314:290, with permission.)

molecular levels. It is hoped that this understanding will lead to the rational development of newer agents that in the long run will have beneficial effects on symptoms and outcomes. In addition, an understanding of normal excitation–contraction coupling allows for an appreciation of the pathophysiology of systolic LV dysfunction.

Cardiac Contraction

Cardiac contraction is a highly complex process that involves the intricate interaction of multiple cellular organelles, including the sarcolemma, contractile proteins, sarcoplasmic reticulum, and the mitochondria. A detailed review of excitation–contraction coupling is outside the scope of this chapter; however, it is pertinent to point out some of the primary components of this pathway because these serve as focal points for therapeutic efforts designed to enhance cardiac contractility. It is well known that the most potent means of increasing the contractility of the normal heart comes from signaling through the beta-adrenergic receptors. Indeed, adrenergic receptors subserve a primary role for the endogenous activation of cardiac contractility in response to stress or exercise. Activation of the beta₁- or beta₂-adrenergic receptors (and perhaps the beta₃-adrenergic receptor) in turn activates G-stimulatory transduction proteins and adenylyl cyclase, with the subsequent production of the ubiquitous second messenger cyclic adenosine monophosphate (cAMP). Subsequent activation of the cAMP-dependent protein kinase results in phosphorylation of multiple cellular proteins, including phospholamban, troponin, and the gated Ca^{2+} channel. When phosphorylated, phospholamban is less avidly bound to the sarcoplasmic reticulum protein Ca^{2+} adenosine triphosphatase (ATPase), resulting in enhanced sarcoplasmic reticulum Ca^{2+} uptake and enhanced diastolic function. Similarly, phosphorylation of the head of troponin also diminishes the sensitivity of the contractile proteins to Ca^{2+}, thereby improving diastolic function. In contrast, phosphorylation of the gated Ca^{2+} channel results in increased transmyocardial Ca^{2+} transport, thereby augmenting both intracellular calcium transport and myocyte contractility. Not surprisingly, the cell can also modify contractility through alternative pathways. Most notably, activation of the G-protein–coupled phosphoinositide pathway results in the cellular production of IP3 and diacylglycerol, the latter having the

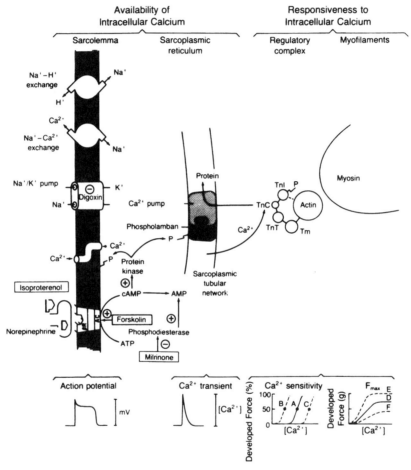

FIG. 3. Four major cellular sites for the regulation of excitation–contraction coupling in the mammalian heart: sarcolemma, sarcoplasmic reticulum, regulatory complex, and myofilament. Cardiac contractility may be altered by changing either the availability of intracellular calcium for activation or the responsiveness of the myofilament to intracellular calcium. Calcium availability is regulated predominantly by sites in the sarcolemma and sarcoplasmic reticulum that can be functionally monitored by means of the action potential and calcium transient, respectively. Responsiveness to intracellular calcium is regulated predominantly by the troponin–tropomyosin complex, attached to actin, and the myofilament actin and myosin. These components can be functionally assessed by the calcium sensitivity and maximal calcium-activated force (F_{max}) of fibers rendered hyperpermeable to calcium. The Ca^{2+} transient is the depolarization-induced increase and decrease in the intracellular calcium concentration: $[Ca^{2+}]$; Ca^{2+} sensitivity is the relation between the intracellular calcium concentration and cardiac activation, expressed as a percentage of peak developed force. Curves A and D are baseline values of the sensitivity of myofilaments to calcium and F_{max}, respectively. Ca^{2+} sensitivity and F_{max} can change independently of each other. Curves B and E show enhancement, and curves C and F depression, of sensitivity and F_{max}, respectively. TnI, troponin I; TnC, troponin C; TnT, troponin T; Tm, tropomyosin; βR, beta-adrenergic receptor; AC, adenylate cyclase; cAMP, cyclic adenosine monophosphate; P, phosphorylation. (Adapted from Morgan JP. Mechanisms of disease: abnormal intracellular modulation of calcium a major cause of cardiac contractile dysfunction. *N Engl J Med* 1991;325:625, with permission.)

ability to modulate cellular Ca^{2+} homeostasis through a protein kinase A-mediated pathway.

Classification of Positive Inotropic Agents

The mechanisms of action of positive inotropic agents are diverse, and an understanding of the signaling pathways and receptors involved allows for rational design and clinical use. Based on the biochemistry of excitation–contraction coupling, it is clear that the inotropic state of the heart can be altered by agents that increase intracellular cAMP, that affect the function of sarcolemma ion pumps/channels, that modulate intracellular calcium by either altering the release of sarcoplasmic calcium or sensitizing the contractile proteins to calcium's actions, or that have pleotrophic properties and multiple mechanisms of action (see Figure 1; Figure 3). Thus, a classification scheme based on mechanism of action would be more rational than grouping inotropic agents by route of administration (i.e., oral vs. parenteral). However, such a classification scheme gives no hints about the possible risk/benefits associated with the drug's clinical use. Therefore, we proposed a classification scheme based on mechanism of action and have divided inotropic agents into four classes (Table 1). Class I agents are those agents that increase intracellular cAMP; class II agents are those that affect sarcolemmal ions pumps/channels; class III comprises those agents that modulate intracellular calcium by altering its release from the sarcoplasmic reticulum, sensitizing contractile proteins to the effects of calcium; and class IV agents are those with multiple mechanisms of action. This scheme has provided a framework for understanding the benefits and limitations of inotropic agents and allowed better characterization of investigational agent being developed.

Class I: Agents that Increase the Intracellular Concentration of Cyclic Adenosine Monophosphate

The autonomic nervous system has a profound effect on the inotropic state of the myocardium. Adrenergic or cholinergic stimulation mediates a complex series of events that eventually alter calcium metabolism and the inotropic state of the myocardium. Adrenergic stimulation of the heart occurs through activation of the beta-adrenergic receptors. The human heart expresses both the $beta_1$ receptor and $beta_2$ receptors, although the former predominate. The beta receptors are associated with a superfamily of signal transduction proteins termed *G-proteins*. The association of the transmembrane beta receptor with G-proteins is cytoplasmic and is vital to signal transduction when the beta receptor is bound by its ligand. The G-proteins are heterotrimeric, consisting of alpha, beta, and gamma subunits that can bind guanosine triphosphate (GTP) and other guanine nucleotides. The beta receptor/G-protein/adenylyl cyclase complex forms the signal transduction machinery for adrenergic stimulation of the myocardium.

These subunits modulate the activity of downstream enzyme systems, including adenylyl cyclase. G-protein systems may be either stimulatory or inhibitory. The stimulatory G_s-protein is responsible for activation of the adenylyl cyclase system, whereas the inhibitory G_i-protein inhibits this system. This inhibition is thought to be activated by cholinergic stimulation of muscarinic receptors and GTP binding to the active site of the $G_{\alpha i}$ protein.

On beta-adrenergic stimulation, the effector enzyme, adenylate cyclase, is activated by the actions of the G-proteins and the hydrolysis of GTP. Cyclic AMP is then generated and is the primary second messenger in the cascade that follows beta-adrenergic stimulation. The increase in cAMP translates into improved contraction and inotropy of the myocardium. The adenylyl cyclase system is coupled to other effector molecules independently and also mediates the function of their membrane-bound receptors, including those for thyroid hormone, glucagon, prostaglandin I_2, calcitonin, and vasoactive intestinal peptide.

Once cAMP is synthesized, its effector function is mediated through the activation of protein kinase systems that phosphorylate and activate downstream effector proteins. In turn, these proteins may alter protein function through posttranslational modification or, alternatively, they may alter the expression of selected candidate genes. For example, cAMP is able to bind the regulatory subunit

TABLE 1. *Classes of inotropic agents by mechanism of action*

Class	Definition
I	Agents that increase intracellular cyclic adenosine monophosphate
	Beta-adrenergic agonists
	Phosphodiesterase inhibitors
II	Agents that affect sarcolemmal ions pumps/channels
	Digoxin
III	Agents that modulate intracellular calcium mechanisms by either:
	A) Release of sarcoplasmic reticulum calcium inositol triphosphate or
	B) Increased sensitization of the contractile proteins to calcium
IV	Drugs having multiple mechanisms of action
	Pimobendan
	Vesnarinone

of various protein kinases, thus liberating the catalytic component and altering cellular processes. At the molecular level, the activation of protein kinases leads to the phosphorylation of serine/threonine residues on target proteins, altering their intrinsic properties. These events lead to further downstream events, eventually affecting the homeostasis of the cell.

In the myocardium, it is thought that events that lead to positive inotropy involve the stimulation of the beta receptor by norepinephrine/epinephrine, leading to molecular changes in the receptor. This is then coupled to events that lead to GTP binding to the catalytic subunit of the G_s-protein complex. The hydrolysis of GTP then allows for the dissociation of the G-protein complex and activation of adenylate cyclase. Formation of cAMP by the hydrolysis of ATP leads to the activation of protein kinases. In particular, protein kinase A is activated, initiating a cascade of events that results in the phosphorylation of the calcium regulatory proteins and culminating in an increase in phosphorylation of the regulatory proteins. This effect can increase sarcoplasmic reticulum calcium uptake and enhance relaxation and contraction. These events are tightly regulated by the actions of phosphodiesterase (PDE), which metabolizes and inactivates cAMP.

On the other hand, events that lead to negative inotropy are also closely linked to the receptor/G-protein/adenylyl cyclase complex. In this case, cholinergic stimulation of muscarinic receptors couples the G_i-protein with inhibition of adenylyl cyclase. The postreceptor mechanisms that are involved in vagal inhibition of myocardial inotropy are less well understood. They appear to be complex, involving an interplay of cyclic guanosine monophosphate (cGMP), cAMP, and protein kinases.

A pathognomonic finding in all patients with CHF is diminished responsiveness to beta stimulation. Seminal investigations by Bristow and colleagues have demonstrated that the insensitivity to adrenergic drive can be explained by downregulation of the beta receptors, decreased activity of adenylate cyclase, and increased activity of PDE and the inhibitory G_i-protein complex. Indeed, patients with established heart failure have a blunted rise in contractile force on beta-adrenergic stimulation and show diminished calcium transients and altered calcium homeostasis.

It is clear that the endogenous catecholamine norepinephrine is much more selective for the $beta_1$-adrenergic receptors than the $beta_2$-adrenergic receptors. However, whether this has anything to do with the selective $beta_1$ downregulation that characterizes the failing human heart remains undefined. In addition, there is an uncoupling of the $beta_2$ receptor from adenylyl cyclase, an effect that may be a result of enhanced functional activity of the G_i-protein. The fact that $beta_2$ receptors are not downregulated in the failing myocardium has led some investigators to hypothesize that $beta_2$-adrenergic receptor stimulation might be more effective than chronic $beta_1$-adrenergic receptor activation in patients with CHF. However, the consequences of chronic $beta_2$ stimulation remain unclear.

Therefore, it is intuitively reasonable that adrenergic agonists or agents targeted to events downstream of the beta-adrenergic receptor might appropriately signal enhanced inotropy. For example, targeted therapy might enhance cAMP production or decrease its breakdown. Alternatively, a pharmacologic agent that could alter the responsiveness of the beta-adrenergic receptor to stimulation or alter the equilibrium of the reaction between the stimulatory G_s-protein and the inhibitory G_i-protein, favoring increased activity of G_s, may be clinically beneficial. Many agents were developed with this rationale in mind. Unfortunately, none has had a favorable impact on the survival of patients with heart failure. In fact, chronic therapy with several adrenergic agonists or PDE inhibitors has been shown to have adverse effects on mortality. One such agent, xamoterol, has shown favorable hemodynamic effects in early phase II and phase III clinical trials. Unfortunately, in a larger phase IV randomized trial, xamoterol was associated with increased mortality (Figure 4). Similarly, oral pharmacologic agents that augment intracellular levels of cAMP by inhibiting the enzyme PDE have also shown benefits in early phase II and phase III trials, but proved harmful in larger phase IV studies.

Although oral adrenergic agonists have not withstood the scrutiny of large, randomized, clinical trials, intravenous inotropic agents remain vitally important in the management of patients with severe and decompensated CHF. These agents include the beta-adrenergic agonists dobutamine and dopamine. There is growing support for these agents in the short-term treatment of patients with decompensated CHF, but their role in the long-term

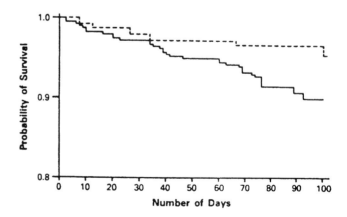

FIG. 4. Three-month survival probabilities from the xamoterol heart failure trial, showing increased mortality with xamoterol. Broken line indicates placebo (n = 164); solid lines, xamoterol (n = 352); $p = 0.02$; hazard ratio 2.54 (confidence interval, 1.06–6.08). (Adapted from Xamoterol in Severe Heart Failure Study Group. Xamoterol in severe heart failure. *Lancet* 1990;336:1–6, with permission.)

management of patients with severe or refractory heart failure remains controversial.

Dobutamine

Dobutamine (Figure 5) is an intravenously administered synthetic catecholamine that increases myocardial contractility without marked tachycardia. This effect is achieved by its selectivity for beta$_1$-adrenergic receptors in the absence of significant effects on beta$_2$ receptors. Dobutamine does possess slight avidity for alpha receptors, which accounts, in part, for its vasodilatory properties. Until the development of dobutamine in 1982, isoproterenol, epinephrine, and norepinephrine were the only adrenergic agonists available for the treatment of CHF. Unfortunately, these nonselective beta agonists were not clinically useful in the management of patients with decompensated heart failure or cardiogenic shock because of their associated tachycardia and vasodilatation. Modification of the structure of isoproterenol led to the discovery of dobutamine, which maintained inotropic properties without significant increases in heart rate. These properties made this compound clinically useful and it was approved in 1978 for the treatment of cardiac failure associated with low cardiac output and elevated filling pressures.

The pharmacologic properties of dobutamine are directly related to its avidity for the beta$_1$-adrenergic receptor. At doses of 2.5 to 15 µg/kg/minute, dobutamine effects a dose-related increase in cardiac contractility and cardiac output. Over a large range of doses, ventricular diastolic pressure tended to fall and there was a balancing effect on peripheral vascular resistance (PVR) and systemic vascular resistance (SVR) because of dobutamine's effect on beta$_2$ and alpha receptors. In animal studies, the inotropic effects of dobutamine outweigh its minor chronotropic effects. The pharmacologic properties responsible for this observation are not completely understood, but may relate to the fact that dobutamine has less avidity for the sinoatrial node than does epinephrine/norepinephrine or isoproterenol. In the presence of beta blockers, dobutamine has been shown to cause a decrease in cardiac output and an increase in PVR and SVR. This relates to the fact that it binds to peripheral alpha receptors in the setting of beta$_1$ and beta$_2$ blockade. At high doses, in excess of 20 µg/kg/minute, dobutamine tends to produce tachycardia and hypotension associated with a reduction in SVR.

Dobutamine requires continuous intravenous infusion to achieve its benefits. It has a short half-life, making it an ideal drug in the management of acutely ill patients. The drug is metabolized in the liver by the enzyme catechol-O-methyl-transferase to an inactive metabolite, 3-O-methyldobutamine, conjugated to an inactive glucuronide, and excreted in the urine. The onset of action of dobutamine is rapid and its beneficial hemodynamic effects can be appreciated quickly, making it an ideal drug for the treatment of severe heart failure.

Dobutamine infusion in the short term can increase contractility and thus increase myocardial oxygen demand, but it may decrease coronary vascular resistance, thus increasing coronary blood flow. The net effect on the

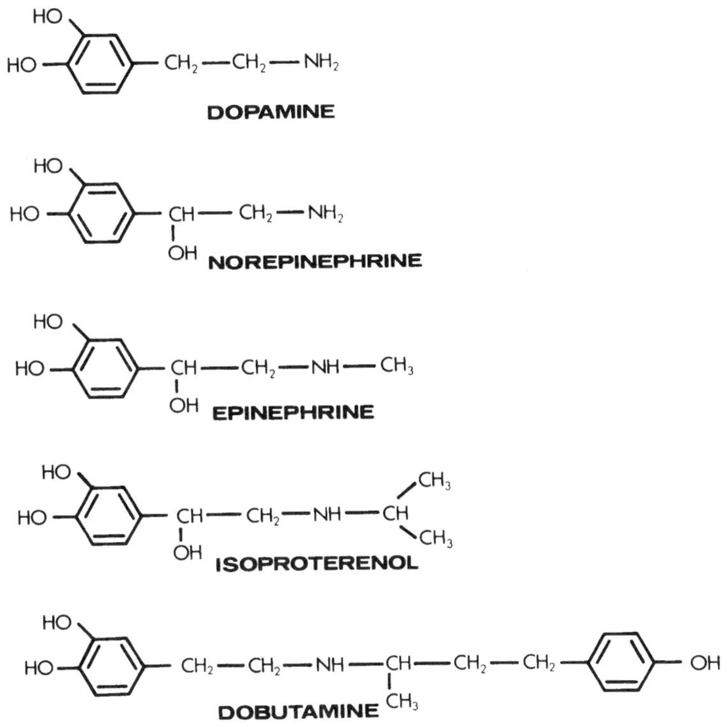

FIG. 5. Chemical structure of various endogenous and synthetic inotropes. (Adapted from Sonnenblick EH, Frishman WH, Lejemtel TH. Dobutamine: a new synthetic cardioactive sympathetic amine. *N Engl J Med* 1979;300:17, with permission.)

myocardium depends on the influence of other factors, including myocardial oxygen supply and demand. Therefore, dobutamine should be used carefully in patients with obstructive coronary artery disease. Dobutamine has been used extensively in patients with shock and low output after myocardial infarctions with favorable effects and demonstrated clinical usefulness. The clinical response to dobutamine correlates with infusion dose and plasma level in patients with varying severities of heart failure. At doses of 2.5 to 15 µg/kg/minute, dobutamine produces predictable increases in cardiac output and decreases in pulmonary capillary wedge pressure as well as LV end-diastolic pressures. The lower doses are associated with minimal effects on SVR or heart rate. However, at doses greater than 15 µg/kg/minute, vasoconstriction, decreased cardiac output, and increased heart rate are observed. These observations have been seen in a range of clinical conditions associated with LV systolic dysfunction, including myocarditis, myocardial infarction, and decompensated human heart failure.

The inotropic properties of dobutamine are associated with relatively minimal toxicity or adverse events. The most serious potential adverse event is the precipitation of arrhythmias. The event rate is reported to be much lower than with dopamine or isoproterenol. Furthermore, early experience with dobutamine-associated arrhythmias occurred at a time when most used higher doses than are common in current practice. A primary concern is the ability of dobutamine to increase heart rate in patients with atrial fibrillation, thereby precipitating supply/demand ischemia in patients with coronary artery disease. This increase in heart rate in the patient with atrial fibrillation is likely due to facilitation of atrioventricular conduction. Other side effects include nausea, headaches, palpitations, and angina; however, these occur in less than 1% of patients. Hypotension may be seen if patients have an enhanced sensitivity to the beta$_2$-adrenergic effects of dobutamine. Finally, it is imperative to recognize that infiltration of dobutamine at the site of venous access can result in tissue necrosis if it is not promptly recognized.

Most physicians agree that dobutamine has a beneficial role in the short-term management of patients with decompensated heart failure or cardiogenic shock. The chronic administration of dobutamine has been more controversial and its benefits less clear. Some clinicians have advocated the intermittent use of dobutamine; however, this technique is also controversial. Clinicians have argued that infusion of dobutamine for longer than 72 hours could in theory cause beta-adrenergic receptor downregulation. This is supported by a reduced effectiveness in patients receiving dobutamine infusions for longer than 96 hours. The investigators speculated that this observation was due to the development of tolerance to constant infusion of dobutamine. Others have postulated that dobutamine infusions improve the contractile state of heart failure, thereby attenuating the neurohormonal augmentation that maladaptively occurs in patients with CHF. Diminished adrenergic drive might result in upregulation of beta receptors and improved long-term hemodynamic responsiveness. This observation has been supported by reports of increased beta receptor density in patients on chronic dobutamine infusion awaiting transplantation and by outcomes studies assessing coronary norepinephrine levels in patients receiving acute infusion of increasing doses of dobutamine. These studies also noted that higher doses of dobutamine are associated with improved hemodynamics and patient outcomes than lower doses, especially in the cohort of patients with more advanced heart failure.

In part, the reluctance of many clinicians to use intravenous inotropic therapy is based on the results of several studies presented at American Heart Association. In one study, Dies et al. reported an increased mortality in patients receiving chronic intermittent dobutamine therapy. However, this study was flawed because (a) doses were far higher than we routinely use; (b) patients were not monitored for electrolyte abnormalities or arrhythmias; (c) the dose of dobutamine was not titrated to changes in a patient's weight; and (d) there was a crossover design for patients who got worse on placebo. More recently, O'Connell et al. reported data from the Flolan study demonstrating increased morbidity and mortality in patients randomized to placebo who entered the study on chronic inotropic therapy. Unfortunately, comparing patients treated with inotropes (Class IV) with those not inotropic dependent (Class III) involves two very different groups of patients, and it would therefore not be unexpected that the inotropic-dependent patients would have worse outcomes. Perhaps the best evidence supporting chronic therapy with dobutamine comes from a study in Europe in which patients were randomized to chronic inotropic therapy or to placebo. In this study, the dobutamine-treated patients demonstrated improvement in New York Heart Association (NYHA) classifications and decreased weight.

Unfortunately, the chronic use of dobutamine in patients with CHF remains controversial. However, there may be subgroups of patients with end-stage myopathic hearts who would benefit from continuous infusion in terms of quality of life and reduction in symptoms. As already noted, there have been no large, randomized, placebo-controlled trials of chronic dobutamine infusion that would allow us to answer this question. Thus, we must make clinical decisions based on anecdotal data from small studies and personal communications. Long-term benefits of dobutamine have been described in a report from Pickworth. Using metaanalysis, he showed that chronic dobutamine was associated with improved symptoms of CHF, improved NYHA functional classification, improved LV ejection fraction (LVEF), and improved exercise tolerance, but, importantly, was not associated with improved survival. In fact, the author states that chronic dobutamine administration had the potential to be arrhythmogenic and might possibly contribute to sudden cardiac death. To prevent some of the unfavorable effects of chronic dobutamine infusion, many centers have gained experience using dobutamine in the out-patient setting as well as with short-term infusions over 72 hours. Unverferth reported sustained clinical improvement in CHF patients who were treated with continuous dobutamine infusions for 72 hours. These effects lasted for up to 10 weeks. Laing et al. reported that 72 hours of continuous dobutamine improved NYHA functional classification, LVEF, and exercise tolerance compared with placebo. Similarly, when dobutamine infusion was examined in a cohort of patients with refractory heart failure, they also benefited from improved symptoms and NYHA functional classification, but mortality in this patient population remained high compared with conventional therapy. However, the dose of dobutamine used in this study was higher than currently recommended. Therefore, the survival benefits of dobutamine in this study cannot be adequately assessed. Large clinical trials using appropriate dosing will be required to resolve this controversy.

The intermittent use of dobutamine also remains controversial. There have been reports of sustained improvements in symptoms of CHF in patients with severe heart failure receiving intermittent infusions of dobutamine. The term "cardiovascular conditioning" has been applied to describe the mechanism of these sustained effects on symptoms and hemodynamics after dobutamine holidays. Unfortunately, long-term effects on survival or clinical efficacy have not been evaluated, and hence existing data to support the long-term benefits are only anecdotal. Therefore, further clinical trials that examine the optimal doses of dobutamine in relation to symptoms and survival should be undertaken in a randomized, placebo-controlled fashion in patients with severe and refractory heart failure. Despite this lack of substantive data, dobutamine continues to be used in out-patient settings, where dobutamine holidays are used in an attempt to improve symptoms and quality of life in patients with CHF.

Dopamine

Dopamine is an endogenous precursor of norepinephrine that has unique pharmacologic properties. At low doses (0.5–2 µg/kg/minute), dopamine stimulates dopaminergic D_1 and D_2 receptors, resulting in peripheral and renal vasodilatation. At higher doses (2–6 µg/kg/minute), beta$_1$- and beta$_2$-adrenergic receptors are stimulated with ensuing inotropy and chronotropy. At even higher doses (7–10 µg/kg/minute), manifestations of alpha-adrenergic stimulation begin to be seen, leading to increases in blood pressure due to increased SVR. In patients with CHF, benefits are obtained at the lower doses as a result of peripheral vasodilatation of the mesenteric, coronary, and renal arteries with accompanying improvements in natriuresis and diuresis. Higher doses are useful in patients with severe LV dysfunction and hypotension associated with cardiogenic shock.

The biologic effects of dopamine result from signal transduction through the dopaminergic receptors located on the cell membranes of numerous organs. Dopamine receptors are grouped in two families: the DA_1- and DA_2-dopaminergic receptors. These receptors resemble the beta-adrenergic receptor in that they have seven membrane-spanning regions and are coupled to adenylate cyclase. The DA_1 receptor mediates the vasoactive properties described previously, whereas the DA_2 receptor mediates predominantly central nervous system effects by altering norepinephrine release and increasing the bioavailability of dopamine. The DA_2 receptor also mediates the tonic inhibition of aldosterone secretion in response to Angiotensin II (AII) stimulation. There has been no long-term, randomized, placebo-controlled trial that has investigated the role of dopamine in the treatment of patients with CHF. However, low-dose dopamine has proved useful in the acute management of patients with exacerbations of chronic CHF and has been used in some centers as adjunctive therapy for patients receiving dobutamine as either chronic out-patient therapy or as a bridge to cardiac transplantation. The vasodilatory properties act synergistically with diuretics to improve diuresis, thereby lowering LV end-diastolic pressure and volume. In addition, dopamine, because of its effects on the resistance vasculature, is very helpful in patients with abdominal discomfort secondary to mesenteric ischemia.

Although intravenous formulations of beta-adrenergic agonists proved useful in the treatment of severe and refractory heart failure in both in-patient and out-patient settings, oral beta agonists have not proved beneficial. These drugs were developed under the same rationale as their intravenous counterparts, that is, to support circulation by improving contractility in patients with LV dysfunction. Unfortunately, the chronic administration of these oral inotropic agents has not proved fruitful. However, it is worthwhile simply to review some of these agents to understand better the biology of inotropic agents in the failing heart.

Levodopa is a precursor of dopamine that is decarboxylated to dopamine after ingestion. This drug has been used in patients with Parkinson's disease, in whom it increased natriuresis and renal blood flow. This observation led to its investigation in the treatment of CHF. Preliminary work demonstrated that levodopa increased cardiac output and decreased SVR, leading to improved clinical end-points. These effects were thought to result from stimulation of beta$_1$ receptors, with improved inotropy, and from stimulation of dopaminergic receptors in vascular smooth muscle, with resultant vasodilation. Prolonged benefit was also demonstrated in a small cohort of patients (n = 14) over a 12-week period of follow-up with levodopa. Unfortunately, a large dose of the drug with frequent dosing (three to four times daily) was required to achieve sustained hemodynamic effects. At these doses, few of the patients were able to tolerate the side effects. To date, however, there has been no controlled trial evaluating the clinical efficacy of levodopa for the long-term management of patients with heart failure.

Doexamine is a synthetic catecholamine that enhances contractility, improving signs and symptoms of CHF. Its other hemodynamic effects include increasing stroke volume and cardiac output while decreasing afterload and SVR. This drug exerts its effects through its avidity for the beta$_2$ receptor. It can also increase renal and visceral blood flow by its agonism for dopamine receptors. Its role in the long-term management of patients with CHF has not been defined.

Fenolopam is another dopamine analog that has been shown to have positive inotropic effects, improve exercise tolerance, and produce vasodilatory effects. Its lack of ability to produce prolonged beneficial effects, however, has halted its development.

A dopamine agonist that received a lot of attention was ibopamine. Ibopamine, an orally active, dopamine-like catecholamine, is converted to epinine after oral administration. This compound is able to bind both DA$_1$ and DA$_2$ receptors, exerting inotropic and vasodilatory effects. Lower doses of the drug activated DA$_1$/DA$_2$ receptors, whereas higher doses also activated alpha receptors peripherally. The hemodynamic effects of ibopamine included an augmentation of cardiac output and stroke volume, and a reduction of filling pressures and afterload, with relatively little effect on heart rate or blood pressure. Preliminary trials suggested ibopamine had beneficial effects on symptoms and exercise tolerance, in addition to decreasing plasma catecholamine levels. The first randomized, double-blinded, placebo-controlled trial to report ibopamine's effects was the Dutch Digoxin-Ibopamine Multicenter Trial (DIMT). This trial examined the effects of ibopamine and digoxin on patients with mild to moderate heart failure. The trial demonstrated an improvement in exercise time in the subgroup of patients with relatively preserved LV function. Importantly, this trial did not demonstrate an increase in arrhythmias, nor did it have a negative impact on mortality. The findings noted in this trial, as well as in a number of other small trials, suggested that ibopamine might be beneficial in the chronic treatment of patients with CHF. Unfortunately, the Second Prospective Study of Ibopamine on Mortality and Ethicacy (PRIME II) trial, evaluating ibopamine in the treatment of patients with NYHA class III/IV CHF, was terminated prematurely in 1995 because the data and safety monitoring committee found an excess mortality in the ibopamine group. As a result, enrollment into the U.S. multicenter ibopamine trial was stopped as well. The PRIME II trial is representative of multiple larger, controlled studies that have demonstrated adverse effects of positive inotropic agents.

The Phosphodiesterase Inhibitors

Phosphodiesterase inhibitors have been extensively evaluated in the treatment of patients with CHF. These agents inhibit the function of PDE and thus lead to increased concentrations of cAMP in cells, an effect that is downstream of the downregulated beta-adrenergic receptors. The PDE system includes at least seven different isoenzymes that are tissue and cell specific. Their association with specific cGMP- and cAMP-dependent signaling systems is now being identified. There are at least three different PDE isoforms with various affinities for cAMP and cGMP. Theophylline is a PDE inhibitor that has been in clinical use. Its hemodynamic effects are complex and its inotropic properties are disappointing. Several relatively cardioselective PDE inhibitors have been developed and studied. The hemodynamic effects of these agents are impressive and are characterized by augmentation of cardiac output and stroke volume as well as vasodilatation, resulting in decreased preload and marked lowering of pulmonary pressures. These acute hemodynamic changes are achieved with little change in mean heart rate and blood pressure. These compounds are grouped chemically and include the bipyridine derivatives amrinone and milrinone; the imidazole derivatives enoximone and piroximone; and the benzimidazole derivatives sulmazole, pimobendan, and adibendan. All these derivatives share similar hemodynamic profiles.

Amrinone and milrinone were the first PDE inhibitors established in clinical trials in the United States. They inhibit the PDE III isozyme, which is primarily found in cardiac and vascular tissue. Amrinone has been studied in both oral and intravenous forms, but is available only in the intravenous preparation. Amrinone can acutely increase contractility, cardiac output, and stroke volume, and decrease filling pressures and lower vascular resistance, leading to lower SVR and PVR. These changes occur without a marked change in the oxygen consumption of the myocardium and mean heart rate, and no net change in lactate production, suggesting a beneficial effect on myocardial energetics. Amrinone also affects the myocardium's handling of calcium by increasing release and uptake from the sarcoplasmic reticulum.

Early clinical studies suggested that amrinone can produce improved exercise performance in patients with CHF. However, the Amrinone Multicenter Trial Group study did not show any statistically significant difference between symptoms, functional classification, ejection fraction, exercise tolerance, or mortality after 12 weeks of treatment. There was also a trend toward more side effects in the amrinone-treated group. Moreover, it can be reasoned that long-term effects of this class of drug will be limited because of the altered function of the receptor/adenyl cyclase/G-protein complex because the efficiency of a PDE inhibitor requires the presence of cAMP. The marked diminution in cAMP synthesis in the failing human heart could preclude a clinical inotropic benefit. Indeed, the primary function of PDE inhibition in a population of patients with cardiac failure might be its vasodilatory (afterload) properties. Although amrinone was not approved for oral use, it was approved for intravenous use in patients with acute heart failure; however, it has not found favor in the management of patients with moderate to severe CHF, in part because of its unpredictable metabolism. This is primarily due to the genetic differences in the enzymes that acetylate amrinone to an inactive metabolite. Thus, plasma levels are difficult to predict. Furthermore, amrinone has been associated with serious and frequent side effects, including jaundice, myositis, pulmonary infiltrates, thrombocytopenia, and polyarteritis. In addition, in a clinical trial comparing amrinone with dobutamine in patients with moderate to severe heart failure, there was no clinical benefit to amrinone over dobutamine; furthermore, the cost of amrinone was substantially higher than that of dobutamine. In addition, the chronic oral administration of amrinone in patients with chronic heart failure was not associated with clinical benefit.

Milrinone is another potent PDE inhibitor with similar hemodynamic effects compared with amrinone. However, in contrast to amrinone, milrinone is associated with a lower incidence of side effects and is better tolerated. The short-term administration of milrinone results in improved cardiac output, exercise tolerance, and maximal oxygen uptake as well as a decrease in PVR and SVR. Oral administration of milrinone was associated with increased mortality and no significant improvement in symptoms compared with placebo. The Milrinone Multicenter Trial Group compared the efficacy of milrinone and digoxin in 230 patients with moderate to severe CHF over a 12-week treatment period. This trial demonstrated that oral milrinone did not seem to offer any advantage over digoxin in terms of exercise tolerance, mortality, or improvement in functional classification. The Prospective Randomized Milrinone Survival Evaluation Trial (PROMISE) trial evaluated the efficacy of milrinone in a prospective, randomized, placebo-controlled fashion in patients with heart failure receiving diuretics, angiotensin-converting enzyme (ACE) inhibitors, and digoxin as background therapy. The study enrolled more than 1,000 patients and followed them for 6 months. The study was stopped prematurely because of an increase in all-cause and cardiovascular mortality in the milrinone-treated group. Again, patients with the most severe heart failure were at greatest risk of death from milrinone (Figure 6). Although oral milrinone is no longer being developed in the United States, the role of intravenous milrinone is evolving. Milrinone is of great benefit in the evaluation of patients for transplantation candidacy because its ability to lower PVR has been shown to be predictive of outcome after trans-

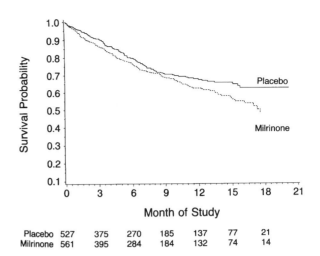

FIG. 6. Kaplan-Meier analysis showing cumulative rates of survival in patients with chronic heart failure treated with milrinone or placebo. Mortality was 28% higher in the milrinone group than in the placebo group ($p = 0.038$). The numbers of patients at risk are shown at the bottom of the figure. (Adapted from Packer M, Carver Jr, Rodeheffner RT, et al. Effect of oral milrinone on mortality in severe chronic heart failure. *N Engl J Med* 1991;325:1468, with permission.)

plantation in patients with pulmonary hypertension and CHF. In addition, there are a substantive number of patients who respond poorly to dobutamine, yet show a substantial hemodynamic response to milrinone. In the acutely ill patient with heart failure, the combination of dobutamine and milrinone has shown hemodynamic benefit, putatively because of synergism between adrenergic stimulation, cAMP production, and PDE inhibition with resulting inhibition of cAMP metabolites. There is growing evidence that this combination can be effective as a bridge to transplantation or device insertion.

Enoximone is another PDE inhibitor that shares a hemodynamic profile similar to that of amrinone and milrinone in patients with CHF. It can produce an increase in cardiac output and can lower PVR and SVR after both oral and intravenous administration. Enoximone's reliable metabolism, better side effect profile, and sustained effects made it a promising drug. Unfortunately, as with all the oral inotropic agents tested in clinical trials, this agent did not stand the test of well designed, large, randomized trials. The Western Enoximone Study Group compared oral enoximone with placebo in patients with mild to moderate CHF. Enoximone failed to show sustained improvement in exercise tolerance or symptoms at 12 weeks. There was no observed difference in terms of mortality at 12 weeks. Interestingly, enoximone did show favorable effects on exercise tolerance and symptoms at 4 and 8 weeks of follow-up. However, these effects were not sustained at the 12-week time point. This raised an interesting prospect for its use in short-term treatment of patients with mild to moderate heart failure. To address this observation, the

Enoximone Multicenter Trial Group was conceived. This study randomized patients with moderate to severe heart failure to receive oral enoximone or placebo. The patients were followed for 6 months, but there were no differences in the symptoms or in exercise tolerance between the enoximone group and placebo group. In addition, there was a trend toward increased mortality in the enoximone group at 4 months. However, as with all of the PDE inhibitors, one must wonder whether the use of lower doses of these agents results in beneficial effects without the associated increase in mortality.

Class II: Agents that Affect Sarcolemmal Ion Pumps/Channels—the Cardiac Glycosides

Digoxin, an extract of the foxglove plant, has been used in the treatment of congestive heart failure since the late 18th century. Indeed, digitalis glycosides remain the most commonly prescribed drugs for heart failure and exert positive inotropic effects as well as having predictable electrophysiologic properties. However, despite their long use, digitalis glycosides have not been used without controversy.

The digitalis glycosides belong to a family of compounds that exert their actions by predictably inhibiting the Na^+/K^+-ATPase pump. Digoxin is a semisynthetic derivative of the glycosides isolated in the *D. lanata* plant, whereas the *D. purpurea* plant contains a number of digitalis glycosides, including digitoxin. It was Stimson who showed that digitalis glycosides exerted positive inotropic effects in the heart. However, it was not until the discovery of the Na^+/K^+-ATPase pump that the mechanism of the positive inotropy was elucidated. The cardiac glycosides all share the property of being selective inhibitors of this electrogenic enzyme pump. This inhibition leads to an increase in the available intracellular calcium concentration, mediated by an associated rise in sodium concentra-

tion. In addition, it is now appreciated that digoxin may have important neurohormonal modulatory effects as well. For example, norepinephrine levels have been shown to decrease after digitalis therapy. Numerous clinical studies have been published that show beneficial effects of digitalis therapy on symptoms, survival, and exercise tolerance. However, these studies were limited by small numbers of patients enrolled, lack of placebo-controlled randomization, and the fact that many of the studies did not objectively assess LV function. The xamoterol trial did allow for evaluation of digitalis in a randomized, double-blind fashion. Improved symptoms were noted in the cohort of patients receiving digoxin compared with those receiving placebo. The captopril–digoxin study was the first randomized, placebo-controlled, double-blinded prospective trial that evaluated the role of digoxin in patients (n = 300) with mild CHF. This study showed improved exercise tolerance as well as increased EF and decreased need for diuretic use in the digoxin treatment group. The PDE inhibitor milrinone was also studied with digoxin in a randomized, double-blinded, placebo-controlled trial. Digoxin use was associated with improved exercise tolerance, increased EF, and a decreased need for diuretics. Because these studies were small, the Randomized Assessment of Digoxin on Inhibitors of the Angiotensin Converting Enzyme (RADIANCE) and Prospective Randomized Study of Ventricular Failure and the Efficacy of Digoxin (PROVED) trials were conceived to assess the efficacy of digoxin in the treatment of patients with mild to moderate CHF from LV systolic dysfunction.

The PROVED trial was designed to demonstrate the efficacy and safety of digoxin in patients with Class I to III CHF. The study was randomized, placebo controlled, and double blinded. The intervention was to withdraw digoxin from patients having stable CHF before randomization, on medical therapy including digoxin and diuretics. All patients had an LVEF less than 35%, NYHA Class

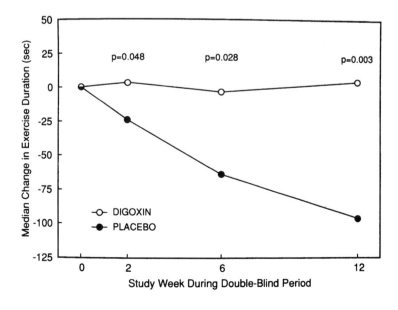

FIG. 7. The change (in seconds) in maximal exercise time of patients continued on digoxin treatment compared with patients receiving placebo. The difference in this change between the two groups was highly significant. The number of study weeks represents the time from double-blinded randomization. (Adapted from Uretsky BF, Young JB, Shahidi FE, et al. Randomized study assessing the effect of digoxin withdrawal in patients with mild to moderate chronic congestive heart failure: results of the PROVED trial. *J Am Coll Cardiol* 1993;22:955, with permission.)

I to III functional status, and were in normal sinus rhythm. After digoxin withdrawal, the patients assigned to the placebo arm showed worsened maximal exercise capacity, increased incidence of treatment failures (increased diuretic requirement, need for hospitalization), reduced LVEF, lower heart rate, and increased body weight compared with the digoxin-treated group (Figures 7, 8).

The RADIANCE trial, on the other hand, included patients with Class II to III CHF who were receiving an ACE inhibitor in addition to digoxin and a diuretic. The design of the study was similar to the PROVED trial in that patients with mild to moderate heart failure were included if they had an LVEF less than 35%, were in normal sinus rhythm, and had an LV internal diameter of at least 60 mm. After randomization, digoxin was maintained or withdrawn and placebo substituted. One hundred seventy-eight patients were randomized in the RADIANCE trial. The mean EF was 28%, the mean digoxin level was 1.1 ng/mL, and coronary artery disease

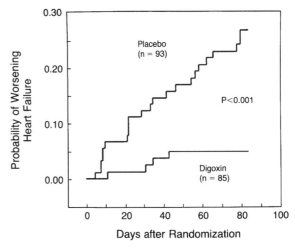

FIG. 9. Kaplan-Meier analysis of the cumulative probability of worsening heart failure in patients continuing to receive digoxin and those switched to placebo. The patients in the placebo group had a higher risk of worsening heart failure throughout the 12-week study (relative risk, 5.9; 95% confidence interval, 2.1–17.2; $p < 0.001$). (Adapted from Packer M, Gheorghiade M, Young JB, et al. Effects of digoxin withdrawal in patients with chronic heart failure treated with converting enzyme inhibitors [RADIANCE]. *N Engl J Med* 1993;329:1, with permission.)

caused 60% of the cardiomyopathies. The patients randomized to placebo had an increased relative risk for development of worsening heart failure compared with the digoxin-treated group (Figure 9). All measures of functional capacity deteriorated in the patients receiving

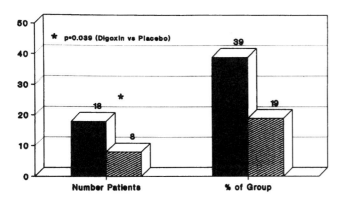

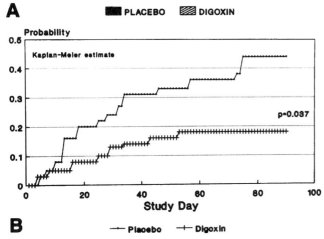

FIG. 8. The number of patients and cumulative incidence (percentage) of treatment failures (A) and time to treatment of heart failure (B) during the double-blinded period. A highly significant increase in the rate and cumulative incidence of treatment failures is observed in the placebo group compared with results in the digoxin group. (Adapted from Uretsky BF, Young JB, Shahidi FE, et al. Randomized study assessing the effect of digoxin withdrawal in patients with mild to moderate chronic congestive heart failure: results of the PROVED trial. *J Am Coll Cardiol* 1993;22:955, with permission.)

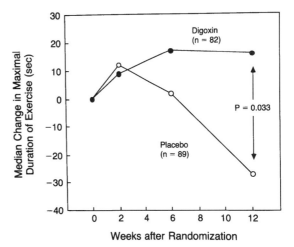

FIG. 10. Median changes in maximal duration of exercise after 2, 6, and 12 weeks in patients continuing to receive digoxin and those switched to placebo. Changes were assessed on a treadmill with a modified Naughton protocol. By the end of the study, exercise capacity had deteriorated significantly in patients in the placebo group ($p = 0.033$). (Adapted from Packer M, Gheorghiade M, Young JB, et al. Effects of digoxin withdrawal in patients with chronic heart failure treated with converting enzyme inhibitors [RADIANCE]. *N Engl J Med* 1993;329:1, with permission.)

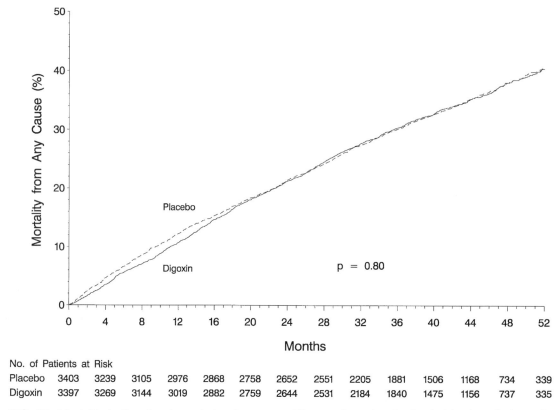

FIG. 11. Mortality in the digoxin and placebo groups. The number of patients at risk at each 4-month interval is shown below the figure. (Adapted from The Digitalis Investigation Group. The effect of digoxin on mortality and morbidity in patients with heart failure. *N Engl J Med* 1997;336:525, with permission.)

placebo compared with those continuing to receive digoxin (Figure 10). In addition, the patients receiving placebo had lower quality-of-life scores as well as lower LVEF, increased heart rate, and increased body weight, and required increased doses of diuretic. Although both PROVED and RADIANCE demonstrated benefit, the results must be viewed with skepticism because of the small size and withdrawal design. Furthermore, early studies in patients post-myocardial infarction suggested an adverse effect of digoxin on long-term survival, and its usefulness in patients with poorly compensated disease remains unclear.

To address more fully the role of digoxin in the treatment of mild to moderate CHF, the National Heart, Lung, and Blood Institute sponsored the Digoxin Investigators Group (DIG) trial. This trial was a randomized, double-blinded, placebo-controlled trial of digoxin in patients with mild to moderate heart failure. The study included patients with an LVEF less than 45% who were randomly assigned digoxin (3,397 patients) or placebo (3,403 patients) in addition to receiving diuretics and ACE inhibitors. During an average follow-up of 37 months, digoxin did not adversely effect patient mortality (Figure 11). In addition, digoxin use was associated with a trend toward a decreased risk of death attributed to worsening heart failure (Figure 12). There were fewer fatal hospital-

izations, as well as fewer hospitalizations for worsening heart failure in the digoxin-treated group compared with placebo (Figure 13). Digoxin was well tolerated and serious complications were uncommon. The DIG trial provides further support for digoxin's continued use in the treatment of CHF. The data also provide evidence that in a large population of patients, digoxin prevents worsening heart failure, improves symptoms, improves exercise capacity, decreases the need for hospitalizations, lowers heart rate, and increases LVEF, and accomplishes this without evidence of increased mortality. Further evaluation of the large database from this study should allow investigators to identify subsets of patients particularly responsive or perhaps unresponsive to digoxin. Furthermore, future analysis should allow for rational use of digoxin in patients with CHF from LV dysfunction when used in conjunction with ACE inhibitors and diuretics and, possibly, beta blockers. However, it is imperative to note that all studies have carefully monitored digoxin levels, with levels never exceeding 1.0 to 1.5 mg/mL. Furthermore, it is important for clinicians to recognize that digoxin can be elevated to toxic levels by comorbidities such as renal dysfunction, cachexia, and heart failure, as well as by advanced age and numerous pharmacologic agents (e.g., quinidine, amiodarone). Therefore, although digoxin is useful, physicians must be judicious in its use.

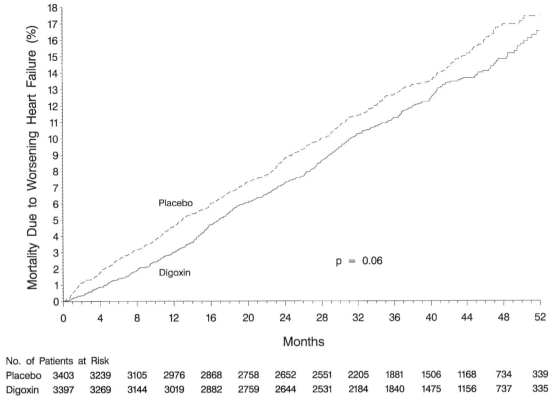

FIG. 12. Mortality due to worsening heart failure in the digoxin and placebo groups. The number of patients at risk at each 4-month interval is shown below the figure. (Adapted from The Digitalis Investigation Group. The effect of digoxin on mortality and morbidity in patients with heart failure. *N Engl J Med* 1997;336:525, with permission.)

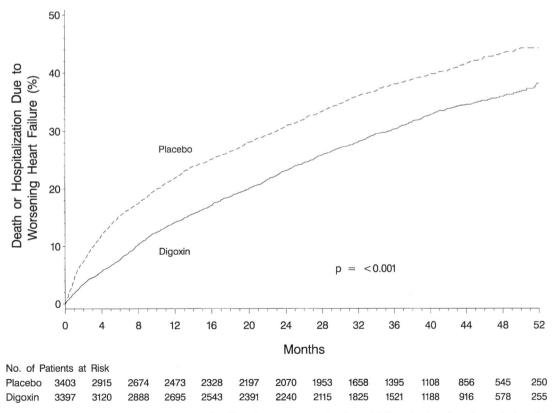

FIG. 13. Incidence of death or hospitalization due to worsening heart failure in the digoxin and placebo groups. The number of patients a risk at each 4-month interval is shown below the figure. (Adapted from The Digitalis Investigation Group. The effect of digoxin on mortality and morbidity in patients with heart failure. *N Engl J Med* 1997;336:525, with permission.)

Class III: Agents that Increase Sensitization of the Contractile Proteins to Calcium

The calcium-sensitizing agents form a class of intriguing compounds. These drugs are able to alter the relationship between the intracellular concentration of calcium and the force generated at any given concentration. They accomplish this by allowing improved interaction of calcium with the contractile proteins, especially troponin. The drugs in this group include pimobendan, sulmazole, simendan, and levosimendan. Sulmazole and pimobendan have both undergone extensive clinical trials in patients with heart failure. They both have PDE III inhibitory properties and both share many of the hemodynamic properties of milrinone and amrinone—that is, they cause an increase in cardiac output, associated with a lowering of ventricular filling pressures. They also are vasodilators and decrease pulmonary vascular resistance and SVR. They have little effect on mean heart rate and mean blood pressure. In small studies, pimobendan was found to have favorable effects on symptoms and exercise tolerance in patients with mild to moderate heart failure. In a study of 52 patients, the lower doses (2.5, 5.0 mg) were found to be more effective than the higher dose (10 mg) in improving exercise tolerance, symptoms, and hemodynamics. A larger trial evaluated these doses in patients with mild to moderate CHF and showed similar results. Again, the lower doses were more effective than the higher dose in achieving the clinical end-points (Figures 14, 15). The 5-mg dose was the most effective in improving quality of

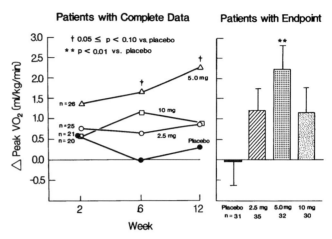

FIG. 15. Graphs show changes in peak VO$_2$ at end-point (*right panel*) and over time for patients with data at every time point (*left panel*). Peak VO$_2$ fell slightly at end-point in patients randomized to placebo. For the 5-mg dose, peak VO$_2$ increased by 2.23 mL/kg/minute at end-point ($p < 0.01$ vs. placebo). Peak VO$_2$ over time was stable for placebo and the 2.5- and 10-mg doses, and showed trends for increases at weeks 6 and 12 for the 5-mg dose. (Adapted from Kubo SH, Gollub S, Bourge R, et al. Beneficial effects of pimobendan on exercise tolerance and quality of life in patients with heart failure. *Circulation* 1992;85:942, with permission.)

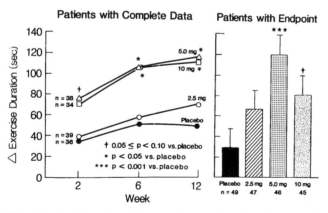

FIG. 14. Graphs show changes in exercise duration at endpoint (*right panel*) and over time for patients with data at every time point (*left panel*). Exercise duration in the placebo group increased by only 29.6 seconds over the 12-week study. The 5-mg/day dose of pimobendan produced a significant increase of 121.6 seconds ($p < 0.001$ vs. placebo). The 10-mg/day dose produced a slightly smaller increase of 81.1 seconds ($p = 0.05$). Over the 12-week study, only the 5- and 10-mg doses demonstrated an increase in exercise duration that was significant compared with placebo at weeks 6 and 12. (Adapted from Kubo SH, Gollub S, Bourge R, et al. Beneficial effects of pimobendan on exercise tolerance and quality of life in patients with heart failure. *Circulation* 1992;85: 942, with permission.)

life, exercise tolerance, and symptoms. Patients also received background therapy that included digoxin, ACE inhibitors, and diuretics. Unfortunately, in a larger prospective trial that evaluated the 2.5- and 5.0-mg dose of pimobendan in 317 patients with Class II to III heart failure, pimobendan was associated with an increased risk or death (19 vs. 11 deaths/100 years at risk). This result did not reach statistical significance, but again raised concern about the role of positive inotropic agents and, in particular, PDE inhibitors in the treatment of heart failure.

Simendan is a PDE III inhibitor that, like pimobendan, has been shown to sensitize contractile proteins to calcium. The levoisomer of racemic simendan was found to be the active form and is in clinical trials. Levosimendan is unique in that it is a selective PDE III inhibitor but does not increase cAMP levels at low concentrations. This drug increases contractility by improving the sensitivity of calcium binding to the contractile proteins, especially troponin C. The molecular/cellular mechanisms that allow for this increased sensitization are poorly understood. Putatively, such an action would improve not only the strength of contraction but the efficiency of contraction.

Class IV: Agents that Have Multiple Mechanisms of Action—Vesnarinone

Vesnarinone (OPC-8212) is an orally active positive inotropic agent. It belongs to the class of agents whose mechanism of action is pleotrophic. Initial clinical observations suggested that vesnarinone increased myocardial contractility and improved hemodynamics and exercise capacity, yet had no effect on myocardial oxygen consumption or heart rate. These observations lead to early randomized, clinical trials that investigated vesnarinone's role in the treatment of patients with moderate to severe heart failure.

Vesnarinone is thought to exert its effects by decreasing delayed outward and inward rectifying potassium currents, thus prolonging diastole. There is evidence that intracellular sodium concentration is increased by prolonged opening of the fast sodium channels. Vesnarinone has also been shown to be a PDE III inhibitor, and thus can increase the inward calcium current and alter intracellular calcium concentrations. This results in a prolonged action potential and a slowing of the heart rate. In fact, vesnarinone has Class III electrophysiologic properties similar to those of sotalol. In addition, vesnarinone has been shown to exert effects on the secretion of various cytokines thought to be important in the development and progression of CHF (i.e., tumor necrosis factor-alpha [TNF-alpha] and interleukin-6 [IL-6]). Cytokine networks are believed to be important in myocardial remodeling, endothelial biology, and regulation of immune responses thought to be involved in the pathogenesis of heart failure. Thus, the attenuation of cytokine production/secretion in autocrine/paracrine networks may play an important role in the modulation and treatment of CHF.

This effect of vesnarinone is interesting in light of the evolving understanding that cytokines play a major role in the development and progression of CHF. TNF-alpha and IL-6 are elevated in the serum of patients with CHF. Torre-Amione et al. have found TNF-alpha mRNA and protein in explanted hearts of patients with CHF but not in nonfailing control hearts. More recently, Kubota et al. have demonstrated that overexpression of TNF-alpha in transgenic mice can recapitulate many of the features of end-stage CHF. Thus, the inhibition of TNF-alpha and IL-6 may be critically important in the attenuation of disease progression and in the everyday therapy of patients with heart failure.

An initial trial of vesnarinone in the United States, in patients with Class II to III heart failure and an LVEF less than 35%, demonstrated an improvement in functional capacity and quality of life. In a larger, multicenter, randomized, placebo-controlled trial in patients with symptomatic heart failure and an LVEF of less than 30%, patients were randomized to receive 60 mg, 120 mg, or placebo. The 120-mg arm was discontinued early because of an associated increase in mortality compared with placebo—another example of the dose-dependent mortality associated with oral inotropic agents. However, when the 60-mg and placebo groups were compared, vesnarinone demonstrated a beneficial effect. Patients receiving vesnarinone had a 50% reduction in the risk of either

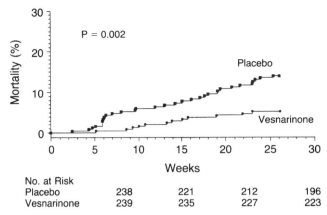

FIG. 16. Cumulative incidence of mortality from any cause, according to treatment group. The values below the figure are the numbers of patients in each group who were alive at baseline and after each 8-week period. (Adapted from Feldman AM, Bristow RM, Parmley WW, et al. Effects of vesnarinone on morbidity and mortality in patients with heart failure: Vesnarinone Study Group. *N Engl J Med* 1993;329:149, with permission.)

dying or for development of worsening CHF during the 6-month trial. There was a 50% decrease in the combined end-point of cardiovascular morbidity and mortality at the 6-month end-point of the trial (Figure 16). In addition, there was a 62% decrease in mortality in the vesnarinone treatment group (Figure 17). More recently, the Vesnarinone in the Severe Heart Failure Trial (VEST trial) randomized nearly 3,800 patients to receive 30 or 60 mg of vesnarinone or placebo. In contrast to the earlier trial, VEST was associated with an increase in mortality with 60 mg and a trend toward increased mortality

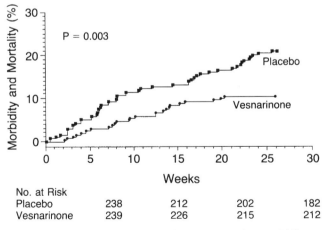

FIG. 17. Cumulative incidence of cardiovascular morbidity or mortality from any cause, according to treatment group. The values below the figure are the numbers of patients in each group who were at risk at baseline and after each 8-week period. (Adapted from Feldman AM, Bristow RM, Parmley WW, et al. Effects of vesnarinone on morbidity and mortality in patients with heart failure: Vesnarinone Study Group. *N Engl J Med* 1993;329:149, with permission.)

with 30 mg of vesnarinone. In contrast to the earlier study, most deaths appeared to be sudden. Several differences exist between the two vesnarinone trials. In contrast to the earlier studies, patients in VEST (a) were not required to be able to exercise, (b) were older, (c) were more likely to be women, and (d) were more severely ill. How these various factors might be responsible for the disparity in the results of these two studies remains unclear; however, further analysis of the large VEST database may provide important clues regarding the use of inotropic therapy in patients with CHF.

Despite over two decades of intense clinical evaluation, the only orally active agent with inotropic properties approved for use in patients with CHF is digoxin. Intuitively, the most logical means of improving signs and symptoms in a patient with systolic dysfunction and CHF would be an inotropic agent. Unfortunately, what is intuitively valid has not been observed in larger, randomized, placebo-controlled clinical trials. Whether it is the ancillary pharmacologic effects of these compounds that cause the detrimental effects of oral inotropes, or our inability to design the perfect inotrope, additional studies are necessary to improve function and survival in patients with heart failure. For example, evidence suggests that by enhancing the sensitivity of the contractile proteins to calcium, we can improve contractility without adversely effecting oxygen consumption. Efforts are now underway to alter the sensitivity of the contractile proteins using targeted gene therapy, an approach that might obviate potentially toxic ancillary effects. Similarly, gene therapy approaches to increasing the number or function of the adrenergic receptors might also have a role in short-term therapy. Furthermore, ongoing and planned clinical trials may provide more than anecdotal support for the use of chronic intravenous inotropic therapy in patients with end-stage disease. Therefore, the future may hold brighter opportunities for mending the broken heart by increasing its ability to contract.

CONCLUSION

Congestive heart failure from systolic LV dysfunction remains a major medical concern. Contractile dysfunction remains the major cause of LV systolic dysfunction, and attempts at improving the contractile function of the heart by oral agents have remained frustrating mainly because of an associated increase in mortality with these agents. Digoxin remains the only oral inotropic agent that is neutral in terms of its effects on patient mortality yet associated with improvement in symptoms and decreased need for diuretics and hospitalizations. On the other hand, the role of oral inotropic agents remains in doubt. It is interesting that the agents associated with the worse outcomes are involved in the generation of cAMP either by stimulating its production (beta agents) or inhibiting its metabolism (PDE inhibitors). Whether other positive

inotropic agents that increase inotropy by other mechanisms will ever be clinically useful, remains to be seen.

The acute use of positive inotropic agents, on the other hand, has a firm place in the management of patients with acute decompensated heart failure and cardiogenic shock. These agents include dopamine, dobutamine, milrinone, and amrinone. The chronic use of these agents remains controversial and may be associated with increased mortality.

The road has been frustrating in the rational development of positive inotropic agents, but the quest for pharmacologic agents that can increase inotropy is attractive and continues with fervor. An improved understanding of the molecular and cellular events that regulate excitation, contraction, and relaxation will allow for further rational development and clinical application of these agents.

ACKNOWLEDGMENTS

The authors thank Tracey Barry and Betsy Cervone for their assistance in the preparation of this manuscript.

SELECTED REFERENCES

Anderson TL. Hemodynamic and clinical benefits with intravenous milrinone in severe chronic heart failure: results of a multicenter study in the United States. *Am Heart J* 1991;121:1956.

Binkley PF, Leier CV. Acute positive inotropic intervention: the catecholamines. *Am Heart J* 1991;121:1866.

Bristow MR, Port JD, Hershberger RE, et al. The β-adrenergic receptor adenylate cyclase complex as a target for therapeutic intervention in heart failure. *Am Heart J* 1989;10:45.

Captopril–Digoxin Multicenter Research Group. Comparative effects of therapy with captopril and digoxin in patients with mild to moderate heart failure. *JAMA* 1988;259:539.

Chaterjee K. Newer oral inotropic agents: phosphodiesterase inhibitors. *Crit Care Med* 1990;18:534.

Chatterjee K, Bendersky R, Parmley WW. Dobutamine in heart failure. *Eur Heart J* 1982;3[Suppl D];107.

Colucci WS, Wright RF, Braunwald E. New positive inotropic agents in the treatment of congestive heart failure. *N Engl J Med* 1986:314:290.

Daly JW. Forskolin, adenylate cyclase, and cell physiology: an overview. *Adv Cyclic Nucleotide Protein Phosphorylation Res* 1984;17:81.

DiBianco R. Acute positive inotropic intervention: the phosphodiesterase inhibitors. *Am Heart J* 1991;121:1871.

Feldman AM. Classification of positive inotropic agents. *J Am Coll Cardiol* 1993;22:1223–1227.

Feldman AM. Inotropic agents and adrenergic agonist as therapy for congestive heart failure. *Curr Opin Cardiol* 1991;6:363.

Feldman AM. Mechanism of increased mortality from Vesnarinone in the Severe Heart Failure Trial (VEST). In: *Program and abstracts of the annual meeting of the American College of Cardiology. March 16, 1997, Anaheim, California* (abst). *JACC* 1997;29(2):710.

Feldman AM, Baughamn KL, Lee WK, et al. Usefulness of OPC-8212, a quinolone derivative for chronic congestive heart failure in patients with ischemic heart disease or idiopathic dilated cardiomyopathy. *Am J Cardiol* 1991;68:1203.

Feldman AM, Bristow MR. The β-adrenergic pathway in the failing human heart: implication for inotropic therapy. *Cardiology* 1990;77[Suppl I]:1.

Feldman AM, Bristow RM, Parmley WW, et al. Effects of vesnarinone on morbidity and mortality in patients with heart failure: Vesnarinone Study Group. *N Engl J Med* 1993;329:149.

Ho KKL, Anderson KM, Kannell WB, Grossman W, Levy D. Survival after onset of congestive heart failure in Framingham study subjects. *Circulation* 1993;88:107–115.

Leier CV. Current status of nondigitalis positive inotropic drugs. *Am J Cardiol* 1992;69:1206.

Leier CV, Webel J, Bush CA. The cardiovascular effects of the continuous infusion of dobutamine in patients with severe cardiac failure. *Circulation* 1977;56:468.

MacGowan GA, Mann DL, Kormos RL, et al. Circulating Il-6 in severe heart failure. *Am J Cardiol* 1997;79:1128.

Miller LW. Outpatient dobutamine for refractory congestive heart failure: advantage, techniques and results. *J Heart Lung Transplant* 1991;10:482.

Morgan JP. Mechanisms of disease: abnormal intracellular modulation of calcium as a major cause of cardiac contractile dysfunction. *N Engl J Med* 1991;325:625.

Mullen JE, Turi ZG, Stme PH, et al, and the MILLIS Study Group. Digoxin therapy and mortality after myocardial infarction. *N Engl J Med* 1984; 314:265.

Packer M, Leier CV. Survival in congestive heart failure during treatment with drugs with positive inotropic actions. *Circulation* 1987;75[Suppl IV]:55.

Pfeffer MA, Braunwald E, Moyé LA, et al. Effect of captopril on mortality and morbidity in patients with left ventricular dysfunction after myocardial infarction: results of the Survival and Ventricular Enlargement Trial. *N Engl J Med* 1992;327:669.

Pickworth KK. Long-term dobutamine therapy for refractory congestive heart failure. *Clin Pharmacokinet* 1992;11:618.

Rahimtoula SH, Tak T. The use of digitalis in heart failure. *Cardiology* 1996;21:781.

Rajfer SI, Goldberg LI. Dopamine in the treatment of heart failure. *Eur Heart J* 1982;3[Suppl D]:103.

Rajteus B, Rossen J, Nemamich J, et al. Sustained hemodynamic improvement during long-term therapy with levodopa in heart failure. *J Am Coll Cardiol* 1987.

Ryan TJ, Bailey KR, McCabe CH, et al. The effects of digitalis in survival in high-risk patients with coronary artery disease: the Coronary Artery Surgery Study (CASS). *Circulation* 1983;67:735.

Simonton C, Chatterjee K, Cody R. Milrinone in congestive heart failure: acute and chronic hemodynamic and clinical evaluation. *J Am Coll Cardiol* 1985;6:453.

Sonnenblick EH, Frishman WH, Lejemtel TH. Dobutamine: a new synthetic cardioactive sympathetic amine. *N Engl J Med* 1979;300:17.

Torre-Amione G, Kapadia S, Lee J, et al. Tumor necrosis factor-alpha and tumor necrosis receptors in the failing human heart. *Circulation* 1995; 92:1487.

Watson DM, Sheng KM, Weston GA. Milrinone: a bridge to heart transplantation. *Anaesthesia* 1991;46:285–287.

Wright RF, Colucci WS, Braunwald E. New positive inotropic agents in the treatment of congestive heart failure. *N Engl J Med* 1986;314:349.

Management of End-Stage Heart Disease, edited
by Eric A. Rose and Lynne Warner Stevenson.
Lippincott–Raven Publishers, Philadelphia ©1998.

CHAPTER 6

Evolution of Heart Failure Treatment: Considering Adrenergic Blocking Agents and Amiodarone

James B. Young

The definitions of heart failure and treatment paradigms have evolved dramatically since the mid-1970s. Before that, therapy for dropsical conditions caused by heart failure evolved slowly. Indeed, movement toward adrenergic blocking agents and amiodarone therapy is a recent phenomenon, despite both agents being available for decades. In 1812 (the year Beethoven wrote his 7th and 8th symphonies, and the United States declared war on Great Britain), Corvisart, in his *Essay on the Organic Diseases and Lesions of the Heart and Great Vessels*, suggested purges, bleeding, leeches, squill (a cardiac glycoside), physical removal of ascites and pleural effusions, puncture of edematous legs, and nitrated drinks for dropsy. The mid-19th century, however, saw more aggressive use of diuretics, although the agents were weak and primitive (primarily mercurial preparations such as calomel or potassium bitartrate). Southey tubes inserted into leg lymphatics were introduced in 1877, with bromides given for sedation and diuretics, including theophylline, theobromine, and urea salts, prescribed. It was not, however, until the 1920s and 1930s that mercurial diuretics began to be used with increasing frequency, usually in conjunction with digitalis preparations. In Arthur Fishberg's 1937 *Heart Disease*, the importance of mercurials, theobromine, theophylline, and urea as diuretics to accompany physical removal of effusions and phlebotomy was emphasized. The carbonic anhydrase inhibitor, acetazolamide (Diamox; Lederle Laboratories, Pearl River, New York), was introduced in 1950 (the year Einstein published his general field theory of relativity), and hexamethonium in 1956 (the year Sabin developed

his polio vaccine). Thiazide diuretics were introduced in 1962, furosemide in 1965, and ethacrynic acid in 1966 (the year DeBakey implanted the first extracorporeal ventricular assist device). Indeed, the first human-to-human cardiac transplantation was performed in 1967, only 2 years after the clinical introduction of furosemide. Despite clinical experience with cardiac glycosides extending back more than two centuries, controversy still exists. The era of the 1970s can be characterized by use of vasodilators for patients with heart failure, and in his 1978 textbook, *The Heart*, J. Willis Hurst recommended decreasing physical and emotional stress, instituting a low-salt diet, and administration of digitalis, diuretics (including thiazide, furosemide, ethacrynic acid, spironolactone, and mercurials) and vasodilators (including nitroprusside, isosorbide dinitrate, and hydralazine) in certain heart failure states. Captopril was introduced in 1980 and enalapril in 1984. The decade of the 1980s can be defined as the era of angiotensin-converting enzyme (ACE) inhibitors, with this treatment closely linked to the "vasodilator in heart failure" strategy introduced a decade earlier. Obviously, early paradigm shifts from diuretic and inotropic agents were counterintuitive in many senses, just as beta blockers would be decades later. Patients with substantive heart failure have relative hypotension, and further blood pressure reduction or interdiction of inotropic drive was disconcerting.

The 1990s have been marked by continued treatment paradigm evolution, with better, but still inadequate, clarification of the role of adrenergic blocking agents and amiodarone in heart failure. Driving all of these paradigm shifts has been greater insight into the pathophysiology of heart failure. Indeed, in the 1970s, focus on hemodynamic elements of heart failure led to use of vasodilating

Kaufman Center for Heart Failure, Cleveland Clinic Foundation, Cleveland, Ohio 44195 compounds that could reduce preload and afterload. In turn, stroke volume would increase while ventricular filling pressures decreased, thereby effecting reduced wall stress, decreased myocardial oxygen demand, and improved mechanical efficiency of the heart.

Subsequently, hemodynamically active drugs that also countermanded the neurohormonal perturbation commonly observed in heart failure began to be used. Blocking essential components of the renin–angiotensin–aldosterone system that were abnormally upregulated proved extremely effective in diminishing heart failure morbidity and mortality. This experience subsequently led to the somewhat counterintuitive concept of blocking beta-adrenergic receptors to effect improvement in patients with heart failure. First given to heart failure patients in the 1970s, beta blockers were accompanied by two decades of drug package inserts cautioning against their use in such individuals. The 1990s, however, has emerged as an era clarifying nuances of this strategy. Indeed, as we enter the 21st century, heart failure treatment paradigms continue to shift, with new emphasis on interruption of alpha- and beta-adrenergic cascades believed important in the pathophysiology of heart failure, as well as renin–angiotensin–aldosterone activity and inflammatory components of the syndrome. Even more complete blockade of the renin–angiotensin–aldosterone pathway has been attempted with angiotensin II receptor antagonists coupled to ACE inhibitors and beta-adrenergic receptor blocking drugs.

Understanding the role of the alpha- and beta-adrenergic systems in heart failure is essential to define the appropriate role of adrenergic blocking drugs, whether it be in patients with mild, moderate, or severely symptomatic heart failure. Teleologically, adrenergic receptors mediate critically important responses after acute systemic injury (usually traumatic) that can precipitate intravascular volume loss and organ hypoperfusion. The receptor-mediated tachycardia, positive inotropism, and vasoconstriction occur in an attempt to maintain reasonable systemic organ perfusion by increasing blood pressure. On the other hand, chronic adrenergic stimulation has adverse effects, such as increasing myocardial workload and wall stress, with decreased coronary perfusion and arrhythmia. Furthermore, excessive activation of these receptors can cause myocyte necrosis or induce myocardial hypertrophy. Table 1 summarizes compensation versus adverse effects of adrenergic receptor stimulation in patients with heart failure.

It is reasonable to couple consideration of amiodarone therapeutics in heart failure to use of adrenergic blocking drugs. Like most of the alpha- and beta-adrenergic blockers, amiodarone has been available for quite some time. Similar to some beta blockers, amiodarone is also a vasodilating, antianginal, and antiarrhythmic agent. The prime rationale for amiodarone in heart failure, however, appears to have been the observation that atrial and ven-

TABLE 1. *"Compensatory" versus "adverse" effects of adrenergic receptor stimulation in heart failure patients*

Compensation benefits	Adverse effects
Increased heart rate	Increased preload/afterload
Positive inotropic action	Increased cardiac work
Vasoconstriction	Decreased coronary perfusion
Sodium/H$_2$O retention	Myocyte necrosis
Blood pressure increase	Congestive states
	Arrhythmias
	Induces myocardial hypertrophy

tricular arrhythmias were adverse components of the syndrome in many patients.

Malignant ventricular arrhythmias are frequently observed in heart failure cohorts. It was the link between heart failure, malignant ventricular arrhythmias, and sudden cardiac death that prompted exploration of a variety of pharmacotherapeutic and mechanical intervention techniques (implantable antiarrhythmia devices) to attenuate mortality thought due to rhythm disturbances. Amiodarone has been hypothesized to provide unique protection against high morbidity and mortality in patients with heart failure. We therefore will consider the role of adrenergic blocking compounds and amiodarone in heart failure, particularly in patients with advanced syndromes, in detail.

ALPHA-ADRENERGIC RECEPTORS IN HEART FAILURE

Ahlquist originally demonstrated two major classes of adrenergic receptors. Both alpha and beta receptor families were found to be present in the human heart. Subclassification of these receptors has been accomplished, and alpha$_1$, alpha$_2$, alpha$_3$, and three subtypes of beta-adrenergic receptors are now delineated. Each pathway elicits a variety of biochemical and physiologic activities that are either antagonistic or additive to the activity of other receptors.

Alpha-Adrenergic Receptor Physiology

Although there are several categories of alpha-adrenergic receptors, only alpha$_1$ receptors demonstrate significant myocardial density. Receptors of the alpha$_1$ subclass are coupled to the guanine-nucleotide regulatory proteins (G-proteins). Stimulation of the alpha$_1$-adrenergic receptor causes activation of phospholipase C, which then promotes the breakdown of phosphoinositol biphosphate into inositol triphosphate and diacylglycerol, which in turn releases calcium from intracellular stores. It is the change in intracellular cytoplasmic calcium concentration that modulates calcium-sensitive regulatory proteins such as protein kinase. This results in activation or suppression of various nuclear transcription factors, enzymes, and cell surface receptors, including the beta-adrenergic receptors. Myocardial alpha$_1$-adrenergic receptor stimulation is also related to phospholipase regulation, as well as to activation of calcium and inhibition of select potassium transmembrane channels. Alpha$_1$-adrenergic stimulation also appears to affect the sodium–calcium exchange pumps. Stimulated alpha$_1$-adrenergic receptor pathways are thus critical modulators of heart rate, contractility, wall tension, and systolic, diastolic, and peripheral vascular compliance. Of importance is the fact that alpha$_1$-adrenergic receptors appear to be central to induction of cardiac hypertrophy. Although the relative abundance of alpha$_1$-adrenergic receptor subtypes is usually lower in human myocardium than in other species, the density of alpha$_1$ receptors increases modestly in settings of heart failure. Alpha$_1$ receptor stimulation likely increases cardiac dysrhythmia, and the presence of ischemia and hypoxia has been demonstrated acutely to upregulate alpha$_1$-adrenergic receptor density.

Use of Alpha-Adrenergic Blocking Agents in Heart Failure

Based on the efficacy of parenterally infused vasodilators in acute and chronic heart failure, prazosin, a peripheral alpha-adrenergic antagonist useful in treating hypertension, was suggested as an effective oral drug treatment for heart failure. This agent caused impedance reduction, with subsequent augmentation of cardiac output, and lowered the left ventricular preload in a fashion similar to combined therapy with hydralazine and isosorbide dinitrate. Miller et al. in 1977 studied a small number of patients with ischemic cardiomyopathy and severe left ventricular dysfunction, demonstrating that 1 hour after prazosin administration, mean arterial blood pressure declined, with concomitant left ventricular filling pressure reduction and cardiac index increase. This observation led to prazosin being one of the therapeutic options studied in the first Vasodilator Heart Failure Trial (V-HeFT-I). V-HeFT compared the effects of placebo versus prazosin, or the combination of hydralazine and isosorbide dinitrate, on survival of men with symptomatic congestive heart failure. Whereas the combination of hydralazine and isosorbide dinitrate seemingly improved survival in this study, prazosin was no better than placebo. Relevant to this, Colucci et al. noted the chronic administration of prazosin in heart failure actually increased plasma norepinephrine, a finding thought counterproductive in patients with heart failure. Furthermore, tachyphylaxis may have been a problem during chronic prazosin therapy. As discussed later, drugs combining alpha- and beta-adrenergic blockade appear to exert antiadrenergic effects that are more complete and beneficial. Nonetheless, the use of isolated alpha$_1$-adrenergic blocking drugs alone in heart failure has in general fallen out of favor. Today, it appears that the primary role for peripheral and centrally acting alpha$_1$ blocking drugs is in the treatment of hypertension or high-normal blood pressure in patients with heart failure receiving, at the least, ACE inhibitors. These drugs may be preferable to calcium channel antagonists when treating hypertension in a setting of left ventricular dysfunction or clinically manifest congestive heart failure (CHF). Table 2 lists the peripheral and centrally active alpha-adrenergic blocking agents that can be used, and compares them with two select direct-acting vasodilators. In patients with advanced heart failure, every effort should be made to achieve an optimal systemic vascular resistance. The lower the pressure, in general the better, as long as orthostatic symptoms are not significant and reasonable renal function is present. Alpha blockers can sometimes be helpful in these difficult situations when added to ACE inhibitors.

TABLE 2. *Direct vasodilators and alpha-adrenergic blockers useful to treat hypertension or high-normal blood pressure in patients with heart failure*

Drug	Initial dose (mg)	Maximum dose (mg)	Major adverse reactions
Direct vasodiators			
Hydralazine	10 mg t.i.d.	75 mg t.i.d.	Headache, nausea, dizziness, tachycardia, lupus-like syndrome
Minoxidil	2.5 mg q.d.	80 mg q.d.	Fluid retention, hair growth, thrombocytopenia, leukopenia
Alpha-adrenergic blockers			
Doxazosin	1 mg q.d.	16 mg q.d.	Postural hypotension, dizziness, syncope, headache, polyarthritis
Terazosin	1 mg q.d.	20 mg q.d.	
Prazosin	1 mg t.i.d.	10 mg t.i.d.	
Centrally acting alpha blockers			
Clonidine tablets	0.1 mg b.i.d.	0.6 mg b.i.d.	Sedation, dry mouth, blurry vision, headache, bradycardia
Clonidine patch	0.1 mg weekly	0.3 mg weekly	Same as clonidine; contact dermatitis
Guanabenz acetate	4 mg b.i.d.	64 mg b.i.d.	Similar to clonidine
Guanfacine hydrochloride	1 mg q.d.	3 mg q.d.	Similar to clonidine

q.d., once a day; b.i.d., twice a day; t.i.d., three times a day.

BETA-ADRENERGIC RECEPTORS IN HEART FAILURE

Beta-Adrenergic Receptor Physiology

Although three subtypes of beta-adrenergic receptors have been described, beta$_3$ activity appears significant only in metabolism and diabetes. Beta-adrenergic receptors produce their effects by interacting with the stimulatory G$_s$-protein. Subsequent stimulation of adenyl cyclase by G$_s$-protein converts adenosine triphosphate to cyclic adenosine monophosphate, which then binds to protein kinase, which mediates phosphorylation at multiple targets. Important activities include stimulation of L-type calcium channels, alpha- and beta-adrenergic cell surface receptors, muscarinic receptors, nuclear transcription factors, and regulatory proteins that are coupled to myocyte contractile elements. Also important is that beta-adrenergic receptor stimulation appears to induce mitogen-activated protein kinase and therefore may be mitogenetic.

Although both beta$_1$- and beta$_2$-adrenergic receptor signaling pathways are linked to G$_s$-protein and adenyl cyclase effects, the receptor subtype coupling strengths are different. In humans, the myocardial beta$_2$-adrenergic receptor is 5 to 15 times more efficiently coupled to production of cyclic adenosine monophosphate. However, the relationship between beta-adrenergic receptor density and inotropic effect is more direct. Normally, beta-adrenergic receptor populations are mixed, with 70% to 80% of surface receptors being the beta$_1$ subtype and the remainder beta$_2$ in characteristics. Bristow et al. have demonstrated that inotropic response of ventricular myocytes from patients with heart failure is blunted during *in vitro* isoproterenol administration compared with the response noted in healthy myocardial tissue. Importantly, similar findings in the clinical laboratory suggest that contractility and tachycardia mediated by adrenergic stimulation are impaired in patients with heart failure. This effect may be due to selective downregulation of beta$_1$-adrenergic receptor subtypes. Indeed, patients with more severe clinical heart failure appear to have greater beta$_1$-adrenergic receptor downregulation. Beta$_2$-adrenergic receptor subtypes are not significantly reduced in density in failing human hearts compared with normal ones. This may reflect the fact that norepinephrine is 10 to 60 times more selective for the beta$_1$- than beta$_2$-adrenergic receptor, or that the beta$_1$-adrenergic receptor is more commonly localized near the sympathetic cleft of the neuron, such that the beta$_1$ receptor is seemingly exposed to greater norepinephrine concentrations over longer periods of time. This downregulation of beta$_1$-adrenergic receptors alters the beta$_1$ and beta$_2$ subtype population such that beta$_2$ receptors increase to approximately 40% of the total beta-adrenergic receptor density. Downregulation of beta-adrenergic receptors does not appear to depend on the etiology of heart failure, with similar findings noted in both ischemic heart failure and idiopathic dilated cardiomyopathy.

In addition to the diminution in beta$_1$-adrenergic receptor density in patients with heart failure, this receptor appears to be inappropriately uncoupled from its signal transduction pathway (as is the beta$_2$-adrenergic receptor). This uncoupling has been associated with phosphorylation of the receptors by phosphokinase systems, referred to as beta-adrenergic receptor kinases. The beta-adrenergic receptor kinase protein appears to be upregulated in the failing ventricle. The implication of relative alterations in beta$_1$- and beta$_2$-adrenergic receptor density and G-protein uncoupling in patients with heart failure relates to the potential for differential beta-adrenergic blocking effects in these patients when various agents are used. Nonselective beta-blocking agents may be better tolerated and effect more positive outcomes in patients with heart failure.

Use of Beta-Adrenergic Blocking Agents in Heart Failure

In general, beta-adrenergic blocking drugs carry regulatory labeling cautioning against their use in heart failure patients. For example, the drug package insert for propranolol, the prototypic beta-adrenergic blocking drug, states that the compound is "contraindicated in cardiogenic shock, sinus bradycardia and greater than first degree block, bronchial asthma and congestive heart failure." Warnings state that patients with congestive heart failure may have worsened symptoms and syndromes when beta blockers are administered. Their use should be avoided in overt congestive heart failure, according to these documents. Similar warnings are found for the other beta-adrenergic blocking compounds used to treat hypertension, angina pectoris, or cardiac arrhythmias. This should be counterposed, however, with clinical observations that beta-adrenergic blocking drugs rather dramatically ameliorate heart failure associated with thyrotoxicosis and tachycardia-induced cardiomyopathy. Indeed, some of the earliest experiences with beta-adrenergic blocking drugs in heart failure were in patients with thyrotoxicosis.

Table 3 summarizes many of the reasons beta-adrenergic blocking drugs might be effective in patients with heart failure. As the foregoing discussion suggests, effects of these agents on prejunctional beta receptor activity with reduction in norepinephrine release might alter one of the primary pathophysiologic events noted in the failing myocardium, downregulation of beta receptor density and activity. Global effects of beta-adrenergic blocking drugs in the heart failure milieu are likely similar to those noted in hypertensive patients (Table 4). There is, with some agents, a reduction in peripheral vascular resistance, reduction in venomotor tone, reduction in plasma volume, resetting of baroreceptor levels, and attenuation of the hypertensive catecholamine response during exercise and stress. Furthermore, renin secretion is inhibited by beta-adrenergic blockade. There is also a reduction in heart rate and restoration of heart rate vari-

TABLE 3. *Reasons beta blockers might be effective in patients with heart failure: potential benefits*

- Effects on prejunctional beta receptors with reduction in norepinephrine release
- Reduction in peripheral vascular resistance
- Reduction in venomotor tone
- Reduction in plasma volume
- Resetting of baroreceptor levels
- Attenuation of the pressure response to catecholamines with exercise and stress
- Inhibition of renin
- Reduction in heart rate
- Restoration of heart rate variability
- Attenuation of potentially malignant ventricular arrhythmias
- Control of atrial arrhythmias
- Reduction of ventricular wall stress
- Amelioration of ischemia

ability. Beta-adrenergic blocking drugs can attenuate potentially malignant ventricular arrhythmias and control problematic atrial rhythm disorders. Also, the combined effects of beta-adrenergic blocking agents reduce ventricular wall stress and ameliorate myocardial ischemia.

Although reports of experiences with beta-adrenergic blocking drugs in heart failure can be found extending back to 1969 and the early 1970s, it was the report by Waagstein et al. in 1975 that first generated wide interest in the potential benefits of beta-adrenergic blockers in heart failure. It should be remembered that this was an era dominated by digoxin and diuretic therapy, and great emphasis was placed on the development of inotropic compounds. As alluded to previously, vasodilator therapy was controversial, and beta-adrenergic drug prescription in this population anathema. Waagstein et al. reported outcome after administration of beta-blocking agents to seven patients with advanced congestive cardiomyopathy who had a relative resting tachycardia (mean heart rate of 98 beats/minute). The patients were on beta blockers for 2 to 12 months (an average of a little more than 5 months), with one patient given alprenolol 50 mg twice daily and the remainder given practolol 50 to 400 mg twice daily. Viral cardiomyopathy was thought to be the etiologic

problem in six of the seven patients. The beta blocker was added to regimens of diuretics and digitalis. Observations in this case series suggested clinical improvement, with treatment resulting in an increase in patient physical activity and reduction in heart size. Noninvasive studies, including phonocardiograms, carotid pulse curves, apex cardiograms, and M-mode echocardiograms, suggested ventricular function improved in all cases. Although uncontrolled and anecdotal, these observations suggested that beta-adrenergic blocking drugs could improve cardiac function in some patients with congestive cardiomyopathy. From a clinical standpoint, this report led to more intense study of the role of catecholamine activity in the pathophysiology of heart failure. Still, this study needed to be juxtaposed to clinical experiences that led to the cautionary drug package insert warnings about using first-generation beta-adrenergic blocking drugs in patients with heart failure. In retrospect, clinical deterioration of patients with heart failure given beta blockers likely occurred because relatively large doses of the drugs were given rapidly. Clearly, clinical status can be acutely worsened with beta blockers, even when these are used in the light of contemporary insight. Still, early observations in patients with heart failure were encouraging, as was the growing experience with beta-adrenergic blocking agents in hypertension and acute myocardial infarction.

In 1979, Swedberg et al. suggested that, in addition to symptomatic improvement, survival might be beneficially affected with beta blockers in heart failure. This initial study was small, with 24 patients having congestive cardiomyopathy compared with 13 control subjects with similar clinical findings and myocardial function selected retrospectively. All patients were receiving diuretics, and beta blockers were then added. The survival rate in patients receiving beta-blocker therapy was 83% at 1 year, compared with 46% in the control group, and 52% at 3 years compared with 10% in the control group. Although interesting, this was a small clinical trial with potential bias toward patients who tolerated the drug.

Swedberg et al. subsequently reported on many of the physiologic parameters tracked during follow-up of patients with cardiomyopathy treated with beta-blocking

TABLE 4. *Pharmacodynamic properties of beta blockers used in randomized heart failure trials*

Agent	Beta₁ selective[a]	Alpha₁ antagonist	Partial agonist activity	Membrane stabilizing activity	Peripheral vascular resistance	Plasma renin activity	Renal blood flow	Glomerular filtration rate	Resting heart rate	Myocardial contractility	Blood pressure
Propranolol	0	0	0	++	↑	↓	↓	↓	↓	↓	↓
Acebutolol	+	0	+	+	↓→	↓→	↓→	↓→	↓→	↓	↓
Bisoprolol	++	0	0	0	↓→	↓→	↓→	↓→	↓	↓	↓
Bucindolol	0	0	+	0	↓	↓→	↓→	→	↓→	↓→	↓
Carvedilol	0	+	0	++	↓	↓→	↓→	→	↓→	↓→	↓
Labetalol	0	+	+	0	↓	↓→	↓→	→	↓→	↓→	↓
Metoprolol	++	0	0	0	↓→	↓→	↓→	↓→	↓	↓	↓
Nebivolol	+	0	0	−	−	−	−	↓	↓	↓	↓

0, no effect; +, modest effect; ++, strong effect; ↑, increase; ↓, decrease; →, no change; −, data not available.
[a]Selectivity seen only with low therapeutic concentration.

drugs for 6 to 62 months. Echocardiographic studies suggested an improvement in both systolic and diastolic left ventricular performance. Indeed, the ejection fraction in this cohort of 28 patients increased from 30% to 42%, with the amplitude of S3 gallop dampened and ventricular rapid filling waves attenuated. Functional New York Heart Association (NYHA) classification improved in 15 patients, remained unchanged in 12, and deteriorated in 1. Ten of the 28 patients died (mostly of sudden cardiac death syndrome) during follow-up. Swedberg et al. also reported on the adverse effects of beta-blocker withdrawal in 15 patients with dilated cardiomyopathy and congestive heart failure who initially improved with therapy. In 6 of the 15 patients, there was a pronounced deterioration of their clinical condition, and in all of the remaining patients there was a significant decrease in ejection fraction. These adverse effects were reversed shortly after restarting beta-blocker therapy.

Coupled to these enticing observations is the now extensive experience with beta-adrenergic blocking drugs used chronically after acute myocardial infarction. It has been over three decades since Snow originally reported his observations regarding the effects of propranolol after acute infarction. Although several early, nonrandomized trials were subsequently performed, none of them demonstrated a significant reduction in mortality. However, large-scale, multicenter, randomized, placebo-controlled trials were mounted in the late 1970s. The routine institution of beta-blocker therapy in the first week after myocardial infarction with long-term continuation of therapy resulted in significant reductions in mortality with timolol, propranolol, and metoprolol. The consistency of mortality reduction after myocardial infarction with beta-blocker therapy has been remarkable. Beta-adrenergic receptor blocking drugs with significant positive intrinsic sympathomimetic actions have not, in general, been associated with significant benefit, and $beta_1$ selectivity may have some importance. Most of these trials were performed in the prethrombolytic era, but in a more contemporary light, beta blockers have proved, over time, their ability to reduce mortality and morbidity substantially in patients with hypertension. Also, routine parenteral administration of atenolol in patients who have or who are at risk for coronary artery disease and must undergo noncardiac surgery was associated with reduction in both acute hospital mortality and incidence of cardiovascular complications and, remarkably, affected these end-points for up to 2 years compared with a placebo-treated group.

Differential Pharmacodynamic Properties of Beta Blockers Used in Randomized Heart Failure Trials

Table 4 summarized important properties of the different beta-adrenergic blocking drugs evaluated in randomized clinical trials of patients with heart failure. Propranolol is listed first as the prototypic compound. Propranolol is a nonselective agent without any intrinsic sympathomimetic agonist activity and no alpha receptor antagonism. It possesses membrane-stabilizing effects as well, which have an unknown clinical effect. Physiologic actions of acute and then chronic administration of this compound have been studied primarily in hypertensive patients. Propranolol is an effective antihypertensive agent that decreases resting heart rate and myocardial contractility. Plasma renin activity falls, and there is a decrease in renal blood flow and glomerular filtration rate with this first-generation drug. Acebutolol is a $beta_1$-selective agent with partial agonist activity and membrane-stabilizing effects. Primarily because of partial receptor agonism, little impact on resting heart rate, peripheral vascular resistance, plasma renin activity, renal blood flow, or glomerular filtration rate is seen. Myocardial contractility is, however, diminished. Bisoprolol is a more potent $beta_1$-selective agent without alpha receptor activity or partial agonist effects. Blood pressure, resting heart rate, and myocardial contractility are diminished as with propranolol. Bucindolol is a nonselective beta-adrenergic agent with partial agonist effects and vasodilatory properties that decrease peripheral vascular resistance. Renal blood flow is diminished with bucindolol. Carvedilol is a nonselective beta-adrenergic antagonist with $alpha_1$ receptor antagonist activities as well. It also has membrane-stabilizing activity. Carvedilol is a very effective blood pressure-lowering agent because of both beta and alpha receptor antagonist properties. Renal blood flow is either increased or unchanged. Resting heart rate and myocardial contractility decrease or remain unchanged. Labetalol is also a nonselective beta-adrenergic agent with $alpha_1$ receptor antagonist properties. Unlike carvedilol, however, it demonstrates partial agonist activity. Labetalol otherwise resembles carvedilol in its physiologic profile. Metoprolol is a $beta_1$-selective agent similar to bisoprolol in most respects.

It has become convenient to characterize these agents in terms of evolving drug generations. First-generation beta blockers include propranolol and timolol, which are nonselective agents, as Table 4 indicates. Second-generation agents, such as metoprolol and bisoprolol, are $beta_1$-receptor–selective agents without ancillary properties. Third-generation agents such as bucindolol, labetalol, and carvedilol have the ancillary property of vasodilation mediated through $alpha_1$ receptor antagonism. Bucindolol appears to have some partial agonist activity, but likely is a more direct vasodilating agent. Agents possessing vasodilatory properties and little inverse agonism will likely be better tolerated because afterload reduction produced by arteriolar dilation might offset the negative inotropic properties of the beta blockers. Agents with more extensive inverse agonism and no vasodilatory properties will likely be tolerated less well than new agents such as bucindolol and carvedilol.

Controlled Clinical Trials
of Beta-Blocker Therapy in Heart Failure

Although many randomized trials have suggested that beta-blocker therapy improves left ventricular function and reduces hospitalization rates in congestive heart failure, mortality effects are less clear. Most individual trials have been too small to test, in a statistically reliable fashion, the hypothesis that mortality is reduced with beta-blocker therapy. Doughty et al. have performed an elaborate and elegant metaanalysis of all published, randomized, placebo-controlled clinical trials of beta-blocker therapy in heart failure in an attempt to gain insight into this question. Table 5 is modified from their presentation and demonstrates that, with few exceptions, these clinical trials have been small. Importantly, not all beta-adrenergic receptor antagonists have been evaluated in clinical heart failure trials. Still, a spectrum of beta$_1$-selective agents and agents with partial agonism, or alpha$_1$ antagonism, have been studied. The more recent experience with carvedilol comprises an important component of these trials and is discussed separately. The metaanalysis of Doughty et al. included 24 randomized, clinical trials involving 3,141 patients with stable congestive heart failure (CHF) (usually not symptomatic NYHA Class IV). A total of 297 deaths were noted over an average follow-up of 13 months. There was a 31% reduction in the risk of death among patients assigned a beta blocker (95% confidence interval, 0.11–0.46; p = 0.0035). This translates into an absolute reduction in mortality from 9.7% to 7.5%. In this metaanalysis, the effect on mortality of vasodilating beta blockers (principally in patients treated with carvedilol) was not statistically greater than that of second-generation agents, principally metoprolol (44% reduction vs. 18%; p = 0.09). Although it suggests that beta-blocker therapy is likely to reduce mortality in patients with heart failure, many difficulties exist with this metaanalysis. For example, the studies extend from 1981 through 1997, a period of time during which medical therapies evolved greatly with respect to heart failure treatment. Furthermore, a heterogenous group of patients with coronary artery disease and idiopathic dilated cardiomyopathy made up the study population. In addition, several of the trials were cross-over studies and therefore limited by trial design weakness. Only mild to moderate heart failure was studied. Still, the trials were blinded and randomized. Typically, the patients included had stable CHF with a mean NYHA functional class at baseline of 2.5 and mean left ventricular ejection fraction of 24%. The average age of patients was 58 years and most (78%) were men. Only the Cardiac Insufficiency Bisoprolol Study (CIBIS) and the Metoprolol in Dilated Cardiomyopathy (MDC) study included mortality as a significant primary end-point identified *a priori*. All of the trials added beta-blocker therapy onto a baseline of, in general, diuretics and ACE

inhibitors or digoxin. Indeed, because more patients were studied between 1990 and 1996, 83% of the patients were receiving ACE inhibitors. Carvedilol was the most frequent agent (53% of patients) in this metaanalysis, with, overall, beta blockers with vasodilating properties (i.e., carvedilol, bucindolol, nebivolol, and labetalol) given to 61% of patients assigned beta-blocker therapy.

The first reported, reasonably large, multicenter, randomized trial of a beta blocker in heart failure that contained a mortality end-point was the MDC study, the results of which were published in 1993. This trial included only patients with dilated cardiomyopathy and had as the primary end-point death or listing for cardiac transplantation. Although this end-point was reduced by 34% in patients receiving metoprolol (p < 0.05), no difference was noted in death rates between the two groups. The trial was criticized because of the nebulousness of "need for cardiac transplantation" as a primary end-point. CIBIS, also a larger study, was designed to assess the beta$_1$-selective receptor antagonist bisoprolol versus placebo when added to standard heart failure therapy. The mean ejection fraction was 25%, with 95% of the patients NYHA symptomatic Class III and 5% Class IV. Patients with ischemic heart disease made up 55% of the study cohort, and 83% of the population was male. There was a 20% risk reduction for total mortality with bisoprolol at 2 years' follow-up, which is not statistically significant. Bisoprolol did significantly improve functional status, fewer patients on bisoprolol required hospitalization for cardiac decompensation (90 events on placebo vs. 61 on bisoprolol; p < 0.01), and more patients on bisoprolol improved at least one NYHA functional class level (p = 0.04).

Carvedilol in Patients with Congestive Heart Failure

The newest beta blocker to gain regulatory approbation for treatment of hypertension is carvedilol. It was also the first to receive approval for heart failure treatment as well. Because this later aspect of approval was controversial, it is important to consider the database for this agent in patients with heart failure. As suggested by Table 4, carvedilol may be more advantageous than pure beta-adrenergic receptor blockers in the treatment of CHF because of its added alpha$_1$-adrenergic blocking activity. Carvedilol is best characterized as a nonselective agent. In hypertensive patients, carvedilol was demonstrated effectively to lower blood pressure as well as block some of the commonly associated events vasodilators can precipitate, including increased heart rate. Unlike pure beta-adrenergic blockers, carvedilol acutely reduces blood pressure and peripheral vascular resistance after a single dose.

Uncontrolled studies of the use of carvedilol in patients with heart failure were initiated in 1988, with

TABLE 5. *Randomized trials of beta-blocker therapy in heart failure patients*

Trial	Year	N	CAD (%)	Baseline ejection fraction	Agent	Follow-up (mo)	End-points	Mortality (%) B-block	Mortality (%) Cont	Change in death rate	VAR
Ikram and Fitzpatrick[a]	1981	17	0	47±13%	Acebutolol	1	LV function Exercise	0	11	−0.47	0.2
Currie et al.[a]	1984	10	40		Metoprolol	1	LV function Symptoms Exercise	0	0	0	0
Anderson et al.	1985	50	0	28±11%	Metoprolol	19	Mortality	20	24	−0.5	2.1
Engelmeirer et al.[a]	1985	25	0	13±6%	Metoprolol	12	LV function Exercise	22	13	0.56	0.8
Sano et al.	1989	22	0	24±3%	Metoprolol	12	LV function	0	14	−0.73	0.4
Leung et al. [a]	1990	12	0	21±8%	Labetalol	2	LV function Symptoms Exercise	0	0	0	0
Pollock et al.	1990	20	37	19±7%	Bucindolol	3	Exercise Symptoms	0	0	0	0
Gilbert et al.[b]	1990	23	0	26±7%	Bucindolol	3	LV function Symptoms Exercise	0	0	0	0
Woodley et al.[b]	1991	50	54	23±6%	Bucindolol	3	LV function Symptoms Exercise	0	0	0	0
Paolisso et al.[b]	1992	10	0		Metoprolol	3	LV function Exercise	0	0	0	0
Waagstein et al. (MDC)	1993	383	0	14±3%	Metoprolol	18	Mortality	12	11	0.71	9.7
Wisenbaugh et al.	1993	29	8	24±7%	Nebivolol	3	LV function	7	0	0.48	0.2
Fisher et al.	1994	50	100	22±6%	Metoprolol	6	LV function Symptoms Exercise Worse disease	4	8	−0.05	0.7
Bristow et al.	1994	139	29	24±7%	Bucindolol	3	Dose titration	4	6	0.53	1.1
Metra et al.	1994	40	0	20±7%	Carvedilol	6	LV function Symptoms Exercise	0	0	0	0
CIBIS	1994	641	55	25±9%	Bisoprolol	23	Mortality	17	21	−6.91	24.4
Olsen et al.	1995	60	28	20±6%	Carvedilol	4	LV function Symptoms Exercise	8	0	0.4	0.2
Krum et al.	1995	49	27	17±7%	Carvedilol	3.5	LV function Symptoms Exercise	9	13	−0.37	1.0
Packer et al. (U.S. Carvedilol) "Dose ranging" (MOCHA) n = 345 "Moderate CHF" (PRECISE) n = 278 "Severe CHF" n = 105 "Mild CHF" n = 366	1996[a,b]	1094	48	23 + 7%	Carvedilol	3.4–6.5	LV function Symptoms Exercise QOL	3	8	−2.44	1.6
AUS–NZ	1997	415	100	26±9%	Carvedilol	20	LV function Symptoms Exercise	10	13	−2.94	10.2
Overview		3,141	46	23±10%		13		7.6%	11.9%	−22.94	61.9

CAD, coronary artery disease; MDC, Metoprolol in Dilated Cardiomyopathy; CIBIS, Cardiac Insufficiency Bisoprolol Study; AUS-NZ, Australia–New Zealand Heart Failure Research Collaborative Group; MOCHA, Multicenter Oral Carvedilol Heart Failure Assessment; PRECISE, Prospective Randomized Evaluation of Carvedilol on Symptoms and Exercise; CHF, congestive heart failure; LV, left ventricular; QOL, quality of life.

[a] Cross-over trial.

[b] Twenty-three common patients (included only once in totals).

Modified from Doughty RN, Rodgers A, Sharpe N, Macmahon S. Effects of beta-blocker therapy on mortality in patients with heart failure: a systematic overview of randomized controlled trials. *Eur Heart J* 1997;18:560–565.

low doses of the drug (usually 6.25–25 mg twice daily) used over a 4- to 6-week observation period in patients with mild to moderate (NYHA Class II–III) caused, primarily, by ischemic heart disease. The drug was reasonably well tolerated (approximately 75% of patients were successfully up-titrated) and improvements were noted in exercise tolerance time, resting ejection fraction, and hemodynamics (Table 6). The first randomized, placebo-controlled trials were reported in 1995. These were studies of between 40 and 60 patients followed for only 3 to 4 months. End-points included left ventricular ejection fraction, exercise tolerance, NYHA functional classification, and patient global self-assessments. Mortality and hospitalization rates were not evaluated (see Table 6). Remarkably, there was a consistent increase in ejection fraction in these trials, with all of them demonstrating substantive and significant improvement (ejection fraction rising from 21% to 32%, 20% to 30%, and 17% to 24%, respectively, in each of these three trials). With the exception of Olsen and colleagues' study, exercise tolerance was improved, and all three of the trials demonstrated reduction in symptomatic classification and improvement in patient global self-assessments.

Most recently, the United States Carvedilol in Heart Failure experience has been presented. Four distinct studies were mounted, with entry criteria based largely on 6-minute walk test distance. Patients ambulating less than 150 m were included in the severe heart failure trial,

those walking 150 to 425 m in a dose–response or moderate heart failure trial, and those walking 425 to 550 m in a mild heart failure study. The Carvedilol in Mild Heart Failure study randomized 366 patients with mildly symptomatic heart failure due to left ventricular systolic dysfunction (treated in general with ACE inhibitors, digoxin, and loop diuretics) to carvedilol, which was up-titrated from 6.25 mg daily to 25 or 50 mg twice daily over a 6- to 8-week period. Patients were then followed for 1 year. Mean ejection fraction for the group was 23%, and mean 6-minute walk distance was 480 m. Eighty-five percent of the population were NYHA symptomatic Class II, with 15% Class III. Clinical progression of heart failure occurred in 21% of placebo patients and 11% of carvedilol-treated patients, reflecting a 48% ($p = 0.008$) reduction in the primary end-point of heart failure progression (relative risk 0.52; 95% confidence interval, 0.32–0.85). The effect was not influenced by age, sex, race, disease etiology, or baseline ejection fraction. Clinical aspects of heart failure improved, but no change in Minnesota Living with Heart Failure Scale or walking distance was noted. Clinical progression of heart failure was defined as death due to heart failure, heart failure hospitalization, or sustained increase in heart failure medications.

The PRECISE (Prospective Randomized Evaluation of Carvedilol on Symptoms and Exercise) trial was a double-blinded, placebo-controlled, randomized study of

TABLE 6. *Effect of carvedilol in congestive heart failure (placebo-controlled trials)*

Study	Total N	Carvedilol N	Follow-up (mo)	End-point effects			Glob. assess.	Hosp.	Mort. (%)
				LVEF	Exercise	NYHA			
Olsen et al. (1995)	60	36	4	++ (21%→32%)	–	++	++	NA	NA
Metra et al. (1994)	40	20	4	++ (20%→30%)	++	++	++	NA	NA
Krum et al. (1995)	49	33	3	++ (17%→24%)	++	++	++	NA	NA
U.S. Mild CHF (Colucci et al., 1996)	366	232	12	++ (22%→32%)	NA	++	++	++	78% (3.7% placebo) (0.9% carvedilol)
PRECISE (Packer et al., 1996b)	278	133	6	++ (23%→31%)	++	++	++	++	43% (7.6% placebo) (4.0% carvedilol)
Severe CHF (Packer et al. 1996a)	105	70	6	++ (23%→30%)	–	–	++	++	47% (5.7% placebo) (2.9% carvedilol)
MOCHA (Bristow et al., 1996)	346	262	6	++ (23%→34%)	–	–	–	++	73% (15.3% placebo) (4.6% carvedilol)
AUS (1997)	415	208	20	++ (28%→34%)	–	–	–	++	28% (13.9% placebo) (10.1% carvedilol)

LVEF, left ventricular ejection fraction (baseline → post treatment); NYHA, New York Heart Association Symptomatic Class; Glob. assess., patient self-assessment of heart failure symptoms; Hosp., number of hospitalizations; ↓ Mort., mortality reduction; +, positive end-point; –, no effect; N, ...; NA, not assessed; CHF, congestive heart failure.

the effects of carvedilol in patients with more moderate to severe heart failure. Two hundred seventy-eight patients with a 6-minute walking distance between 150 and 450 m and an ejection fraction less than 35% were randomized to carvedilol or placebo. As with the Carvedilol in Mild Heart Failure trial, patients were to be on standard triple therapy. Indeed, 90% of patients were on digoxin, 98% on a loop diuretic, and 96% on an ACE inhibitor. Mean ejection fraction was 22%, mean patient age 60 years, and 73% of the population was female. Mean 6-minute walk distance was 346 m. Thirty-six percent of the population was NYHA functional Class II, 52% functional Class III, and 4% functional Class IV. Compared with placebo, patients receiving carvedilol had a greater frequency of symptomatic improvement and lower risk of clinical deterioration, as evaluated by changes in NYHA class or by a global assessment of heart failure judged either by the patient or clinician. In addition, carvedilol significantly increased ejection fraction and decreased combined morbidity/mortality risk ($p = 0.029$). However, there was little effect noted on the primary end-point of exercise tolerance as judged by submaximal exercise testing and quality-of-life scores. Findings were the same in ischemic and nonischemic patients. Though this patient group was more ill than that studied in the Carvedilol in Mild Heart Failure trial, severely ill and congested patients were not in general included in the PRECISE program. Taken alone, this study suggests that, in addition to carvedilol's favorable effects on clinical aspects of heart failure, survival may be improved. As with the Carvedilol in Mild Heart Failure trial, it is important to emphasize that carvedilol was added to triple heart failure therapy.

The MOCHA (Multicenter Oral Carvedilol Heart Failure Assessment) trial was designed to establish the safety and efficacy of three separate dosing schedules of carvedilol. Carvedilol 6.25, 12.5, or 25 mg was given twice daily, with patients followed for approximately 6 months. Three hundred forty-six patients were randomized after meeting entry criteria that included an ejection fraction less than 35% and a 6-minute walk between 150 and 450 m. Exercise tolerance was the primary end-point. The mean 6-minute walk distance for the trial group was 357 m; 46% of the patient population were NYHA symptomatic Class II, with 52% Class III and 2% Class IV. No carvedilol dose had a detectable impact on submaximal exercise, but dose-related increases in ejection fraction of 5%, 6%, and 8% with low, medium, and high doses, respectively, were noted versus placebo ($p < 0.001$). Crude mortality rates were lower with increasing carvedilol doses (6%, 6.7%, and 1.1%) than placebo (15.5%; $p < 0.001$). For all carvedilol groups, the mortality risk was lowered by 73% when compared to placebo ($p < 0.001$), and the hospitalization rate was 58% versus 64% in the placebo group ($p = 0.01$). Although the primary end-point of exercise tolerance was not affected in

a statistically significant fashion by carvedilol, dose-related improvements in left ventricular function and reductions in mortality and hospitalization rates were observed.

Finally, a combined United States Carvedilol Clinical Trial analysis was performed to assess the effect of carvedilol on mortality. The pooled analysis from four distinct trials (three summarized earlier) randomized 1,094 patients with heart failure of mild to moderate severity to placebo or carvedilol. Mortality in the placebo group was 7.8% versus 3.2% in the carvedilol group (a 65% risk reduction; $p > 0.001$), and carvedilol was associated with a 27% reduction in risk of hospitalization for cardiovascular causes (19.6% vs. 14.1%; $p = 0.036$). The conclusions were that carvedilol reduces risk of death as well as risk of hospitalization for cardiovascular causes in patients with heart failure who are receiving background treatment with digoxin, diuretics, and an ACE inhibitor. There are weaknesses, however, with this program and study design. It has been pointed out that conclusions were based on a total of only 53 deaths occurring during a median follow-up of less than 7 months. Furthermore, the run-in design of the protocol resulted in censoring of events in the treated group during the 2-week period when patients were all receiving carvedilol in an attempt to determine their ability to tolerate the drug. Seven deaths occurred during the run-in period and were not tabulated in the initial mortality statistics for the carvedilol group, although they would have accounted for a significant percentage of deaths overall. Because many patients were withdrawn abruptly from short-term exposure to carvedilol, it could be argued that deaths in the placebo group, particularly those occurring early after carvedilol withdrawal, were in actuality due to withdrawal of this drug rather than placebo administration. Finally, this was a pooled analysis of four distinct clinical trials, none of which was individually empowered to detect a significant mortality benefit independently. Mortality was tabulated as a safety parameter for each individual trial, and then pooled for this analysis. Still, the compendium of data suggests that multiple factors important in the heart failure milieu are benefited during heart failure treatment. When all of these issues are taken together (improvement in left ventricular ejection fraction, reduction in functional symptomatic classification, improvement in patient and physician global assessment of clinical heart failure severity, decrement in hospitalization rates, and decreased mortality), there is a convincing argument that this adrenergic blocking compound is important in patients with heart failure.

Finally, results from the 20-month follow-up analysis of the Australia–New Zealand Heart Failure Collaborative Research Group also demonstrated mortality decrement with carvedilol. In 415 patients randomized to either carvedilol or placebo, ejection fraction rose from 28% to 34%. Mortality decreased 28% (13.9% in the placebo group and 10.1% in the carvedilol group). It appears, then, that the two largest carvedilol treatment programs, the United States Combined Clinical Trials and the Australia–New Zealand Collaborative effort, are consistent with respect to their observations regarding clinical benefit.

Some insight into reasons for the benefits of carvedilol is also available. In a substudy of patients entering the Australia–New Zealand Heart Failure Research Collaborative evaluation, effects of this treatment on left ventricular size and function were determined by using quantitative two-dimensional echocardiography; 123 patients from 10 centers participating in this study were also in the echocardiographic substudy. Evaluations were performed before randomization and then repeated at the 6- and 12-month treatment marks. After 12 months of carvedilol therapy, heart rate was 8 beats per minute lower in the carvedilol group than the placebo group, whereas left ventricular end-diastolic and end-systolic volumes were increased in the placebo group, but reduced in the carvedilol group. At 12 months, the left ventricular end-diastolic volume index was 14 mm/m^2 less in the carvedilol than in the placebo group ($p = 0.0015$), left ventricular end-diastolic volume index was 15.3 mL/m^2 less ($p = 0.0001$), and left ventricular ejection fraction was 5.8% greater ($p = 0.0015$) in the active treatment group. These findings suggest that carvedilol has a beneficial effect on parameters regulating left ventricular remodeling.

The compendium of data regarding carvedilol appears to support its use in symptomatic patients with mild to moderate CHF. Inadequate data are available to support its use in either asymptomatic or severely symptomatic and congested patients. Furthermore, at this time, clinical trial data support this drug being used only as an adjunctive agent in addition to the combination of ACE inhibitors, digoxin, and diuretic.

Initiating Beta-Adrenergic Blocking Agent Therapy in Patients with Heart Failure

Clinical trial experience has given us insight into the manner in which beta-blocker therapy can be used in patients with heart failure. It is difficult at this time to determine whether any given beta blocker is superior to another in terms of survival impact because no direct beta-blocker comparison trials have yet been completed. With respect to left ventricular function, both selective and non-selective agents have proved beneficial. However, as discussed, many theoretical reasons exist to suggest that a nonselective, third-generation beta-adrenergic blocking drug may be advantageous with respect to survival outcome. Third-generation agents, such as carvedilol with its beta- and alpha-adrenergic blocking actions, in theory provide more complete cardiac protection.

Up-titrating patients on beta-blocking agents can be tricky. Indeed, many patients may feel substantively worse during the early weeks of drug titration. Initiation of beta-adrenergic blocker therapy can result in immediately significant negative inotropic and chronotropic effects. Improvement in ventricular function usually occurs only after prolonged therapy. When starting beta-blocker therapy, patients should be clinically stable and on background medications consisting of diuretics, digoxin, and ACE inhibitors. Furthermore, patients should not have recently required hospitalization for decompensated heart failure, be hypotensive, or have volume-overloaded states. Thus, most patients diagnosed with severe or "end-stage" heart failure would not be considered for beta-blocker therapy until clinical status had improved to some stability. Starting doses for metoprolol, labetalol, carvedilol, and bucindolol, the most commonly used beta blockers for heart failure (although bucindolol is not yet clinically available), are quite low (6–12 mg of metoprolol, 6 mg of labetalol, 3.125 mg of carvedilol, and 6 mg of bucindolol). Since the lowest available dose of metoprolol is a 50-mg tablet, low doses are sometimes difficult to achieve. Pharmacists can compound lower doses as necessary, or the pediatric elixir can be used when properly concentrated. An example of one titration scheme well studied is that used for carvedilol. When starting this drug, 3.125 mg is given twice daily for 2 weeks without regard to patient weight or age. Patients should be observed for several hours after the initial dose administration and with each increase in dose strength. An alternative strategy might be to take the first dose at bedtime. If the initial dose is tolerated, subsequent doses can be increased to 6.25 mg twice daily for 2 weeks. Dosing should then be doubled every 2 weeks or so, to the highest level tolerated by the patient. These are, in general, the target doses used in clinical trials (25 or 50 mg twice daily). Efficacy appears to be dose related and titration up to the highest tolerated dose is encouraged. Vasodilator side effects such as orthostatic hypotension or worsening renal function (rising blood urea nitrogen or creatinine) should prompt reconsideration of the global strategy. Beta-blocker dosing intervals might be altered or doses of diuretics or ACE inhibitors reduced. If symptoms are severe, the beta blocker should be discontinued. Mild worsening of heart failure symptoms may be addressed by increasing certain heart failure medications, particularly diuretics. Again, the beta blocker should be discontinued when symptoms are severe. When problematic bradycardia or heart block appears, the dose of the beta blocker should be reduced or the drug stopped. Sometimes it is the combination of digoxin or amiodarone with beta blockers that causes the bradycardia or heart block. Digoxin toxicity should be ruled out and amiodarone use reconsidered. After even severe decompensation has occurred with initiation of beta blockers, reintroduction of these agents might be possible after stabilizing the patient, optimizing volume status, and adjusting concurrent drug doses.

AMIODARONE IN PATIENTS WITH ADVANCED CONGESTIVE HEART FAILURE

Like propranolol, amiodarone has been available for many years, but only relatively recently studied in heart failure. Amiodarone is a benzofuran derivative chosen for evaluation in cardiovascular conditions because of its highly potent coronary vasodilating effects. Initial focus of interest in this drug was as an antianginal agent. Indeed, the first report of amiodarone's antianginal efficacy appeared in 1967, with its antiarrhythmic properties not elucidated until later. Detailed electrophysiologic properties were clarified in 1970 along with the first clinical experiences with its antiarrhythmic properties. Today's use of oral amiodarone as a potent and versatile antiarrhythmic drug springs from several seminal reports that detailed observations regarding control of tachyarrhythmias.

Actions Making Amiodarone Attractive in Heart Failure

Drug properties that were responsible for amiodarone's antianginal action included reduction in heart rate, vasodilation with systemic blood pressure reduction, increased myocardial blood flow, and a partial inhibition of the effects of catecholamines. These activities are distinct from the antiarrhythmic actions of the drug. Still, other chemical compounds having the same antianginal profile do not demonstrate antiarrhythmic properties, as does amiodarone. Importantly, amiodarone has been shown to be a noncompetitive inhibitor of alpha- and beta-adrenergic–mediated vascular activity. These actions are dissimilar to beta-adrenergic receptor blocking drugs. For example, amiodarone does not bind to the catecholamine recognition site of the beta-adrenergic receptor, but rather appears to induce a significant decrease in the number of beta-adrenergic receptors. The noncompetitive beta-adrenergic antagonist properties of amiodarone appear related to inhibition of the coupling of beta receptors with the regulatory units of adenyl cyclase, which can be a result of a decrease in the number of receptors at the myocardial cell surface. Amiodarone also increases energetic myocyte reserves and inhibits myocardial depletion of glycogen induced by ephedrine, theophylline, and dihydrophenol. Collectively, these effects support, from a pharmacodynamic standpoint, the use of amiodarone in patients with angina pectoris, in particular. Intravenous amiodarone causes a dose-dependent decrease in cardiac contractility, but because of the concomitant reduction in systemic vascular resistance induced by vasodilation, cardiac output is usually increased. It is known that cardiac failure is rarely worsened by amiodarone, even when patients with severe cardiomyopathy are being treated.

Table 7 summarizes the principal effects of amiodarone that make it an attractive agent in patients with congestive heart failure.

TABLE 7. *Reasons amiodarone might be effective in patients with heart failure: potential benefits*

- Heart rate reduction
- Arteriolar vasodilation with afterload reduction
- Reduced myocardial oxygen consumption
- Increased myocardial blood flow
- Inhibition of catecholamine effects (noncompetitive inhibitor of various alpha- and beta-adrenergic cardiac phenomena)
- Inhibition of myocardial glycogen depletion
- Control of atrial arrhythmias
- Control of potential malignant ventricular arrhythmias

Prevention of Sudden Cardiac Death in Patients after Myocardial Infarction and in Those with Congestive Heart Failure

It is important to consider the effects of amiodarone on mortality in both acute myocardial infarction survivors and patients with heart failure. There is a direct link between infarction and left ventricular dysfunction. In both patient sets, an increasing prevalence of potentially malignant ventricular arrhythmia is observed as ventricular dysfunction worsens and ejection fractions fall. Furthermore, almost one half of all deaths in patients with significant CHF are sudden cardiac deaths and, hypothetically, represent malignant ventricular arrhythmia that might respond to empiric antiarrhythmic therapy (drug or arrhythmia terminating device). This hypothesis might be looked at skeptically, however, because of data suggesting that the elimination of ventricular arrhythmias alone with pharmaceutical agents does not necessarily translate into mortality reduction. Table 8 summarizes select, controlled, clinical trials of amiodarone after myocardial infarction or as adjunctive heart failure therapy.

In patients who have survived acute myocardial infarction, the combination of ventricular ectopy and diminished left ventricular ejection fraction is a harbinger of high sudden death rates during follow-up. Indeed, as few as ten premature ventricular contractions per hour indicate high risk for sudden cardiac death after myocardial infarction. A number of well designed, mortality endpoint, placebo-controlled clinical trials have investigated potent Type I antiarrhythmic agents. These trials consistently demonstrate that these drugs are more harmful than helpful. Indeed, the inverse relationship between baseline left ventricular ejection fraction and outcome of antiarrhythmic therapy has now become well recognized. Most antiarrhythmic agents demonstrate attenuated efficacy as ejection fraction falls with increased likelihood of inducing proarrhythmia. However, because of the aforementioned amiodarone effects, this agent might be a safer and more effective drug to use in these specific populations. Indeed, some clinical trial evidence (see Table 8) suggests that amiodarone may be effective in reducing the incidence of sudden cardiac death syndrome in survivors of

TABLE 8. *Amiodarone in heart failure/myocardial infarction: controlled clinical trials*

Acronym	Title	Year	Design	N	Amiodarone dose	Mean EF	CAD	Mean age	Follow-up (mo)	Findings
BASIS (Burkart et al.)	Basel Antiarrhythmic Study of Infarct Survival	1990	MI survivors with low 3/4B arrhythmia randomized, to placebo, amiodarone, or individualized antiarrhythmic therapy	312	1,000 mg × 5 d 200 mg q.d.	43±16%	100% Post acute MI	61	12	Amiodarone associated with better survival than individualized or no antiarrhythmic therapy.
GESICA (Doval et al.)	Group Study of Heart Failure Argentina	1994	Placebo-controlled study of amiodarone in moderate to severe CHF assessing mortality as a primary end-point	516	600 mg × 14 d 300 mg q.d.	20±8%	38% Post MI	59	13	Mortality was significantly reduced with amiodarone (42%) compared with placebo (53%). Suggested amiodarone can be used in some CHF patients.
CHF-STAT (Singh et al.)	Congestive Heart Failure Survival Trial of Antiarrhythmic Therapy	1995	Survival study of amiodarone vs. placebo in CHF patients with 10 premature ventricular contractions/hours	674	800 mg × 14 d 400 mg × 50 wk 300 mg q.d.	25±8%	70% Post MI	65	45	Amiodarone overall did not improve survival compared with placebo. Did not support hypothesis that amiodarone was helpful generally in CHF.
CAMIAT (Cairns et al.)	Canadian Myocardial Infarction Amiodarone Trial	1997	Patients 6–45 days postinfarction with no EF entry criteria but EKG ventricular arrhythmia followed for combined end-point of arrhythmic death or resuscitated ventricular fibrillations all-cause mortality and cardiac mortality secondary end-points	1,202	10 mg/kg × 14d 400 mg × 10 wk 800 mg × 24 wk 200 mg q.d.	—	100% Post acute MI	64	24	Primary end-point benefited with amiodarone but toxicity great (42% of treatment group stopped amiodarone by 2 years) and all-cause mortality not reduced.
EMIAT (Julian et al.)	European Myocardial Infarction Amiodarone Trial	1997	Patients 5–21 days postinfarction with EF <40% randomized with mortality as primary end-point	1,486	800 mg × 14 d 400 mg × 14 wk 200 mg q.d.	30%	100% Post acute MI	60	21	Primary end-point, death, not reduced by amiodarone, but combined end-point of arrhythmic death/ resuscitated cardiac arrest reduced slightly. Toxicity of drug significant in this study.

EF, ejection fraction; CAD, coronary artery disease, CHF, congestive heart failure; EKG, electrocardiogram; MI, myocardial infarction.

acute myocardial infarction, particularly when heart failure is present. The observations made in these clinical trials, however, must be explored carefully, because results have not been quite as clear-cut as hoped. Furthermore, amiodarone is a toxic compound associated with difficulties during administration.

In the Basel Antiarrhythmic Study of Infarct Survival (BASIS) (Table 7), 1,220 consecutive survivors of acute myocardial infarction were screened for inclusion to determine the effects of prophylactic antiarrhythmic treatment on postinfarct complex ventricular ectopy. Three hundred twelve patients with Lown Class III or IVB arrhythmia were randomized to one of three groups: treatment with low-dose amiodarone (200 mg/day), treatment with individualized antiarrhythmic therapy, or no *ad hoc* prophylactic antiarrhythmic therapy. End-points were total mortality and arrhythmic events, defined as sudden cardiac death syndrome, sustained ventricular tachycardia, and ventricular fibrillation. This was a small trial, but 30 deaths occurred at the 1-year mark and the probability of survival when given amiodarone was significantly greater than that of control patients (13% in the control group, 10% with patients treated in individualized antiarrhythmic drug therapy, and 5% in patients treated with amiodarone; $p < 0.01$). In these patients, left ventricular dysfunction was not uncommon. The mean ejection fraction for the study cohort was 43%. Although this was a small trial, observations were intriguing. Particularly interesting was that the dose of amiodarone used was small compared with other trials. Still, because of the serious toxicity of amiodarone, risk–benefit ratios must be carefully examined, and that issue prompted larger clinical trials in both heart failure and postmyocardial infarction populations.

The GESICA (Grupo Estudio de la Sobrevida Insuficiencia Cardiaca en Argentina) study was a randomized trial of low-dose amiodarone in severe CHF. In this trial, 516 patients with CHF and no substantive symptomatic ventricular arrhythmias (other than nonsustained ventricular tachycardia) were randomized to either 300 mg/day of amiodarone or placebo, in addition to their optimized standard therapeutics. Total mortality at the 24-month point was the primary end-point, with subgroup mortality, sudden death, death due to progressive heart failure, and hospital admission due to CHF secondary end-points. Drug dosing began with 600 mg of amiodarone daily for 2 weeks and then 300 mg daily for the duration of the study. Although the trial was randomized, parallel, and placebo controlled, it was only single blinded. There was a 28% risk reduction for the amiodarone group with respect to total mortality ($p = 0.024$). Interestingly, risk reduction was the same for sudden cardiac death (with benefit seen early) as for progressive CHF-related deaths (benefits seen late). The combined end-point of death and hospitalizations for CHF was also significantly reduced in the amiodarone group (risk reduction of 31%; $p = 0.0024$).

In the Congestive Heart Failure Survival Trial of Anti-Arrhythmic Therapy (CHF-STAT), patients with NYHA symptomatic functional Class III or IV CHF and ten or more ventricular premature beats per hour on ambulatory monitoring were randomized to receive amiodarone or placebo in addition to standard heart failure therapies. Six hundred seventy-four patients were randomized to either placebo or amiodarone therapy in a parallel-group, placebo-controlled, double-blinded fashion. Amiodarone was administered as 800 mg daily for 2 weeks, then 400 mg daily for the remaining year, and 300 mg daily subsequently. Sixty-six percent of the population had an ejection fraction less than 34%, with the remainder of the group having ejection fractions ranging between 30% and 40%. Approximately 70% of enrolled patients had ischemic heart disease, with randomization being stratified for presence or absence of this diagnosis and ejection fraction below or above 30%. The primary end-point was total mortality and cardiac sudden death episodes. No significant difference in overall mortality with respect to the primary end-point was demonstrable ($p = 0.6$). At the 2-year point, the sudden cardiac death rate was 15% in the amiodarone group and 19% in the placebo group ($p = 0.43$). Amiodarone was effective in suppressing ventricular arrhythmias and increased the ejection fraction by 42% at the 2-year mark (left ventricular ejection fraction was 35% in the amiodarone group vs. 29% in the placebo group; $p < 0.001$). There was the suggestion that the overall mortality rate was better among patients with nonischemic cardiomyopathy in the amiodarone group (relative risk, 0.56; 95% confidence interval, 0.36–0.87; $p = 0.01$). This should be contrasted to the findings in GESICA, which suggested that patients with ischemic and nonischemic heart failure were equally benefited. Despite a relatively low dose of amiodarone, study medication was stopped because of side effects in 27% of amiodarone-treated patients compared with 23% of the placebo group. Although amiodarone was effective in suppressing ventricular arrhythmia and improving ventricular function, it did not reduce the incidence of sudden death or prolong survival among patients with heart failure in general.

The Canadian Myocardial Infarction Amiodarone Trial (CAMIAT) was a randomized clinical trial of outcome after myocardial infarction in patients with frequent or repetitive premature ventricular beats (Table 7). Although the study did not require heart failure for randomization, 16% of the patient population had pulmonary edema at the time of their myocardial infarction. Patients were required to have had an acute myocardial infarction that was 6 to 45 days old and more than 10 premature ventricular depolarizations per hour or nonsustained ventricular tachycardia on ambulatory monitoring. This was a placebo-controlled, parallel-group, double-blinded, randomized study. Mean patient age was 64 years, and 18% of the population was female. Amiodarone was given as a 10-mg/kg loading dose, twice daily over 2 weeks, then 400 mg daily for 12 weeks. At the 12-week mark, the dose was reduced to 300 mg daily, and at the 8-month mark again reduced to 200 mg daily. The primary endpoints were resuscitated ventricular fibrillation, arrhythmic death, other cardiac death, and noncardiac vascular death. Resuscitated ventricular fibrillation or arrhythmic death occurred in 6% of the placebo group and in 3.3% of the amiodarone group, a risk reduction of 48.5% (95% confidence interval, 0.05–0.72; *p* =.016). Although the findings suggested that amiodarone reduced the risk of ventricular fibrillation or arrhythmic deaths in myocardial infarction survivors with frequent premature ventricular contractions, especially those with CHF, the sample size was not great enough to address definitively the question of all-cause mortality. Conclusions from this study should be tempered by the fact that there are many limitations associated with definitions of arrhythmic death, that total mortality was not reduced in the trial, that the analysis was not based on intention-to-treat principles, and that there were many dropouts.

The European Myocardial Infarction Amiodarone Trial (EMIAT) also studied the effect of amiodarone on mortality in myocardial infarction survivors, but this clinical trial required presence of left ventricular dysfunction for entry. Entry criteria included being 5 to 21 days post acute myocardial infarction and an ejection fraction less than 40%, but no arrhythmia documentation was required for randomization. The primary end-point was all-cause mortality, with secondary end-point being the combination of cardiac mortality and arrhythmic death. The trial was a parallel-group, placebo-controlled, double-blinded study. Amiodarone was given in the dose of 800 mg for 14 days, 400 mg for 14 days, and then 200 mg of the remainder of the study. All-cause mortality and cardiac mortality did not differ between the two groups. A 35% risk reduction in arrhythmic deaths was observed (95% confidence interval, 0.00–0.58%; *p* = 0.05). The most striking observation was a reduction in the combined end-point of arrhythmic death and resuscitated cardiac arrest, with 59 events in the placebo group versus 30 in the amiodarone group (risk reduction of 0.55; *p* = 0.006). Critically evaluated, findings of this study also do not support systematic prophylactic use of amiodarone in all patients with depressed left ventricular function after myocardial infarction. Because this study did not demonstrate substantive proarrhythmia (observations similar to those in the GESICA, CHF-STAT, and CAMIAT studies), and reduction in arrhythmic death was observed, an argument can be made for using amiodarone in patients similar to the ones studied in these trials when antiarrhythmic therapy is indicated for either atrial fibrillation or symptomatic ventricular arrhythmias. This should be weighed against the fact that in CAMIAT, thyroid function abnormalities developed in 3.1% of the amiodarone group (vs. 0.5% in the placebo group), and three patients receiving amiodarone died from pulmonary

fibrosis. As with CAMIAT and CHF-STAT, substantial numbers of patients in the treatment group were withdrawn early from the study drug.

Amiodarone Toxicity and Side Effects

As should be evident from the foregoing discussion, one of the greatest concerns about chronic amiodarone therapy in patients with heart failure is drug toxicity and problematic side effects. Substantial numbers of patients in clinical trials to date have been unable to tolerate the medication. Amiodarone toxicity includes pulmonary fibrosis, thyroid dysfunction, corneal microdeposits, neurologic findings, dermatologic difficulties, and gastrointestinal and hepatic problems. Most adverse effects appear to depend on dose or dose duration, and some improvement ensues with reduced doses. Pulmonary toxicity is the significant exception. There is evidence to suggest that the pneumonitis and subsequent interstitial pulmonary fibrosis developing during amiodarone therapy is an immune-mediated difficulty. The pulmonary fibrosis causes dyspnea, cough, chest pain, and low-grade fever. Rales can frequently be heard, as can pulmonary friction rubs. Leukocytosis and eosinophilia have been reported. Chest radiographs reveal a diffuse interstitial or patchy alveolar infiltrate. It can be challenging to differentiate between amiodarone-induced pulmonary toxicity and worsening CHF.

Thyroid dysfunction is probably the most often noted difficulty with amiodarone. Thyroxine and thyroid-stimulating hormone levels are increased and triiodothyronine levels decreased. In general, clinical hypothyroidism or hyperthyroidism is not seen. However, changes in hormone levels make the diagnosis of physiologically significant thyroid dysfunction difficult. It has been suggested that thyroid-stimulating hormone levels over 26 units indicate hypothyroidism, and thyroxine levels over 2 mg/dL or triiodothyronine over 200 mg/dL can be used for diagnosing hyperthyroidism. Preexisting thyroid disease and older age appear to be risks for amiodarone-induced hypothyroidism. Withdrawing amiodarone usually is effective in normalizing thyroid function.

Corneal microdeposits can be found in virtually everyone on long-term amiodarone therapy. Visual complaints, however, are rare. Neurologic findings include tremor, sleep disturbances, and, sometimes, proximal muscle weakness during periods of high loading dose. Peripheral neuropathy and extrapyramidal tract difficulties can also be observed. Skin photosensitivity is quite common during amiodarone therapy, and can range from lower thresholds for sunburn to substantive erythema and edema of sun-exposed skin. Often, sun-exposed areas acquire a blue-gray pigmentation after prolonged amiodarone therapy. This difficulty may only partially resolve after stopping the drug. Loss of appetite and nausea may also occur during loading-dose administration, with constipation frequent during chronic therapy. Biochemical alterations of hepatic function are also commonly noted during high-dose loading of amiodarone, but these are rarely significant. Still, amiodarone-induced hepatitis has caused death in some patients.

Amiodarone Therapy in Patients with Heart Failure Remains Controversial

Table 8 summarizes reasons amiodarone could be beneficial in heart failure. Still, data do not support routine administration of this drug as part of the basic heart failure treatment program. Although benefit can be seen, toxicity is problematic. It is possible that doses, even the low doses, have been too high. Amiodarone has been given in the heart failure and postmyocardial infarction trials in doses of 200 to 400 mg daily after a significantly higher dose load. Mahmarian et al. demonstrated in a small pilot project that 100-mg and even 50-mg daily doses might achieve desired antiarrhythmic and hemodynamic activity in patients with heart failure. Possibly these lower dosages could effect end-points of mortality reduction and improvement in clinical morbidity without the substantive toxicity associated with the high degree of drug intolerance. Based on the clinical trials reviewed, amiodarone therapy should be reserved for those patients in whom an antiarrhythmic drug is required, rather than prescribed in routine fashion for heart failure. Fortunately, clinical trial observations did not result in the same troubling findings that have been noted in heart failure cohorts treated with Vaughn Williams Class I antiarrhythmics.

SUMMARY

Treatment paradigms for CHF have shifted dramatically over the past several decades. Initially, therapy was based on a diuretic–digoxin combination, subsequently evolving to prescription of vasodilators, which changed to the more specific use of vasodilators that also interdicted neurohumoral perturbation. The broad-spectrum use of adrenergic blocking agents, specifically alpha- and beta-adrenergic blocking drugs, has fluctuated in terms of enthusiasm regarding their use. Initially, alpha-adrenergic blocking agents were used as vasodilators. Inability to sustain long-term benefit with these agents forced reconsideration of them as integral elements of heart failure treatment protocols. Likewise, beta-adrenergic blocking therapy has waxed and waned in terms of enthusiasm, with more recent information supporting their prescription to attenuate heart failure morbidity and mortality. Because of the seeming problem with sudden cardiac death and potentially malignant atrial and ventricular arrhythmias in heart failure, amiodarone is an intriguing option. Amiodarone and beta-adrenergic receptor blocking drugs have a great deal in common, particularly their

ability to interdict adverse adrenergic activity. It appears that alpha$_1$-adrenergic blocking drugs should be used only as adjunctive therapy to assist with lowering blood pressure in situations when ACE inhibitors are performing inadequately with respect to this end-point. Beta-adrenergic drugs, particularly metoprolol and third-generation compounds such as carvedilol, might be considered useful in patients with mild to moderate congestive heart failure who are well stabilized on ACE inhibitors, diuretics, and digoxin. Amiodarone likely should not be prescribed routinely for treatment of heart failure or to survivors of acute myocardial infarction. However, amiodarone may be the best antiarrhythmic option available when such a compound is desired.

SELECTED REFERENCES

Ahlquist R. A study of the adrenotropic receptors. *Am J Physiol* 1948;153: 586–600.

Anderson JL, Lutz JR, Gilbert EM, et al. A randomized trial of low-dose beta-blockade therapy for idiopathic dilated cardiomyopathy. *Am J Cardiol* 1985;55:471–475.

Australia–New Zealand Heart Failure Research Collaborative Group. Effects of carvedilol, a vasodilator-beta-blocker, in patients with congestive heart failure due to ischemic heart disease. *Circulation* 1995; 92:212–218.

Australia–New Zealand Heart Failure Research Collaborative Group. Effects of carvedilol in patients with congestive heart failure due to ischemic heart disease: final results from the Australia–New Zealand Heart Failure Research Collaborative Group Trial. *Lancet* 1997;349: 375–380.

Bristow MR, Gilbert EM, Abraham WT, et al. Carvedilol produces dose-related improvements in left ventricular function and survival in subjects with chronic heart failure (MOCHA). *Circulation* 1996;94:2807–2816.

Bristow MR, O'Connell JB, Gilbert EM, et al., for the Bucindolol Investigators. Dose–response of chronic β-blocker treatment in heart failure from either idiopathic dilated or ischemic cardiomyopathy. *Circulation* 94;89:1632–1642.

Burkart F, Pfisterer M, Kiowski W, Follath F, Burchhardt D. Effect of antiarrhythmic therapy on mortality in survivors of myocardial infarction with asymptomatic complex ventricular arrhythmias: Basel Antiarrhythmic Study of Infarct Survival (BASIS). *J Am Coll Cardiol* 1990; 16:1711–1718.

Cairns JA, Connolly SJ, Roberts R, Gent M, for the Canadian Amiodarone Myocardial Infarction Arrhythmia Trial Investigators. Randomized trial of outcome after myocardial infarction in patients with frequent or repetitive ventricular premature depolarizations: CAMIAT. *Lancet* 1997;349:675–682.

CIBIS Investigators and Committees. A randomized trial of beta-blockade in heart failure: the cardiac insufficiency bisoprolol study (CIBIS). *Circulation* 1994;90:1765–1773.

Cohn JN. Current therapy of the failing heart. *Circulation* 1988;78: 1099–1107.

Cohn JN. The management of chronic heart failure. *N Engl J Med* 1996;335:490–498

Cohn JN, Franciosa JA. Vasodilator therapy of cardiac failure. *N Engl J Med* 1977;297:254–258.

Colucci WS, Packer M, Bristow MR, et al. Carvedilol inhibits clinical progression in patients with mild symptoms of heart failure. *Circulation* 1996;94:2800–2806.

Colucci WS, Williams GH, Braunwald E. Increased plasma norepinephrine levels during prazosin therapy for severe congestive heart failure. *Ann Intern Med* 1980;93:452–453.

Currie PJ, Kelly MJ, McKenzie A, et al. Oral beta-adrenergic blockade with metoprolol in chronic severe dilated cardiomyopathy. *J Am Coll Cardiol* 1984;3:203–209.

Doughty RN, MacMahon S, Sharpe N. Beta-blockers in heart failure: promising or proud? *J Am Coll Cardiol* 1994;23:814–821.

Doughty RN, Rodgers A, Sharpe N, MacMahon S. Effects of a beta-blocker therapy on mortality in patients with heart failure: a systematic overview of randomized controlled trials. *Eur Heart J* 1997;18:560–565.

Doval HC, Nul DR, O'Grancelli HO, Perrone SV, Bortman GR, Curiel R, for Grupo de Estudio de la Sobrevida en la Insuficiencia Cardiaca en Argentina (GESICA). Randomized trial of low-dose amiodarone in severe congestive heart failure. *Lancet* 1994;344:493–498.

Eichhorn EJ, Heesch CM, Barnett JH, et al. Effect of metoprolol on myocardial function and energetics in patients with nonischemic dilated cardiomyopathy: a randomized, double-blind, placebo-controlled study. *J Am Coll Cardiol* 1994;24:1310–1320.

Engelmeier RS, O'Connell JB, Walsh R, Rad N, Scanlon PJ, Gunnar RM. Improvement in symptoms and exercise tolerance by metoprolol in patients with dilated cardiomyopathy; a double-blind, randomized, placebo-controlled trial. *Circulation* 1985;72:536–546.

Fisher ML, Gottlieb SS, Plotrick GD, et al. Beneficial effects of metoprolol in heart failure associated with coronary artery disease: a randomized trial. *J Am Coll Cardiol* 1994;23:943–950.

Gagnol JP, Devos C, Clinet M. Amiodarone: biochemical aspects and haemodynamic effects. *Drugs* 1985;29[Suppl 3]:1.

Gilbert EM, Anderson JL, Deitchman D, et al. Chronic β-blocker-vasodilator therapy improves cardiac function in idiopathic dilated cardiomyopathy: a double-blinding randomized study of bucindolol versus placebo. *Am J Med* 1990;88:223–229.

Ikram H, Fitzpatrick D. Double-blind trial of chronic oral beta-blockade in congestive cardiomyopathy. *Lancet* 1981;2:490–493.

Julian DG, Camm AJ, Frangin G, Janse MJ, Munoz PJ, Schwartz P, for the European Myocardial Infarct Amiodarone Trial Investigators. Randomized trial of effect of amiodarone on mortality in patients with left-ventricular dysfunction after recent myocardial infarction. EMIAT. *Lancet* 1997;349:667–674.

Krum H, Sackner-Bernstein J, Goldsmith RL, et al. Double-blind, placebo-controlled study of the long-term efficacy of Carvedilol in patients with severe chronic heart failure. *Circulation* 1995;92:1499–1506.

Leung W, Lau C, Wong C, Cheng C, Tai Y, Lim S. A double-blind cross-over trial of labetalol in patients with dilated cardiomyopathy. *Am Heart J* 1990;119:884–890.

Mahmarian JJ, Smart FW, Moye LA, et al. Exploring the minimal dose of amiodarone with antiarrhythmic and hemodynamic activity. *Am J Cardiol* 1994;74:681–686.

Metra M, Nardi M, Giubbini R, DeiCas L. Effects of short- and long-term carvedilol administration on rest and exercise hemodynamic variables, exercise capacity and clinical conditions in patients with idiopathic dilated cardiomyopathy. *J Am Coll Cardiol* 1994;24:1678–1687.

Miller RR, Awan NA, Maxwell KS, Mason DT. Sustained reduction of cardiac impedance and preload in congestive heart failure with the antihypertensive vasodilator prazosin. *N Engl J Med* 1977;297:303–307.

Olsen ST, Gilbert EM, Renlund DG, et al. Carvedilol improves left ven-

tricular function and symptoms in chronic heart failure: a double-blind randomized study. *J Am Coll Cardiol* 1995;25:1225–1231.

Packer M, Bristow MR, Cohn JN, Colucci WS, Fowler MB, Gilbert EM, Shusterman NH for the U.S. Carvedilol Heart Failure Study Group. Effect of carvedilol on morbidity and mortality in chronic heart failure. *N Engl J Med* 1996a;334:1349–1355.

Packer M, Colucci WS, Sackern-Bernstein JD, et al. Double-blind, placebo-controlled study of the effects of carvedilol in patients with moderate to severe heart failure. *Circulation* 1996b;94:2793–2799.

Paolisso G, Gambardella A, Marazzo G, et al. Metabolic and cardiovascular benefits deriving from β-adrenergic blockade in chronic congestive heart failure. *Am Heart J* 1992;123:103–110.

Pollock SG, Lystash J, Tedesco C, Craddock G, Smucker SM. Usefulness of bucindolol in congestive heart failure. *Am J Cardiol* 1990;66:603–607.

Sano H, Kawabata N, Yonezawa K, Hirayana H, Sakuma I, Yasuda H. Metoprolol was more effective than captopril for dilated cardiomyopathy in Japanese patients. *Circulation* 1989;80[Suppl]:118(abst).

Singh SN, Fletcher RD, Gross Fisher S, et al. Amiodarone in patients with congestive heart failure and symptomatic ventricular arrhythmia. *N Engl J Med* 1995;333:77–82.

Swedberg K, Hjalmarson A, Waagstein F, Wallentin I. Adverse effects of beta-blockade withdrawal in patients with congestive cardiomyopathy. *Br Heart J* 1980;44:134–142.

Swedberg K, Hjalmarson A, Waagstein F, Wallentin I. Beneficial effects of long-term beta-blockade in congestive cardiomyopathy. *Br Heart J* 1980;44:117–133.

Swedberg K, Hjalmarson A, Waagstein F, Wallentin I. Prolongation of survival in congestive cardiomyopathy by beta-receptor blockade. *Lancet* 1979;1:1374–1376.

Teo KK, Yusuf S, Furburg CD. Effects of prophylactic antiarrhythmic drug therapy in acute myocardial infarction: an overview of results from randomized controlled clinical trials. *JAMA* 1993;270:1589–95.

Waagstein F, Bristow MR, Swedberg-Camerini F, et al., for the Metoprolol in Dilated Cardiomyopathy (MDC) Trial Study Group. Beneficial effects of metoprolol in idiopathic dilated cardiomyopathy. *Lancet* 1993;342:1441–1446.

Waagstein F, Hjalmarson A, Varnauskas E, Wallentin I. Effect of chronic beta-adrenergic receptor blockade in congestive cardiomyopathy. *Br Heart J* 1975;37:1022–1036.

Wisenbaugh T, Katz I, Davis J, et al. Long-term (3 month) effects of a new beta-blocker (nebivolol) on cardiac performance in dilated cardiomyopathy. *J Am Coll Cardiol* 1993;21:1094–1100.

Woodley SL, Gilbert EM, Anderson JL, et al. β-Blockade with bucindolol in heart failure due to ischemic vs idiopathic dilated cardiomyopathy. *Circulation* 1991;84:2426–2441.

Young JB, Pratt CM. Hemodynamic and hormonal alterations in patients with heart failure: toward a contemporary definition of heart failure. *Semin Nephrol* 1994;14:427–440.

Management of End-Stage Heart Disease, edited
by Eric A. Rose and Lynne Warner Stevenson.
Lippincott–Raven Publishers, Philadelphia ©1998.

CHAPTER 7

Arrhythmias in End-Stage Heart Failure

William G. Stevenson and Michael O. Sweeney

Arrhythmia management is an important component of caring for the patient with advanced heart failure. In patients with Class III or IV heart failure, 28% to 48% of deaths are classified as sudden; arrhythmias are an important although not the only cause. At the time of referral for evaluation for cardiac transplantation, 11% of patients have already been resuscitated from a cardiac arrest; another 5% of patients have had sustained ventricular tachycardia without cardiac arrest (Table 1). Supraventricular arrhythmias and bradyarrhythmias are also frequent problems; 20% to 50% of patients have atrial fibrillation, and approximately 8% of patients require permanent pacemakers for bradyarrhythmias. When ventricular dysfunction is advanced, supraventricular arrhythmias can precipitate severe decompensation or cardiac arrest. Supraventricular tachycardias that produce inappropriately rapid heart rates over long periods can further depress ventricular function or cause chronic dilated heart failure.

FACTORS CONTRIBUTING TO ARRHYTHMIAS IN HEART FAILURE

Tachyarrhythmias are due to reentry or to automatic firing (automaticity) of myocytes or Purkinje fibers. The likely mechanism of a ventricular arrhythmia is influenced by the underlying heart disease. Patients with heart failure due to coronary artery disease ("ischemic cardiomyopathy") usually have an infarct region that can be the substrate for reentrant ventricular tachycardia (see later). Acute myocardial ischemia inducing polymorphic ventricular tachycardia and ventricular fibrillation is also a risk. In "nonischemic cardiomyopathy," which is idiopathic, postviral, or due to chronic aortic or mitral regurgitation, myocardial infarct scars and epicardial coronary

Cardiovascular Division, Brigham and Women's Hospital, Boston, Massachusetts 02115

artery disease are absent. Myocardial ischemia can occur, however, because of high intraventricular and right atrial pressures and inadequate capillary supply in hypertrophied muscle. In all causes of heart failure, sympathetic nervous system activity, which promotes many arrhythmias, is increased, and parasympathetic tone, which usually has a salutary effect, is diminished.

Chronic heart failure from any cause is accompanied by myocardial hypertrophy, associated with several electrophysiologic abnormalities. Potassium currents (IK1 and Ito) that contribute to repolarization are diminished, prolonging action potential duration and, hence, the QT interval in the surface electrocardiogram. Prolongation of refractoriness is not uniform throughout the myocardium; the heterogeneity may facilitate reentry. Action potential prolongation and abnormal intracellular calcium cycling is present and increases susceptibility to spontaneous membrane depolarizations, called afterdepolarizations. Afterdepolarizations have been linked to polymorphic ventricular tachycardia, torsade de pointes, and to arrhythmias induced by digitalis toxicity. Electrical coupling between myocytes is diminished because of a reduction in gap junction surface area and interstitial fibrosis. This slows conduction velocity and contributes to heterogeneous recovery after depolarization—factors that promote reentry. Interstitial fibrosis is prominent in the volume- and pressure-overloaded atria, promoting atrial fibrillation. Myocardial stretch, which may in theory occur with bulging of a ventricular aneurysm or sudden elevations in intracardiac filling pressures, may also promote arrhythmias.

Potassium and Magnesium

Chronic diuretic therapy depletes potassium and magnesium stores. Serum magnesium levels can be normal despite total body magnesium depletion. Beta-adrenergic stimulation from circulating or exogenously administered

TABLE 1. *Cardiac arrhythmia history in 770 consecutive patients with advanced heart failure*[a]

Age (years)	51±12
Male/female	611/159
Coronary artery disease	52%
Left ventricular ejection fraction	0.21±0.07%
Prior cardiac arrest[b]	11%
Ventricular tachycardia	3.4%
Ventricular fibrillation	4.6%
Bradyarrhythmia	0.7%
Unknown rhythm	0.9%
Torsades de pointes	1.4%
Sustained ventricular tachycardia without arrest	5.2%
Syncope	16.3%
Atrial fibrillation	22%
Holter ECG (n=492)	
Nonsustained ventricular tachycardia >3 beats	63.2%
PVC/hr	
<5	22.4%
5–40	29.1%
>40	48.6%

[a]Patients discharged from University of California, Los Angeles, Medical Center Cardiomyopathy Service from 1983 to 1993.
[b]From Stevenson WG, Middlekauff HR, Saxon LA. Ventricular arrhythmias in heart failure. In: Zipes DP, Jaife J, eds. *Cardiac electrophysiology: from cell to bedside.* Philadelphia: WB Saunders, 1995:848–863.

catecholamines drives potassium into cells, and can further lower serum potassium. Hypokalemia hyperpolarizes myocardial tissue, increases automatic firing of Purkinje fibers, and slows repolarization, prolonging the QT interval. Hypokalemia increases the risk of ventricular fibrillation during acute myocardial ischemia, promotes digitalis-induced arrhythmias, and can precipitate torsade de pointes (see later). Maintenance of adequate serum potassium and magnesium levels is important. Correction of hypokalemia often requires correction of hypomagnesemia as well.

The electrophysiologic effects of hypomagnesemia are not well understood, but increased susceptibility to torsade de pointes is likely. In patients with heart failure with normal or low serum magnesium concentrations, acute intravenous administration of magnesium reduces ventricular ectopic activity. Oral administration of 3.2 g of magnesium chloride daily for 6 weeks reduced ventricular ectopic activity and nonsustained ventricular tachycardia, and increased serum potassium in one study of 21 patients. Magnesium supplementation is reasonable when chronic diuretic therapy is required, but the effect of this practice on sudden death is not yet known.

Although electrolyte depletion is clearly important, hyperkalemia is probably a more common cause of cardiac arrest in patients with end-stage heart failure. Potassium supplementation, angiotensin-converting enzyme inhibitors, potassium-sparing diuretics (e.g., spironolac-

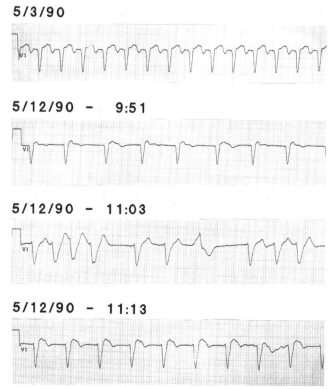

5/3/90

5/12/90 – 9:51

5/12/90 – 11:03

5/12/90 – 11:13

FIG. 1. Single-channel electrocardiogram tracings from a patient with idiopathic dilated cardiomyopathy in whom hyperkalemia developed. The patient was receiving captopril and large doses of diuretics and potassium supplementation. On 5/3/90, sinus tachycardia with first-degree atrioventricular (AV) block is present. On 5/9/90, the potassium-sparing diuretic amiloride was added to his regimen. The first tracing on 5/12/90 shows a slower junctional rhythm. The 11:03 tracing was recorded after he complained of weakness and an irregular pulse was noted; serum potassium was 7.0 mEq/L. Runs of irregular wide QRS complexes are present without P waves. Intravenous calcium gluconate was administered and the tracing in the bottom panel was recorded 10 minutes later. There is an improvement in intraventricular conduction with narrower, more regular QRS complexes. P waves immediately follow the QRS complexes, suggesting either a junction rhythm or marked first-degree AV block.

tone, amiloride, triamterene), and low cardiac output with diminished renal perfusion are important causes. Hyperkalemia shortens action potential duration, depolarizes cells, suppresses automaticity, and slows conduction velocity. The typical electrocardiographic sequence of developing hyperkalemia proceeds from peaked T waves, to junctional rhythm, QRS prolongation, and finally asystole or a wide QRS sinusoidal tachycardia (Figures 1, 2). Thus, cardiac arrest may present as either a bradyarrhythmia or ventricular tachycardia.

Hypermagnesemia is uncommon, occurring in patients with severely impaired renal function who receive large supplemental doses of magnesium. Hypotension and respiratory depression can result.

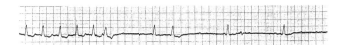

FIG. 2. A sudden bradyarrhythmia at the onset of cardiac arrest in a patient with idiopathic dilated cardiomyopathy.

THERAPIES FOR TACHYARRHYTHMIAS

Antiarrhythmic Drugs in Heart Failure

The risks of antiarrhythmic drug therapy (Table 2) are increased in patients with heart failure; these drugs should be avoided unless clearly required for arrhythmia control. The volume of distribution and clearance of antiarrhythmic drugs is reduced; drug accumulation to toxic levels is more likely to occur. Drug administration should be individualized. In most cases, therapy should be initiated at low doses during electrocardiographic monitoring in hospital. Serum levels should be monitored. When there is a change in hemodynamic status that might impair renal or hepatic drug excretion, serum drug levels should be reevaluated.

With the possible exceptions of quinidine, and amiodarone during chronic oral therapy, all antiarrhythmic drugs have negative inotropic effects. Sodium channel blockade (Class I drug effect) reduces intracellular sodium, diminishing sodium–calcium exchange, which consequently diminishes intracellular calcium. With some drugs, the direct negative inotropic effect of sodium channel blockade is offset to some extent by vasodilation, prominent with intravenous administration of procainamide or quinidine, or by prolongation of action potential duration, which increases the time for calcium entry during systole. Ravid and coworkers observed exacerbation of chronic stable heart failure by antiarrhythmic drugs in 10% of 167 patients during 491 antiarrhythmic drug trials. Despite negative inotropic effects, heart failure may improve if an arrhythmia that is aggravating heart failure, such as rapid atrial flutter, is brought under control.

Aggravation of Arrhythmias—Proarrhythmia

All antiarrhythmic drugs have the potential to cause a new arrhythmia, or exacerbate a preexisting arrhythmia. The risk is greatest in patients with severely depressed ventricular function. Drugs that prolong the QT interval can cause torsade de pointes (see later). Any drug can potentially increase the frequency of a previously infrequent tachycardia or cause the tachycardia to become incessant. This type of proarrhythmia is most frequent with drugs that slow conduction velocity, such as the Class IC drugs flecainide and propafenone.

Proarrhythmic responses can also occur during treatment of supraventricular tachycardias. An antiarrhythmic drug may increase the ventricular rate during atrial flutter or fibrillation; rarely, this may lead to cardiac arrest. Antiarrhythmic drugs can also aggravate bradyarrhythmias, which is the most common adverse cardiac effect of amiodarone. Negative inotropic and proarrhythmic effects may contribute to the increased mortality produced by therapy with Class I drugs and d-sotalol in myocardial infarction survivors and by Class I drugs in heart failure patients with atrial fibrillation.

TABLE 2. *Antiarrhythmic drugs in heart failure*

	Potential for aggravating heart failure	Potential for bradyarrhythmias	Torsade de pointes	Total proarrhythmia	Major route of elimination	
					Elimination	Half-life (hr)
Class I						
Quinidine	±	+	2%	7%	Hepatic	5.9
Procainamide	+	+	+	4%	Renal/hepatic	3–5
Disopyramide	+++	+	+	5%	Renal/hepatic	4–10
Lidocaine (i.v.)	+	+	-	Low	Hepatic	1–2
Mexiletine	++	+	-	6%	Hepatic	10–17
Tocainide	++	+	-	16%	Renal/hepatic	11
Flecainide	++	++	-	7%	Renal/hepatic	20
Propafenone	+++	++	-	5%	Hepatic	5–8
Moricizine	++	+	-	11%	Hepatic	1–3
Class III						
Amiodarone						
Chronic oral therapy	±	+++	1%	5%	Hepatic	7 wk
Acute intravenous	++	+++	1%	1%	Hepatic	
Sotalol	+++	+++	2–4%	4.5%	Renal	12
Ibutilide (i.v.)[a]	±	+	3–8%	3–8%	Hepatic	3–6
Bretylium (i.v.)	?	+	?	3%	Renal	8

i.v., intravenous.

[a]Approved for conversion of atrial fibrillation or atrial flutter only.

Modified from Stevenson WG, Friedman PL. Drug treatment of ventricular tachycardias. In: Smith TW, ed. *Cardiovascular therapeutics.* Philadelphia: WB Saunders, 1995.

Amiodarone

Amiodarone is the favored antiarrhythmic drug for chronic therapy in patients with advanced heart failure because of its efficacy against a variety of ventricular and supraventricular arrhythmias, low potential for proarrhythmia, and absence of negative inotropic effects during chronic oral therapy. Chronic oral therapy produces blockade of potassium, sodium, and calcium channels, and blunts the response to sympathetic stimulation. Sinus node automaticity is depressed and atrioventricular (AV) nodal conduction is slowed. Refractoriness is prolonged in all cardiac tissues. Depending on the loading dose, these effects take 2 to 5 days to develop and increase further over weeks. Amiodarone also has mild vasodilator properties.

From a cardiac standpoint, chronic oral therapy with amiodarone is relatively safe in heart failure. In randomized trials in patients with heart failure and in survivors of myocardial infarction, amiodarone therapy either had no impact on mortality, improved survival, or reduced sudden death without altering total mortality. The incidence of proarrhythmia is low. In patients who have had sustained ventricular tachycardia, amiodarone therapy occasionally precipitates more frequent or incessantly slower ventricular tachycardia. Amiodarone rarely induces torsade de pointes, and has often been administered to patients who have had torsade de pointes to other antiarrhythmic drugs. In advanced heart failure, however, torsade de pointes and sudden death have been observed during amiodarone therapy in patients who have had torsade de pointes provoked by other agents; the drug should be avoided in these patients. The major cardiac adverse effect is bradyarrhythmia, which occurs in 1.7% to 4% of patients. Amiodarone should be avoided if sinus or AV node disease is present and the patient does not have a permanent pacemaker. In patients with advanced heart failure, a resting sinus rate below 70 to 80 beats/minute may be an indication of increased risk for bradyarrhythmia during amiodarone therapy. The presence of bundle branch block is not a contraindication to amiodarone therapy. In patients with implantable defibrillators, amiodarone can increase the energy required for successful defibrillation, and occasionally renders the defibrillator ineffective. Repeat testing of defibrillation is recommended after amiodarone therapy is initiated.

Because of its large volume of distribution and long half-life, amiodarone therapy is usually initiated with a loading dose, typically 800 to 1600 mg daily. Large oral doses (e.g., 50 mg/kg/day) can produce vasodilation and hypotension, evident within 2 hours of administration. Heart rate typically slows after 2 to 5 days. In advanced heart failure, heart rate may initially slow without a compensatory increase in stroke volume, causing a fall in cardiac output, increase in filling pressures, and exacerbation of heart failure. A relatively low initial loading dose of 600 mg/day is usually well tolerated, but antiarrhythmic effects may not become evident for 1 to 2 weeks. During long-term oral therapy, amiodarone is hemodynamically well tolerated; left ventricular ejection fraction and heart failure symptoms often improve, possibly because of slowing of heart rate or antiischemic or vasodilatory effects (see Chapter 6). One small study found impaired ventricular relaxation after 2 to 12 weeks of amiodarone therapy.

Noncardiac toxicities are a major concern during long-term amiodarone therapy and are a major reason that therapy is discontinued in 5% to 40% of patients (Table 3). Acute pneumonitis or pulmonary fibrosis occurs in 1% to 3% of patients. Pulmonary toxicity is dose related and uncommon at chronic maintenance doses of less than 300 mg daily. It often presents with chest radiograph findings indistinguishable from those of heart failure. The risk may be greater in patients with diminished pulmonary diffusing capacity. Although routine pulmonary function tests are advocated by some, these measures fluctuate with the severity of heart failure and do not reliably identify pulmonary toxicity. Patients receiving amiodarone may be at increased risk for development of adult respiratory distress syndrome after cardiac surgery. Amiodarone therapy does not appear to increase the risk of pulmonary complications after cardiac transplantation. Amiodarone does depress the donor heart sinus node, increasing the duration of temporary pacing required in the postoperative period.

Hyperthyroidism or hypothyroidism occurs in 2% to 25% of patients; they are important potential causes of heart failure or arrhythmia exacerbation. Amiodarone blocks peripheral deiodination of thyroxine (T_4) to triiodothyronine (T_3), resulting in a decrease in T_3 and increases in serum T_4 and reverse T_3. Thyroid-stimulating hormone (TSH) remains in the normal range after an initial, transient increase. A serum TSH level within the normal range is usually sufficient to exclude hyper-

TABLE 3. *Amiodarone in heart failure: severe adverse reactions*

Reaction	Amiodarone (%)	Placebo (%)
Pulmonary toxicity	1.7	0.3
Pulmonary fibrosis	1.2	0.9
Hypothyroidism or hyperthyroidism	1.2	0.6
Atrioventricular block	1.7	1.5
Hepatitis	1.2	0.6
Ataxia or gait disturbance	4.7	1.7
Gastrointestinal upset	6.0	4.7
Skin discoloration	0.01	<0.01

Modified from Singh SN, Fletcher RD, Singh BN, et al. Amiodarone in patients with congestive heart failure and asymptomatic ventricular arrhythmia. *N Engl J Med* 1995;333: 77–82.

thyroidism or hypothyroidism; serum T_4 and T_3 levels are not reliable for screening. Assessment of TSH every 6 months is prudent. Hepatitis occurs in approximately 1% of patients.

Drug interactions are an important consideration with amiodarone therapy. Digoxin clearance is reduced by approximately 30%. Warfarin is potentiated by approximately 50%. In general, the doses of digoxin and warfarin should be reduced by 50% when amiodarone is initiated, and then followed closely.

Antiarrhythmic Drugs for Acute Intravenous Use

Antiarrhythmic agents available for acute intravenous administration include lidocaine, procainamide, quinidine, bretylium, amiodarone, and ibutilide (see Table 2). As discussed previously, the Class I antiarrhythmic drugs lidocaine and procainamide have negative inotropic effects. Lidocaine is usually well tolerated hemodynamically, but acutely terminates only 8% to 30% of sustained ventricular tachycardias induced at electrophysiologic study. The efficacy of procainamide is somewhat higher, but this agent has potent vasodilatory properties that often produce hypotension. Bretylium is a Class III drug with an efficacy for controlling ventricular tachycardia that is comparable to that of intravenous amiodarone. Potent ganglionic blocking effects produce hypotension in 30% of patients. Ibutilide is a Class III drug approved only for acute termination of atrial fibrillation or flutter. It causes torsade de pointes in 3% to 8% of patients and has not been studied in heart failure populations.

Intravenous Amiodarone

The initial effects of amiodarone administered intravenously are somewhat different than those observed after chronic oral therapy (see later). Acute, intravenous administration of amiodarone promptly depresses sinus and AV node function, but there is no change in ventricular or atrial refractory periods. Despite the lack of demonstrable effects on refractoriness, ventricular tachycardia or ventricular fibrillation is often suppressed; the mechanism is not clear.

The usual dose is 150 mg followed by a continuous infusion of 1 mg/minute for 6 hours, then 0.5 mg/minute as a maintenance infusion. The 150-mg bolus may be repeated for breakthrough arrhythmias, but the total dose should not exceed 2,000 mg in a 24-hour period. Phlebitis occurs commonly if the maintenance infusion is administered through a peripheral vein; administration through a central vein is the preferred route. For intravenous administration, amiodarone is dissolved in benzyl alcohol and the solvent Tween-80. This preparation has potent vasodilating and negative inotropic effects, in part mediated by the vehicle. Acute administration produces hypotension in approximately 25% and bradyarrhythmias in approximately 5% of patients. Transient support with an inotropic agent, volume expansion, or temporary pacing is sometimes required. Proarrhythmia in the form of polymorphic ventricular tachycardia occurs in no more than 1% of patients.

Implantable Defibrillators in Heart Failure

Implantable cardioverter–defibrillators (ICDs) are an important nonpharmacologic option for treating malignant ventricular arrhythmias in patients with heart failure. In high-risk populations, including patients with and without heart failure, ICDs reduce sudden death rates to less than 3% at 2 years. There are several advantages compared with antiarrhythmic drugs. ICDs do not cause any long-term organ toxicities or proarrhythmia. Patient compliance is guaranteed with ICD therapy. Current ICDs also provide protection from bradyarrhythmias with backup pacing.

Early ICD systems mandated general anesthesia and thoracotomy for placement of extrapericardial high-voltage electrodes and epicardial rate-sensing electrodes, and a separate abdominal incision for placement of the bulky (110–150 cc) and heavy (200–240 g) pulse generators; the operative mortality rate was in the range of 2% to 5%. Advances in ICD technology have rendered the operative risk minimal. Successful defibrillation can now be achieved in 98% of patients using nonthoracotomy lead systems and a biphasic pulsing waveform. Small (45–60 cc, 100–130 g) pulse generators permit single-incision (infraclavicular) surgical approaches under conditions of local anesthesia and light conscious sedation. Intraoperative defibrillation threshold testing is now routinely performed using transient light general anesthesia with intravenous induction agents (such as propofol or etomidate) identical to transthoracic cardioversion. With current surgical approaches, the ICD operative mortality rate is less than 1%. However, in patients with heart failure, the implant and defibrillation testing procedure can exacerbate heart failure. Rarely, hemodynamic collapse with slow recovery follows successful termination of ventricular fibrillation by high-energy internal pulses during the implantation procedure. In the overall ICD population, this phenomenon is extremely uncommon (<1%). However, it may be as high as 5% to 6% in patients with severe left ventricular dysfunction awaiting transplantation. The cause of this phenomenon is unknown, but anecdotal observation suggests it is independent of anesthetic technique, electrode configuration, pulsing waveform, and duration of defibrillation threshold testing. ICD implantation should not be attempted during an exacerbation of heart failure.

Although it is widely perceived that the energy required for successful defibrillation (defibrillation threshold) increases with the severity of ventricular dysfunction and heart failure, this is not well supported by the available data in humans. In retrospective analyses using various electrode configurations, pulsing waveforms, and methods of defibrillation, threshold determination, factors predictive of increased energy requirement have included myocardial mass, left ventricular ejection fraction, concomitant drug therapy (particularly amiodarone), gender, and technical variables (e.g., electrode polarity, electrode surface area, electrode position, and waveform shape). More recently, Raitt et al. analyzed patients with identical electrode configurations and pulsing and found that left ventricular mass and resting heart rate were independent predictors of defibrillation threshold. With current systems, adequate defibrillation is achieved in almost all patients regardless of the severity of heart failure and degree of left ventricular dysfunction.

Rarely, episodes of ventricular tachycardia or ventricular fibrillation transiently increase in frequency after ICD implantation. Rapid atrial fibrillation or flutter may increase heart rate above the programmed tachycardia detection rate of the ICD, resulting in spurious tachycardia therapies. Antitachycardia pacing during supraventricular tachycardia may initiate ventricular tachycardia and cause the patient to receive painful, inappropriate shocks. For repetitive inappropriate shocks, arrhythmia detection can be temporarily suspended by placing a magnet over the ICD. When the magnet is removed, detection is immediately reenabled. Nonfatal complications of lead dislodgement, lead fracture, or infection occur in 6% to 20% of patients.

Although sudden death rates are impressively low in ICD recipients, it is not yet clear if this will translate to an increase in survival in patients with advanced heart failure. Sweeney et al. analyzed sudden death and survival in 291 consecutive patients evaluated for cardiac transplantation; 179 patients did not receive antiarrhythmic treatment, and the remainder received treatment for ventricular arrhythmias with an ICD (59 patients) or antiarrhythmic drugs (53 patients). Actuarial sudden death rates were lowest in the ICD group, intermediate in the no antiarrhythmic treatment group, and highest in the drug treatment group (12-month sudden death rates of 9.2%, 16.0%, and 34.7%, respectively). However, total mortality and nonsudden death rates did not differ among groups. There were no differences in baseline clinical variables, medical therapies for heart failure, and actuarial rates of transplantation between groups. Kim and coworkers reported a 2-year sudden death rate of 6% for patients with left ventricular ejection fractions less than 30%; total mortality was 17%. Occasionally, recurrent ventricular fibrillation that is successfully terminated by the ICD is followed after some brief period by death from cardiogenic shock, leading to "not-so-sudden" death or "arrhythmia-related nonsudden death." Thus, a survival benefit from sudden death pre-

vention may be reduced by high nonsudden and arrhythmia-related nonsudden death rates. Although the sudden death rates are relatively low, they are higher in ICD patients with severe ventricular dysfunction compared with those observed in larger series including patients without heart failure. It is likely that many sudden deaths in patients with heart failure with ICDs are due to electromechanical dissociation, similar to that which can follow acute defibrillation threshold testing (see earlier), and to catastrophic noncardiac events such as pulmonary emboli or stroke. In summary, ICDs can alter the mode of cardiac death in patients with advanced heart failure. This reduction in sudden death due to malignant ventricular tachyarrhythmias translates to extension of survival in some patients, but does not alter the underlying disease process. In some cases, an ICD allows survival of transplantation from the outpatient waiting list.

MANAGEMENT OF SPECIFIC ARRHYTHMIAS

Sustained tachycardias are those that require an intervention for termination, such as cardioversion, or that produce severe symptoms, such as syncope or pulmonary edema before terminating spontaneously. Acutely, hemodynamic stability must be restored, aggravating factors removed or corrected, and the need for long-term therapy assessed. A number of common precipitating factors, including toxicities of antiarrhythmic and inotropic drugs, and electrolyte abnormalities induced by diuretic drugs or renal insufficiency, should be immediately considered (Table 4). After restoration of sinus rhythm, the

TABLE 4. *Common provocative factors for arrhythmias in advanced heart failure*

Ventricular tachycardia
  Myocardial ischemia
  Hyperkalemia
  Hypokalemia, hypomagnesemia
  Antiarrhythmic drugs
  Hypoxia
  Inotropic agents
  Beta-adrenergic agonists
  Phosphodiesterase inhibitors
  Digitalis toxicity
Atrial arrhythmias
  Hypokalemia, hypomagnesemia
  Elevated atrial pressures
  Inotropic agents (see above)
Bradyarrhythmias
  Hyperkalemia
  Apnea/hypoventilation
  Digitalis
  Antiarrhythmic drugs
  Myocardial ischemia
  Calcium channel blockers
  Beta-adrenergic blockers

need for chronic therapy is determined by the type of arrhythmia.

Sustained Monomorphic Ventricular Tachycardia

Approximately 9% of patients referred for evaluation for cardiac transplantation have survived one or more episodes of sustained monomorphic ventricular tachycardia (see Table 1; Figure 3). Slow ventricular tachycardias may be hemodynamically well tolerated, but fast tachycardias usually cause hemodynamic collapse and cardiac arrest, frequently degenerating to ventricular fibrillation. The likely mechanism depends on the underlying heart disease. The most common cause is reentry in an infarct or region of scar, in which case tachycardias can usually be initiated by programmed electrical stimulation, allowing evaluation in the electrophysiology laboratory. Rarely, digitalis toxicity causes sustained monomorphic ventricular tachycardia. Sustained monomorphic ventricular tachycardia is common in patients with prior myocardial infarction, and is relatively rare in patients with idiopathic

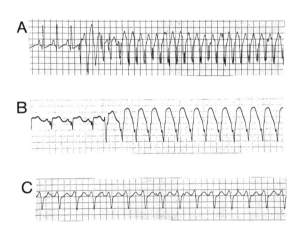

FIG. 3. Three examples of sustained monomorphic ventricular tachycardia from patients with heart failure. **A:** The spontaneous onset of rapid (220 beats/minute), sustained monomorphic ventricular tachycardia in a patient with prior myocardial infarction. Tachycardia produced syncope, requiring cardioversion. **B:** Spontaneous onset of relatively slow (120 beats/minute), sustained monomorphic ventricular tachycardia in a patient with prior myocardial infarction. Tachycardia was hemodynamically tolerated and was terminated by an intravenous injection of procainamide. **C:** Slow, sustained monomorphic ventricular tachycardia that was a possible proarrhythmic response to amiodarone. Over a 1-year period, the patient had several episodes of ventricular tachycardia at 150 to 180 beats/minute, requiring cardioversion. After 2 weeks of amiodarone therapy, ventricular tachycardia was markedly slowed to 100 beats/minute, but was incessant and immediately recurred after each cardioversion. Atrioventricular dissociation is evident from the presence of P waves deforming the T waves after the first, fourth, seventh, and ninth QRS complexes. (From Stevenson WG, Stevenson LW. Evalution and management of arrhythmias in heart failure. In: Parmley WW, Chatterjee K, eds. *Cardiology*. Vol. 3. Philadelphia: JB Lippincott, 1993:5.)

dilated cardiomyopathy. Chagas' disease and sarcoidosis cause nonischemic cardiomyopathies that are more frequently associated with ventricular tachycardia.

Electrocardiographic criteria for distinguishing monomorphic ventricular tachycardia from supraventricular tachycardia with aberrancy are not always reliable in patients with advanced heart failure. Marked ventricular enlargement is often associated with unusual conduction abnormalities; supraventricular QRS complexes may resemble those of ventricular tachycardia. In general, the diagnosis should be confirmed unequivocally at electrophysiologic study with attention to excluding the more easily treatable arrhythmias: supraventricular tachycardia conducted with aberrancy and bundle branch reentry tachycardia.

In bundle branch reentry ventricular tachycardia, the reentry wavefront propagates up one bundle branch, down the contralateral bundle branch, and through the interventricular septum (Figure 4). Substantial disease of the cardiac conduction system is usually required for this type of reentry to occur. More than 80% of patients have a prolonged QRS duration during sinus rhythm with a pattern of incomplete left bundle branch block, and a prolonged His-V interval. Because one of the bundle branches forms part of the circuit, the tachycardia QRS resembles right or left bundle branch block, and may appear similar to that during sinus rhythm. Bundle branch reentry should be particularly suspected in patients with no prior myocardial infarction. This mechanism accounts for up to 36% of sustained monomorphic ventricular tachycardias in nonischemic cardiomyopathy, but only 5% of the tachycardias in patients with prior myocardial infarction. The tachycardia rates range from 140 to 240 beats/minute, often causing syncope or degenerating to ventricular fibrillation. Confirmation of the tachycardia mechanism requires recording the His bundle electrogram or right bundle electrogram during electrophysiologic study and obtaining evidence that these are linked to the tachycardia circuit. Radiofrequency catheter ablation of the right bundle branch is curative. In 20% to 30% of patients, placement of a permanent pacemaker is needed because of impaired conduction through the remaining His-Purkinje system. In some patients, coexistence of other reentrant ventricular tachycardias requires additional therapy.

When sustained monomorphic ventricular tachycardia is not due to bundle branch reentry, which can be treated with ablation, recurrence rates exceed 40% over 2 years despite therapy with Class I antiarrhythmic drugs or sotalol. In studies including patients with a spectrum of ventricular function, most ventricular tachycardia recurrences are not fatal. However, patients with heart failure and those who have previously been resuscitated from cardiac arrest are at greater risk for a fatal recurrence. Class I antiarrhythmic drugs are usually avoided as initial therapy because of their low effi-

Sinus Rhythm

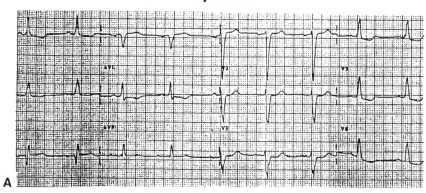

Bundle Branch Reentry VT

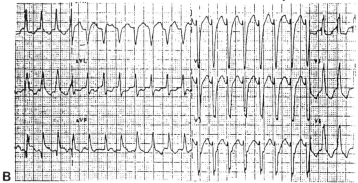

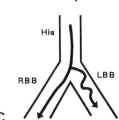

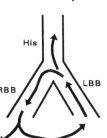

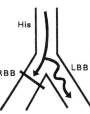

Sinus rhythm   Bundle Branch Reentry   After RBBB Ablation

FIG. 4. Panels **(A)** and **(B)** show 12-lead electrocardiograms from a patient with heart failure many years after inferior wall myocardial infarction in whom bundle branch reentry ventricular tachycardia developed. In panel **(A)**, sinus rhythm is present with evidence of old inferior wall myocardial infarction and interventricular conduction abnormality. Panel **(B)** shows sustained tachycardia that has a morphology similar to the sinus rhythm QRS complexes. Atrioventricular dissociation is present (*arrows*), excluding supraventricular tachycardia as the mechanism. At electrophysiologic study, this was confirmed to be bundle branch reentry tachycardia. The mechanism is illustrated in panel **(C)**. The reentrant wavefront circulates down the right bundle branch (*right BB*), through the interventricular septum, and up the left bundle branch (in the illustration, the posterior division of the left bundle branch is the retrograde limb of the tachycardia. This bundle of His is depolarized passively, but is close to the circuit. Ablation of the right bundle branch was curative [not shown]). (From Stevenson WG, Sweeney MO. Pharmacologic and nonpharmacologic treatment of ventricular arrhythmias in heart failure. *Curr Opin Cardiol* 1997;12:242–250, with permission.)

cacy and negative inotropic effects. Sotalol may have greater efficacy, but its beta-adrenergic blocking effects limit therapy in advanced heart failure. The major therapeutic options are amiodarone or an ICD.

Amiodarone versus Implantable Defibrillators as Chronic Therapy

The Antiarrhythmics Versus Implantable Defibrillators (AVID) trial found better overall survival in patients who received an ICD rather than amiodarone or sotalol. All patients had been resuscitated from sustained ventricular tachycardia or ventricular fibrillation. The specific impact on sudden death and in patients with advanced heart failure has yet to be reported.

Selection of initial therapy should take into consideration the expected longevity from the standpoint of progressive ventricular dysfunction, the nature and frequency of the ventricular arrhythmia, and the risks of the therapies (Table 5). Amiodarone is favored for patients

TABLE 5. *Amiodarone versus implantable defibrillators as initial therapy for survivors of VT/VF with heart failure*

Favor amiodarone
    Incessant or very frequent VT
    Implantable defibrillator contraindication
        Active infection
        Decompensated heart failure
    High risk for heart failure deterioration
Favor implantable defibrillator
    Amiodarone contraindication
        Increased risk of bradyarrhythmias
            Resting heart rate <60/min
            Atrioventricular block
        History of torsade de pointes
        Hyperthyroidism
        Liver disease

VT, ventricular tachycardia; VF, ventricular fibrillation.

who have a very limited life expectancy because of progressive pump failure, including bedridden patients with Class IV symptoms, in whom an ICD is not likely meaningfully to extend survival and the implantation procedure may precipitate hemodynamic deterioration. The frequency of ventricular tachycardia episodes is another important consideration. ICDs terminate ventricular tachycardia either by a shock, which is usually painful, or by antitachycardia pacing, which is well tolerated. Shocks are acceptable if episodes of tachycardia are infrequent, but frequent shocks are not well tolerated. Antitachycardia pacing is well tolerated and acceptable therapy for frequent episodes of ventricular tachycardia, but not effective for all tachycardias. With daily or more frequent episodes of antitachycardia pacing, unacceptable symptoms, or pacing-induced acceleration of tachycardia requiring a shock for termination, often occur. Therapy with amiodarone is a better initial option if tachycardia episodes are frequent. If episodes of ventricular tachycardia do recur, they are usually less frequent and slower. For patients who have good functional capacity despite severe ventricular dysfunction and infrequent episodes of sustained ventricular tachycardia, an ICD is an excellent option. If episodes of ventricular tachycardia become frequent and symptomatic, amiodarone can then be added. Defibrillation safety margin verification should be performed after amiodarone loading and at least yearly to ensure that amiodarone has not increased the energy required for defibrillation above that delivered by the defibrillator, particularly for patients who required relatively high energy for defibrillation when the device was initially implanted.

Recurrent Episodes of Sustained Monomorphic Ventricular Tachycardia

Ventricular tachycardia that occurs frequently despite therapy with amiodarone, or when amiodarone is contraindicated, is a difficult problem. If episodes increase after amiodarone loading, the drug may be having a proarrhythmic effect; other therapy should be sought. An ICD can be considered provided the patient is an acceptable candidate and the tachycardia can be terminated by pacing. Beta-adrenergic stimulation reduces the electrophysiologic effects of antiarrhythmic drugs, including amiodarone, and is an important trigger of ventricular arrhythmias. Therapy with a beta-adrenergic blocker may reduce episodes of ventricular tachycardia, but is often not tolerated in advanced heart failure. Whether newer beta-adrenergic blockers that possess vasodilating properties, such as carvedilol and bucindolol, will be useful for reducing arrhythmias has not yet been determined. Combinations of antiarrhythmic drugs can also be considered. Selection of therapy is by necessity empiric. Drugs that have been administered concomitantly with amiodarone include mexiletine, procainamide, quinidine, flecainide, and sotalol. As with a single drug, drug combinations can also be proarrhythmic. For selected patients, arrhythmia surgery and catheter ablation can be considered (see later). In some cases the only option is cardiac transplantation.

When cardioversion or antitachycardia pacing terminates ventricular tachycardia for only brief periods, tachycardia is termed *incessant*. Possible provocative factors should be immediately considered (see Table 4). If digitalis toxicity is suspected, digoxin–Fab fragments (Digibind; Burroughs Wellcome Co., Research Triangle Park, North Carolina) should be administered. Hyperkalemia should be considered and excluded or treated immediately with intravenous administration of calcium or sodium bicarbonate. Rarely, incessant idiopathic ventricular tachycardia is the cause of a tachycardia-induced dilated cardiomyopathy (see later). In these cases, tachycardia has been present and unrecognized for months or years.

Antiarrhythmic drugs are an important cause of incessant ventricular tachycardia. It may be possible to support the patient hemodynamically with inotropic agents or intraaortic balloon counterpulsation (adequate synchronization can often be achieved if the tachycardia is relatively slow) until the drug is excreted. When the precipitating factor is a Class I antiarrhythmic drug, lidocaine, hypertonic saline, beta-adrenergic blockers, or intravenous amiodarone may be helpful. If amiodarone is the precipitating drug and has been administered for several weeks, it may take days or weeks for the effect to dissipate; in most cases other means of control must be sought. The addition of another antiarrhythmic drug or intravenous amiodarone is sometimes beneficial, but can also further aggravate the problem. Ventricular tachycardia may become less well tolerated because of rate acceleration or negative inotropic effects of the drug.

When correction of provocative factors is not effective and incessant tachycardia continues after cardioversion, antiarrhythmic drug therapy must be considered. Intravenous lidocaine is not often effective, but is usually relatively well tolerated and, if ineffective, washes out relatively quickly once it is discontinued. Intravenous procainamide is more effective than lidocaine, but has a greater risk of producing hypotension. Intravenous administration of amiodarone or bretylium probably has greater efficacy than lidocaine or procainamide; in one study, incessant ventricular tachycardia that had not been controlled by lidocaine or procainamide was brought under control in most patents within 7 hours. If ventricular tachycardia persists after administration of an intravenous drug, electrical cardioversion should be performed because the drug may prevent or delay reinitiation of ventricular tachycardia despite failure acutely to terminate tachycardia. Antitachycardia ventricular pacing with a temporary pacing wire or an implanted defibrillator or pacemaker can sometimes be used to terminate tachycardia, allowing external shocks to be avoided. Antitachycardia pacing should be attempted by experienced personnel, always prepared to deliver an external countershock should pacing accelerate tachycardia or produce ventricular fibrillation. Occasionally, pacing at a rate faster than the sinus rate after tachycardia termination prevents arrhythmia recurrences.

Radiofrequency Catheter Ablation of Ventricular Tachycardia

If ventricular tachycardia is relatively slow (typically < 200 beats/minute) and hemodynamically tolerated for at least brief periods of time, radiofrequency catheter ablation can be considered. This approach is investigational and usually reserved for patients who have failed other therapies, but can be life saving. Efficacy in selected patients ranges from 50% to 70%; major complications of stroke, myocardial infarction, cardiac perforation occurred in 3% of 123 patients in four recent series.

Arrhythmia Surgery

Arrhythmia surgery is an option for selected patients. The major determinant of survival is left ventricular function. If heart failure is due to a large, anterior wall ventricular aneurysm, with well preserved contraction at the base of the ventricle, aneurysmectomy combined with subendocardial resection or cryoablation of surrounding fibrotic regions can be considered. Efficacy in abolishing spontaneous episodes of ventricular tachycardia is 8% to 11%. Operative mortality ranges from 5% to over 20%, depending on the severity of ventricular dysfunction. Three-year survival rates range from approximately 70% to 80%, with pump failure the major source of mortality.

Polymorphic Ventricular Tachycardia

When the QRS morphology is continually changing during tachycardia, the arrhythmia is termed "polymor-

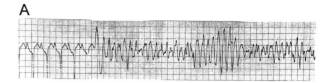

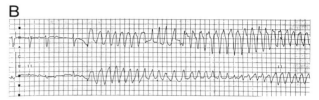

FIG. 5. Examples of spontaneous initiation of sustained polymorphic ventricular tachycardias from two patients with heart failure are shown. **A:** Initiation of rapid polymorphic ventricular tachycardia in a patient hospitalized for evaluation of heart failure. Resuscitation attempts were unsuccessful and autopsy revealed fresh thrombotic occlusion of the proximal left anterior descending coronary artery. **B:** Shows an example of torsade de pointes in a patient with heart failure in whom renal failure developed while receiving procainamide, resulting in marked accumulation of N-acetyl procainamide. The QT interval from the 12-lead electrocardiogram (not shown) was 0.6 seconds. Note that the tachycardia initiation is by a typical long–short sequence created by a pause after the third supraventricular beat from the left. The next supraventricular beat is followed by the first beat of polymorphic ventricular tachycardia. (From Stevenson WG, Stevenson LW. Evalution and management of arrhythmias in heart failure. In: Parmley WW, Chatterjee K, eds. *Cardiology.* Vol. 3. Philadelphia: JB Lippincott, 1993:7.)

phic" (Figure 5). The most common causes are acute myocardial ischemia/infarction and torsade de pointes associated with QT interval prolongation (see Figure 5). Less commonly, sustained polymorphic ventricular tachycardia is due to reentry in an area of scar, or digitalis intoxication. If a transient or reversible factor can be identified and addressed, such as acute myocardial infarction or a cause of torsade de pointes, long-term therapy for arrhythmia prevention is not required.

Torsade de Pointes

Polymorphic ventricular tachycardia associated with QT interval prolongation is known as torsade de pointes (see Figure 5B). It can be due to a provocative agent (acquired) or a congenital abnormality of ionic channels. This arrhythmia has been linked to development of afterdepolarizations, to which the hypertrophied myocardium may be predisposed. Anything that prolongs the QT interval can cause torsade de pointes (Table 6). It is rare with amiodarone despite the frequent development of marked QT prolongation. The QT interval preceding the episode is usually, but not always, greater than 0.48 second. Slow heart rates or long R-R intervals, such as pauses created by premature ventricular beats or during atrial fibrilla-

TABLE 6. *Common causes of QT prolongation and torsade de pointes in heart failure*

Electrolyte abnormalities
  Hypokalemia
  Hypomagnesemia
Bradycardia
Drugs
  Antiarrhythmics
    Amiodarone
    Disopyramide
    N-acetylprocainamide (NAPA)
    Procainamide
    Quinidine
    Sotalol
    Ibulitide
  Antibiotics
    Ampicillin
    Erythromycin
    Pentamidine
  Others
    Astemizole
    Bepridil
    Cisapride
    Haloperidol
    Phenothiazine
    Probucol
    Tricyclic antidepressants
    Vesnarinone

tion, further prolong the QT interval and characteristically precede initiation of the arrhythmia, which is therefore referred to as "pause dependent."

Episodes of torsade de pointes can usually be suppressed by administration of intravenous magnesium sulfate as a 1- to 2-g bolus over 1 to 2 minutes. If ventricular ectopy persists or recurs, a 3- to 20-mg/minute continuous infusion can be administered. If renal function is impaired, careful attention is necessary to avoid toxic serum magnesium concentrations that produce neuromuscular depression. If magnesium is not effective, overdrive atrial or ventricular pacing or isoproterenol infusion should be added in an attempt to shorten the QT interval. All potential precipitating factors should be corrected or removed.

Patients with advanced heart failure who have had torsade de pointes should be viewed as being susceptible to arrhythmia and should not receive other drugs that prolong the QT interval. Although amiodarone has been considered an exception, one small study found a markedly high mortality in patients with advanced heart failure treated with amiodarone after having torsade de pointes to another agent. Thus, torsade de pointes in patients with advanced heart failure may be a marker for marked electrical instability and a high sudden death risk even after the precipitating factors are corrected.

The Ventricular Fibrillation Survivor

Of 770 patients with advanced heart failure, 5% had been resuscitated from ventricular fibrillation in the absence of acute myocardial infarction (see Table 1). Patients with ventricular fibrillation due to acute myocardial infarction do not require further specific arrhythmia evaluation because the risk of recurrence is similar to that in myocardial infarction survivors without cardiac arrest. If clear, causative factors are absent, the severity of coronary artery disease should be defined and invasive electrophysiologic study considered. If sustained ventricular tachycardia is inducible, this is the likely cause of the arrest, and management is as for monomorphic ventricular tachycardia (see previous discussion). If ventricular tachycardia is not inducible, but severe coronary artery disease with the potential for ischemia is present, transient myocardial ischemia is the likely cause of ventricular fibrillation. Revascularization should be considered, if possible. If revascularization is not feasible, medical therapy for ischemia should be optimized and amiodarone or an ICD considered. Amiodarone possesses antianginal effects, probably because of heart rate slowing and coronary artery vasodilation, and reduces the incidence of ventricular fibrillation during acute ischemia in animal models. ICDs can effectively terminate ischemia-induced ventricular fibrillation. Rarely, a rapid supraventricular tachycardia precipitates cardiac arrest; this should also be sought at electrophysiologic study. In some patients, the cause of ventricular fibrillation is not clear. Despite absence of inducible ventricular arrhythmia at electrophysiologic study, the risk of recurrence is high; up to 48% of such patients receive a shock from an implanted ICD or have recurrent cardiac arrest during follow-up. Implantation of an ICD should be considered.

Electrical Storm and Recurrent Cardiac Arrest

"Electrical storm" refers to recurrent episodes of rapid monomorphic or polymorphic ventricular tachycardia producing repeated cardiac arrest. This tends to occur early after myocardial infarction, cardiac surgery, or defibrillator implantation, or as a proarrhythmic response to antiarrhythmic drug therapy. Potentially correctable precipitating factors should be considered (see Table 4). Intravenous magnesium should be administered for the possibility of torsade de pointes, as discussed earlier. Any beta-adrenergic agonists that could be aggravating arrhythmias of a variety of causes should be withdrawn when possible. Intravenous lidocaine followed, if ineffective, by intravenous amiodarone or bretylium should be considered early in the management (see earlier).

A number of other therapies are occasionally effective in refractory cases. Some tachycardias are sympathetically mediated and respond to beta-adrenergic blockers, but these drugs often are not tolerated hemodynamically. Endotracheal intubation, assisted ventilation, and general anesthesia sometimes quiet the arrhythmia. Percutaneous left stellate ganglion blockade has been successful in achieving control in some anecdotal cases. Overdrive ventricular pacing is sometimes helpful. In some cases, mechanical support with a ventricular assist device followed by cardiac transplantation is the only option. Although ventricular tachycardia was considered a contraindication to left ventricular assist because of the concern that impaired right ventricular filling would produce hemodynamic collapse, this has not in general been the case.

Syncope

Syncope is a very serious symptom in patients with heart failure and is a marker for an increased risk of sudden death, which was 45% at 1 year in one study. The most common identifiable cardiac cause is ventricular tachycardia (Table 7). Other common causes are orthostatic hypotension aggravated by excessive diuresis and vasodilating medications, and bradyarrhythmias. Unless syncope can be clearly attributed to orthostatic hypotension or a noncardiac cause, a careful evaluation for arrhythmias is warranted, including electrophysiologic testing. Even if this does not establish a cause, the risk of sudden death is high. Implantation of an ICD that also provides back-up bradycardia pacing has been suggested, but the value of this approach has not been determined and this indication has not been specifically approved by the U.S. Food and Drug Administration (FDA).

Ventricular Ectopic Activity and Nonsustained Ventricular Tachycardia

Ventricular premature beats and nonsustained ventricular tachycardia are found in over 60% of patients with advanced heart failure referred for possible cardiac transplantation (see Table 1). In patients with heart failure and

TABLE 7. *Causes of syncope in patients with heart failure*

Cause	Patients (N = 60)
Cardiac etiology of syncope	29 (48)[a]
Ventricular tachycardia	21 (35)
Symptomatic nonsustained VT	8
Inducible VT at electrophysiologic testing	6
Recorded during syncope	5
Torsade de pointes (drug induced)	2
Bradyarrhythmia	5 (8)
Supraventricular tachycardia	1 (2)
Valvular stenosis	2 (3)
Other causes of syncope	31 (52)
Orthostatic hypotension	9 (15)
Situational	3 (5)
Neurologic	1 (2)
Undetermined	18 (30)

VT, ventricular tachycardia.
[a]Numbers in parentheses are percentages.
From Middlekauff HR, Stevenson WG, Stevenson LW, Saxon Syncope in advanced heart failure: high risk of sudden death regardless of origin of sync. *J Am Coll Cardiol* 1993;21: 110–116.

in myocardial infarction survivors with depressed ventricular function, frequent ventricular ectopic activity and nonsustained ventricular tachycardia are markers for increased mortality. Attempts to further stratify sudden death risk using electrophysiologic testing, signal-averaged electrocardiography, and heart rate variability have limited usefulness in patients with advanced heart failure. The sudden death risk is relatively high regardless of the test outcome, and the impact of antiarrhythmia treatment strategies is not clear.

Suppression of ventricular ectopic activity does not necessarily improve survival or reduce sudden death. In myocardial infarct survivors, Class I antiarrhythmic drug therapy and d-sotalol increase mortality and sudden death. There are few data regarding the use of these drugs in nonischemic cardiomyopathy, but avoidance is prudent. Beta-adrenergic blockers reduce sudden death in myocardial infarction survivors, but often are not tolerated in patients with advanced heart failure. It is not yet clear if these drugs reduce sudden death in nonischemic cardiomyopathy.

Amiodarone can be used safely to treat symptomatic ventricular ectopy and nonsustained ventricular tachycardia in heart failure, but it is not clear that this reduces sudden death. The GESICA (Grupo Estudio de la Sobrevida Insuficiencia Cardiaca en Argentina) trial randomized patients with Class III or IV heart failure to receive amiodarone 300 mg daily or no antiarrhythmic therapy. Presence of ventricular ectopy was not a criterion for entry. Amiodarone reduced 2-year mortality from 41% to 33.5%, with a favorable trend toward a reduction in sudden death (15% in the control group vs. 12% in the amiodarone group) that did not reach statistical significance. Benefit was confined to patients who had resting heart rates of 90 beats/minute or greater; there was no benefit in patients with slower heart rates. In patients with mild to moderate heart failure (predominantly functional Class II) and frequent ventricular ectopy, the Veterans Administration cooperative trial (Congestive Heart Failure Survival Trial of Anti-Arrhythmic Therapy [CHF-STAT]) found no effect of amiodarone (400 mg/day for 1 year followed by 300 mg/day) on survival or sudden death. Interestingly, there was a trend that did not reach statistical significance toward reduced mortality in patients with nonischemic cardiomyopathy. Drug withdrawal due to a side effect occurred in 27% of amiodarone-treated patients, but also in 23% of the placebo group. In some patients, lower doses than studied in these trials (≤200 mg/day) suppress symptomatic ventricular ectopy; the effect on survival is unknown, but a reduction of side effects would be expected.

More recently, the Multicenter Automatic Defibrillator Implantation Trial (MADIT trial) suggested a possible role for electrophysiologic testing and ICDs in myocardial infarction survivors with depressed ventricular function. Myocardial infarction survivors with nonsustained ventricular tachycardia and a left ventricular ejection fraction less than 36% (mean, 25%–27%) underwent electrophysiologic study. Those who had inducible ventricular tachycardia that was not suppressed by intravenous infusion of procainamide (196 patients) were randomized to receive either an ICD or antiarrhythmic drug therapy (amiodarone in most). Those treated with an ICD had better survival. Whether these results are applicable to patients with advanced heart failure is not clear.

Supraventricular Arrhythmias: Atrial Fibrillation and Flutter

Atrial fibrillation occurs in 20% to 50% of patients with advanced heart failure. Adverse hemodynamic effects could be due to rapid or slow heart rates, loss of coordinated atrial contribution to ventricular filling, and heart rate irregularity. It is not clear if mechanisms other than those related to heart rate are clinically relevant in advanced heart failure. Ventricular rates persistently faster than 100 to 110 beats/minute can depress ventricular function and aggravate heart failure. Faster rates over long periods can be the primary cause of heart failure (see later). In some patients, conversion of atrial fibrillation to sinus rhythm or control of the ventricular rate markedly improves ventricular function. Patients with atrial fibrillation and congestive heart failure have a risk of stroke due to embolization of cardiac thrombus as high as 18% annually if they are not anticoagulated. Chronic anticoagulation with warfarin is indicated. With current management, patients who have atrial fibrillation do not appear to have substantially increased mortality compared with patients without atrial fibrillation.

Whether conversion of atrial fibrillation to sinus rhythm is beneficial in chronic dilated heart failure is not clear, although this is a common clinical impression. Because of the potential hemodynamic and thromboembolic risks, however, it is reasonable to attempt restoration of sinus rhythm, particularly for recent-onset atrial fibrillation. Class I antiarrhythmic agents may increase mortality and should be avoided. Amiodarone is a useful agent, although it is not approved by the FDA for treatment of atrial fibrillation. Of 25 patients with persistent atrial fibrillation and New York Heart Association functional Class III or IV heart failure treated with amiodarone by Middlekauff and coworkers, sinus rhythm could be restored either spontaneously or by electrical cardioversion in 84% and was maintained during follow-up in 87% of those converted. Bradyarrhythmias are the major cardiac risk. A maintenance dose of 200 mg/day is often possible, reducing the likelihood of serious side effects during long-term therapy. Drug interactions with digoxin and warfarin must be anticipated, as discussed earlier.

When sinus rhythm cannot be maintained, attention should focus on adequate control of the ventricular rate at rest and with exertion. Inotropic drugs, including phosphodiesterase inhibitors and beta-adrenergic agonists, may increase the ventricular rate and make adequate control difficult. If digoxin alone is ineffective, a careful trial of beta-adrenergic blocking agents can be considered for patients who can tolerate the negative inotropic effects of these drugs. The calcium channel blocking agents verapamil and diltiazem reduce the ventricular rate, but also possess negative inotropic effects. In addition, these drugs may increase sympathetic nervous system activation, which may be detrimental during long-term therapy. Amiodarone depresses AV conduction and often controls the ventricular rate when it does not effectively maintain sinus rhythm. Whether this benefit justifies the risk of long-term side effects is unknown. When pharmacologic therapy does not sufficiently control the ventricular rate, radiofrequency catheter ablation of the AV junction and placement of a rate-responsive ventricular pacemaker should be considered. Patients should be carefully monitored for torsade de pointes and hemodynamic deterioration for the first few days after AV junction ablation. It is not clear if the occasional hemodynamic deterioration is due to the ventricular activation sequence produced by pacing, or use of too slow a pacing rate. In some patients it is possible to modify AV conduction to achieve rate control without producing complete heart block, but there is as yet limited long-term follow-up for this approach; the heart rate remains irregular.

Occasionally atrial flutter is a major problem with a difficult-to-control ventricular rate. Therapy with amiodarone can be attempted. Atrial flutter can usually be abolished by radiofrequency catheter ablation. Atrial fibrillation recurs in 25% of patients after successful flutter ablation, but may be easier to manage than flutter.

TACHYCARDIA-INDUCED CARDIOMYOPATHY

Incessant tachycardia of any cause can cause progressive ventricular dilation and dysfunction. The tachycardia may be asymptomatic until marked ventricular dysfunction is present, and the patient presents with dilated cardiomyopathy. In general, heart rate is persistently above 120 beats/minute for most of any 24-hour period. Control of the arrhythmia is usually followed by a gradual improvement in ventricular function over weeks to months.

BRADYARRHYTHMIAS

Advanced heart failure is often accompanied by sinus or AV node dysfunction, leading to bradyarrhythmias. Bradyarrhythmias can also occur due to hyperkalemia, acute myocardial ischemia, digitalis toxicity, and antiarrhythmic drug therapy, particularly amiodarone and sotalol (see Table 4). The possibility of bradyarrhythmias should be considered when drugs that suppress sinus or AV node function are administered. Bradyarrhythmias caused 41% of unexpected cardiac arrests in hospitalized patients with advanced heart failure in one series. In patients with dilated cardiomyopathy, Schoeller and coworkers found that first-degree AV block and episodes of AV Wenckebach conduction during 24-hour electro-cardiogram recordings identified patients with an increased risk of sudden death. Occasionally, a persistent bradycardia aggravates heart failure. Some bradyarrhythmic cardiac arrests have been hypothesized to be mediated by vagal reflexes or release of endogenous adenosine. Administration of aminophylline, a competitive antagonist of adenosine, has been reported to reverse some bradyarrhythmias during inferior wall infarction or cardiac arrest. Sleep disturbances with periods of peripheral oxygen desaturation are common in heart failure, and can precipitate vagally mediated reflex bradycardia. Whether treatment of sleep apnea would prevent some bradyarrhythmic cardiac arrests is unknown.

SELECTED REFERENCES

Bashir Y, Sneddon JF, Staunton A, et al. Effects of long-term oral magnesium chloride replacement in congestive heart failure secondary to coronary artery disease. *Am J Cardiol* 1993;72:1156–1162.

Chelimsky-Fallick C, Middlekauff HR, Stevenson WG, et al. Amiodarone therapy does not compromise subsequent heart transplantation. *J Am Coll Cardiol* 1992;20:1556–1561.

Falk RH. Proarrhythmia in patients treated for atrial fibrillation or flutter. *Ann Intern Med* 1992;117:141–150.

Fenelon G, Wijns W, Andries E, Brugada P. Tachycardiomyopathy: mechanisms and clinical implications. *Pacing Clin Electrophysiol* 1996; 19:95–106.

Gettes LS. Electrolyte abnormalities underlying lethal ventricular arrhythmias. *Circulation* 1992;85:70–76.

Kim SG, Fisher JD, Choue CW, et al. Influence of left ventricular function on outcome of patients treated with implantable defibrillators. *Circulation* 1992;85:1304–1310.

Kim SG, Roth JA, Fisher JD, et al. Long-term outcomes and modes of death of patients treated with nonthoracotomy implantable defibrillators. *Am J Cardiol* 1995;75:1229–1232.

Kowey PR, Levine JH, Herre JM, et al. Randomized, double-blind comparison of intravenous amiodarone and bretylium in the treatment of patients with recurrent, hemodynamically destabilizing ventricular tachycardia or fibrillation. *Circulation* 1995;92:3255–3263.

Packer M. Hemodynamic consequences of antiarrhythmic drug therapy in patients with chronic congestive heart failure. *J Cardiovasc Electrophysiol* 1991;25:240–247.

Ravid S, Podrid PJ, Lampert S, Lown B. Congestive heart failure induced by six of the newer antiarrhythmic drugs. *J Am Coll Cardiol* 1989;14: 1326–1330.

Raitt MH, Johnson G, Dolack GL, et al. Clinical predictors of the defibrillation threshold with the unipolar implantable defibrillation system. *J Am Coll Cardiol* 1995;25:1576–1583.

Schoeller R, Andresen D, Büttner P, Oezcelik K, Vey G, Schröder R. First- or second-degree atrioventricular block as a risk factor in idiopathic dilated cardiomyopathy. *Am J Cardiol* 1993;71:720–726.

Stevenson WG, Middlekauff HR, Saxon LA. Ventricular arrhythmias in heart failure. In: Zipes DP, Jaife J, eds. *Cardiac electrophysiology: from cell to bedside.* Philadelphia: WB Saunders, 1995:848–863.

Stevenson WG, Stevenson LW, Middlekauff HR, Saxon LA. Sudden death prevention in patients with advanced ventricular dysfunction. *Circulation* 1993;88:2953–2961.

Stevenson WG, Sweeney MO. Pharmacologic and nonpharmacologic treatment of ventricular arrhythmias in heart failure. *Curr Opin Cardiol* 1997;12:242–250.

Sweeney MO, Ruskin JN, Garan H, et al. Influence of the implantable cardioverter/defibrillator on sudden death and total mortality in patients evaluated for cardiac transplantation. *Circulation* 1995;92:3273–3281.

Tomaselli GF, Beuckelmann DJ, Calkins HG, et al. Sudden cardiac death in heart failure: the role of abnormal repolarization. *Circulation* 1994;90: 2534–2539.

Zipes DP, Roberts D. Results of the international study of the implantable pacemaker cardioverter–defibrillator: a comparison of epicardial and endocardial lead systems: The Pacemaker–Cardioverter–Defibrillator Investigators. *Circulation* 1995;92:59–65.

Management of End-Stage Heart Disease, edited by Eric A. Rose and Lynne Warner Stevenson. Lippincott–Raven Publishers, Philadelphia ©1998.

CHAPTER 8

Permanent Pacemaker Therapy for Improvement of Cardiac Function in Advanced Heart Failure

Leslie A. Saxon

The primary indication for permanent pacemaker placement is symptomatic bradycardia, and over 160,000 pacemakers are implanted annually in the United States. Most of these pacemakers are transvenous and support the heart rate by either pacing the right atrial appendage and right ventricular apex (dual-chamber pacemakers) or the right ventricular apex alone (single-chamber pacemakers).

Conduction system disease consisting of varying degrees of atrioventricular (AV) block or bundle branch block accompanies myocardial disease in advanced heart failure, and approximately 10% of patients require pacemakers for rate support. Expansion of the traditional indications for pacemakers in patients with advanced heart failure is an area of active investigational interest. Pacemakers may be of therapeutic value in advanced heart failure by (a) optimizing AV contraction and (b) improving the timing and efficiency of ventricular contraction. The expanded use of pacemakers for these functions has far-reaching therapeutic and economic ramifications, particularly given the growing population of patients with advanced heart failure who remain symptomatic on optimal medical therapy.

DUAL-CHAMBER PACING WITH PROGRAMMED SHORT ATRIOVENTRICULAR DELAY

Background

First-degree AV block has been identified as a risk factor for cardiac death in idiopathic dilated cardiomyopathy and is observed in an estimated 30% of patients with advanced heart failure. The presence of first-degree block may worsen hemodynamic status by causing a delayed and ineffective atrial contraction, resulting in abbreviation of the diastolic filling time and diastolic mitral regurgitation. However, in many patients with advanced heart failure, atrial mechanical contraction is ineffective because of atrial dilatation and chronic mitral regurgitation. Moreover, the importance of atrial transport function to overall cardiac performance in patients with advanced heart failure is debated. It has traditionally been held, on the basis of acute pacing studies performed in patients with coronary artery disease, that the contribution of atrial transport function to overall cardiac function increases as left ventricular function worsens. In the presence of an effective mechanical atrial contraction, ventricular filling depends on the diastolic filling properties of the left ventricle, including left ventricular diastolic pressure and volume. Hemodynamic studies performed in patients with advanced heart failure at rest, during atrial and ventricular pacing, have identified two types of responses to the loss of atrial transport. One group of patients with significant elevations in ventricular filling pressure and volume have been described who experience little augmentation of cardiac output with atrial versus ventricular pacing. In this group, the heart may be acting on the flat rather than steep portion of the ventricular function curve, where myocardial fiber stretch is maximal. In another group of patients with less significant elevations in ventricular filling pressure and volume, atrial transport appears to contribute significantly to cardiac output. In this group, the heart may be acting on the steep portion of the ventricular function curve. To complicate matters further, marked variability in the contribution of

Department of Cardiac Electrophysiology, University of California at San Francisco, San Francisco, California 94143-1354 atrial transport to cardiac performance has been observed between patients with similar ventricular filling pressures and degrees of ventricular dilatation.

Shortening the time to atrial contraction by dual-chamber pacing with a programmed short AV delay may in theory improve cardiac function by a number of mechanisms, including pacing-related (a) increases in right and left ventricular diastolic filling times by prevention of mitral valve preclosure resulting from premature elevation of ventricular end-diastolic pressure over left atrial pressure, as observed with delayed atrial contraction; and (b) optimization of ventricular preload at the onset of ventricular contraction by decreasing diastolic mitral regurgitation resulting from mitral valve preclosure.

Review of Published Data

Table 1 summarizes the results of acute and chronic pacing studies in the published literature evaluating the effects of short AV delay pacing on cardiac function in patients with advanced heart failure. Hochleitner et al. performed an uncontrolled dual-chamber pacing study in 17 patients with decompensated heart failure due to dilated cardiomyopathy, 7 of whom were awaiting cardiac transplantation. First-degree AV block was present in half of the study subjects, and no subject had a history of symptomatic bradycardia. Permanent dual-chamber pacemakers were implanted and programmed to an AV delay of 100 milliseconds. Marked improvement in subjective and objective measures of cardiac function were observed throughout a 5-year follow-up interval. In the year before pacemaker implantation, all patients had required multiple hospital admissions for exacerbation of

heart failure, and no patients required hospitalization for worsening heart failure after pacemaker placement. Median survival time after implantation was 22 months, with no patient dying of progressive pump dysfunction. Marked improvement in left ventricular ejection fraction was observed, and the degree of cardiac dilatation was reported to be reduced. The finding of decreased ventricular chamber size was attributed to decreases in wall stress caused by early excitation of the right ventricular apex with ventricular pacing. In subsequent studies, right ventricular apical pacing has not been demonstrated to reduce wall stress or prevent dilatation in the failing ventricle. On the contrary, right ventricular apical pacing has been associated with decreases in regional left ventricular ejection fraction and increased hemodynamic deterioration in patients with advanced heart failure with pacemakers implanted for bradycardia indications. Nonetheless, the dramatic improvements observed in this critically ill group of patients prompted a number of other investigators to design further acute and chronic controlled studies.

Brecker et al. performed an acute study with a randomized cross-over design to evaluate short AV delay pacing in 12 patients with ischemic and idiopathic dilated cardiomyopathy in association with AV valve regurgitation. Five of 12 patients had first-degree AV block and 4 of 12 patients permanent pacemakers implanted for complete heart block. The duration of mitral and tricuspid regurgitation, ventricular filling times, and cardiac output were assessed by Doppler echocardiogram at rest and with cardiopulmonary exercise testing. Compared with baseline, programmed AV intervals of only 6 to 31 milliseconds resulted in small but statistically significant

TABLE 1. *Short atrioventricular delay pacing in advanced heart failure*

Study	No. Patient	AV delay (msec)	NYHA (nonpaced/ paced)	Left ventricular function (nonpaced/paced)	Study design (acute/chronic)	Follow-up (mo)
Hochleitner et al., 1990, 1992	17	100	IV/II	19±3%/30±4% LVEF $p = 0.001$	Chronic, uncontrolled	72
Kataoka et al., 1991	1	100	IV/III	10%/29% LVEF	Acute and chronic, uncontrolled	4
Brecker et al., 1992	12	6–31	III	3.9 L/min/5.0 L/min Cardiac output[a] $p = 0.01$	Acute, blinded cross-over	—
Guardigli et al., 1994	10	100	IV	40.2%/43.6% LVEF $p = 0.001$	Acute and chronic, uncontrolled	2
Linde et al., 1995	10	50–120	III/IV	1.9±0.6 L/min/2.2±1.1 L/min Cardiac output $p = 0.10$	Chronic, uncontrolled	6
Gold et al. 1995	12	100	III/III	18±4%/16±6% LVEF $p = $ NS	Acute and chronic, randomized cross-over	2–3
Nishimuru et al., 1995	15	60–240	III	3.0±1 L/min/3.9±0.43 L/min Cardiac output[a] $p = 0.005$	Acute	—
Shinbane et al., 1997	9	50–200	IV	4.8±2 L/min/5.0±2 L/min Cardiac output[a] $p = 0.29$	Acute randomized	—

AV, atrioventricular; NrHA, New York Heart Association; LVEF, left ventricular ejection fraction.
[a]Cardiac output obtained at the "optimal" AV delay.

improvements in cardiac output, exercise duration, peak oxygen consumption, and subjective symptoms of breathlessness. Improvement in forward cardiac output was attributed to improvement in diastolic filling time resulting from pacing-induced diminution of presystolic and systolic AV valve regurgitation.

Nishimura et al. performed an elegant hemodynamic study of temporary dual-chamber pacing in 15 patients with advanced heart failure due to ischemic and dilated cardiomyopathy (mean left ventricular ejection fraction, 19%). First-degree AV block was present in eight patients, and six patients had significant mitral regurgitation. Left atrial and ventricular pressures were measured directly and cardiac output calculated by the thermodilution technique. Doppler mitral inflow velocity was recorded simultaneously with left atrial and left ventricular pressures at AV delays ranging from 60 to 240 milliseconds. In contrast to earlier studies, no significant change in left atrial pressure or cardiac output was observed with short AV delay pacing compared with baseline normal sinus rhythm. More important, there was a wide variation in cardiac output response to the short AV delay pacing between patients. Patients with baseline first-degree AV block had measured improvement in cardiac output with optimization of AV delay guided by pressure and Doppler measurements, but there was clearly no universal AV delay that resulted in improvement in all subjects with first-degree AV block or mitral regurgitation. Patients without AV block had longer diastolic filling times with short AV delay pacing, but cardiac output fell because of atrial contraction occurring with the onset of ventricular contraction. Patients with ineffective atrial contraction did not benefit from any paced AV delay because there was no contribution from atrial contraction to mitral flow velocity or atrial or ventricular pressure.

Two additional, well-designed, blinded, cross-over, acute and chronic studies of short AV delay pacing in patients with advanced heart failure were performed by Gold et al. and Shinbane et al. These studies did not find improvement in any measure of heart failure status or left ventricular function with short AV delay pacing.

Discussion

Current data do not support the indiscriminate use of dual-chamber pacemakers with short AV delay programming as therapy for improvement of cardiac function in advanced heart failure. In spite of early enthusiasm generated by uncontrolled studies, subsequent, carefully performed acute and chronic studies suggested that there is no universal AV delay for optimization of the atrial contribution to ventricular filling in advanced heart failure. A subset of patients with advanced heart failure with first-degree AV block and diastolic or systolic AV valve regurgitation may benefit from dual-chamber pacemaker implantation with AV interval programming guided by careful acute hemodynamic and Doppler assessment.

MULTISITE VENTRICULAR PACING

Background

In advanced heart failure, structural changes in ventricular muscle resulting from ventricular hypertrophy, prior dense infarct scar, or myocardial fibrosis compromise electrical activation and mechanical contraction. Electrical excitation wavefronts may be delayed in the atria and ventricles because of direct pathologic involvement of the conduction system or inhomogenous spread of excitation wavefronts across scarred tissue. Manifest bundle branch block is present in roughly 20% of patients with advanced heart failure, but virtually all patients have some degree of atrial and ventricular conduction delay.

Pacemakers capable of pacing the right or left atrium followed by the simultaneous activation of the right and left ventricles may improve ventricular function by (a) reestablishing normal ventricular activation patterns and narrowing QRS duration, (b) promoting early recruitment of ventricular muscle mass critical to effective contraction, (c) resynchronizing intraventricular septal motion, and (d) decreasing volume and pressure dissipation to ventricular segments incapable of effective mechanical contraction.

Review of Published Data

Several uncontrolled studies, presented in abstract form, have reported dramatic improvements in cardiac function with implantation of pacemakers incorporating a left ventricular epicardial apical pacing electrode and custom-made Y adapter, allowing for simultaneous pacing of the right and left ventricular apices. These studies were performed in hospitalized patients with advanced heart failure succumbing to progressive pump dysfunction on intravenous inotropes. In these initial reports, all patients had manifest bundle branch block, and QRS duration was shortened with simultaneous biventricular apical pacing. Most patients survived to hospital discharge with improvements in functional class and exercise duration. However, the reliability of left ventricular capture with these custom-made pacing systems was poor, and several patients required revision of the pacing systems.

Cazeau et al. reported on eight patients with advanced heart failure due to ischemic and dilated cardiomyopathy who underwent either revision of standard pacing systems (four patients) or implantation of new biventricular pacing systems for refractory heart failure. An acute hemodynamic study was performed before permanent pacemaker placement to determine the optimal atrial and right ventricular pacing site (right ventricular apex vs. right ventricular outflow tract). For chronic pacing, the left ventricular lead was placed on the lateral left ventricular wall through the coronary sinus vein (two patients) or the posterolateral wall of left ventricular epicardium, with exposure to the left heart obtained by limited thoracotomy. Of the eight patients who were scheduled to undergo implantation of a chronic biventricular pacing system, one died before surgery of pump failure, one succumbed to intractable ventricular fibrillation during the operative procedure, and two patients died within 3 months of implant. Of the four surviving patients, two lost left ventricular capture, requiring surgical revision of the left ventricular lead. At a mean follow-up of 6 months, all four patients had observed improvements in functional class. In this study, neither atrial nor biventricular lead placement was standardized; each patient received a customized system shown to result in improved hemodynamics during the acute study. The placement of the left ventricular lead was highly variable, and was unreliable for maintenance of chronic left ventricular capture.

In an effort to determine optimal biventricular pacing sites, Saxon et al. performed an acute operative study with epicardial pacing electrodes placed on the left ventricular apex, right ventricular apex, and right ventricular outflow tract. These sites were paced separately and simultaneous biventricular pacing was performed between the left ventricular apex and right ventricular outflow tract or left ventricular apex and right ventricular apex. A total of 11 patients with depressed ventricular function undergoing elective coronary bypass or aortic valve replacement were studied. The narrowest paced QRS duration was obtained with simultaneous biventricular apical pacing. Improvement in left ventricular fractional area change above baseline values (measured by transesophageal echocardiography) was obtained with simultaneous biventricular apical pacing and not with simultaneous right ventricular outflow tract and left ventricular apical pacing. Simultaneous left and right ventricular apical pacing resulted in a complete resequencing of left ventricular activation/contraction as assessed by phase-analysis comparison of baseline and paced echocardiographic images.

There is an ongoing multicenter study of simultaneous biventricular apical pacing in stable patients with functional Class II to III advanced heart failure (The Vigor Congestive Heart Failure Trial) that is sponsored by Guidant Corporation (Minneapolis, Minnesota). Patients are eligible for enrollment with idiopathic or ischemic cardiomyopathy, bundle branch block, and left ventricular ejection fraction less than 30%. A dual-chamber biventricular pacemaker capable of simultaneous right and left ventricular pacing is being used, incorporating an endocardial right atrial and right ventricular apical lead and an epicardial left ventricular lead. Patients are randomized at implantation to a paced or nonpaced mode for the initial study interval, and thereafter all patients undergo atrial-sensed biventricular pacing. Placement of the left ventricular epicardial apical lead has been standardized, and access to the left ventricular apex is achieved through a small thoracotomy incision. The study end-points include peak oxygen consumption measured with cardiopulmonary exercise testing, the 6-minute walk test, and left ventricular ejection fraction. Cost and health care utilization data will also be collected.

Figure 1 illustrates a 12-lead electrocardiogram in normal sinus rhythm and with atrially sensed biventricular pacing in a Vigor-CHF patient with a left ventricular ejection fraction of 10% due to idiopathic dilated cardiomyopathy. In normal sinus rhythm, the QRS morphology in lead V_6 (placed over the left ventricular apex) is upright and consistent with late activation of the left ventricle. In paced rhythm, a marked shift in the frontal plane axis and lead V_6 QRS morphology is observed with biventricular pacing, indicating that the predominant left ventricular activation wavefront is proceeding away from the left ventricular apex, consistent with pacing-induced early left ventricular apical activation. Figure 2 is a nuclear blood pool scan obtained in this patient at rest with phase imaging applied to assess the activation/contraction sequence. The areas in light gray demonstrate earliest cardiac activation/contraction. The phase histogram on the left side of the image is a measure of the duration of atrial and ventricular contraction. Gross inspection of the cardiac image indicates marked inhomogeneity of biventricular activation/contraction, with the entire right ventricle (shown in light gray) activated before the left ventricle and intraventricular septum (shown in dark gray). A portion of the septum and left ventricular apex demonstrates late contraction timing with atrial contraction. The image on the right was recorded with the pacemaker programmed to dual-chamber biventricular pacing. Inspection of the phase histogram shows a decrease in the biventricular activation/

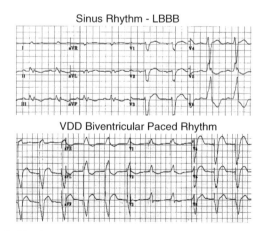

FIG. 1. Twelve-lead electrocardiograms in normal sinus rhythm with left bundle branch block and atrial-paced, ventricular-sensed (VDD) simultaneous biventricular pacing. See text for explanation.

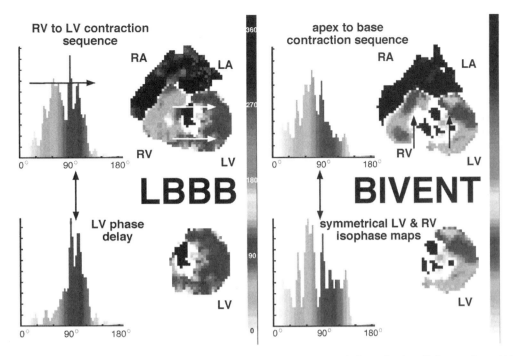

FIG. 2. Nuclear blood pool scan with phase-color imaging in normal sinus rhythm (*left panel*) and VDD simultaneous biventricular pacing (*right panel*). See text for explanation.

contraction time with a clear separation of atrial (shown in dark gray) from right and left ventricular contraction (shown in lighter gray). The cardiac image demonstrates early activation/contraction of the left ventricular apex consistent with simultaneous right and left ventricular contraction and biventricular activation proceeding from apex to base. In this acute study, a modest increase in left ventricular ejection fraction was demonstrated with biventricular pacing (10%–17%).

There are two additional studies of chronic biventricular pacing for advanced heart failure currently enrolling patients in Europe, Pacing Therapies-Congestive Heart Failure (PATH-CHF) (Guidant Corporation) and InSync (Medtronic, Inc., Minneapolis, Minnesota).

Discussion

Biventricular pacing appears to improve ventricular function in patients with decompensated advanced heart failure and intraventricular conduction delay. In acute studies, biventricular pacing results in preexcitation of the ventricular apices and global resynchronization of biventricular contraction. The ongoing controlled studies of patients with biventricular pacing will determine if improvement in objective measures of heart function are achieved with this therapy. If the results of these studies are favorable, identification of an advanced heart failure population beyond those with intraventricular conduction delay who may benefit from biventricular pacing is critical before recommending this therapy to the larger population of patients with heart failure.

Advances in chronic pacing lead technology are also needed so that the left ventricle can be paced reliably with a transvenous lead deployed through the coronary sinus into the left ventricular coronary sinus branch veins, to allow for a minimally invasive implant procedure. Further studies are needed to determine if simultaneous biventricular apical pacing is superior to simultaneous pacing at other sites on the right or left ventricle, and to determine if simultaneous biventricular pacing is superior to pacing the right and left ventricles in sequence.

ABLATION OF THE ATRIOVENTRICULAR NODE AND RATE-RESPONSIVE VENTRICULAR PACING IN ESTABLISHED ATRIAL FIBRILLATION

Background

Atrial fibrillation is present in 15% to 30% of patients with advanced heart failure. Low-dose amiodarone therapy has been shown to have a low incidence of serious side effects and to be superior to placebo therapy in maintaining normal sinus rhythm. However, a significant percentage of patients are either intolerant of chronic amiodarone therapy or experience recurrent atrial fibrillation. In these patients, controlling the resting and activity related ventricular rate response to atrial fibrillation with medical therapy can be difficult. Medical therapy with AV nodal blocking agents such as the calcium or beta blockers often requires dosages that encounter patient intolerance because of the cardiodepressant effects of these medications. In addition, none of the medical therapies can achieve ventricular rate regularity, which may be beneficial in patients with advanced heart failure with atrial fibrillation. The irregular ventricular response present in atrial fibrillation results in beat-to-beat variability in ventricular filling, intensity of left ventricular contractility, and blood pressure. In advanced patients with heart failure, these beat-to-beat changes may result in further increases in sympathetic tone and salt and water retention.

Radiofrequency catheter ablation of the AV node and implantation of a rate-responsive ventricular pacemaker have been shown to be safe and effective procedures for creating AV block and providing physiologic ventricular rate support. In a general population of patients with a rapid ventricular response to atrial fibrillation, improvements in quality of life and health care costs have been demonstrated with ablation of the AV node and permanent pacemaker implantation. In patients with compromised ventricular function and atrial fibrillation, improvement in cardiac function may occur after AV node ablation and pacing because of (a) reversal of tachycardia-mediated cardiomyopathy with attainment of ventricular rate control, or (b) optimization of ventricular dynamics by establishing rate regularity.

Review of Published Data

Table 2 summarizes studies in the literature that include patients with depressed ventricular function and atrial fibrillation to assess the effects of establishing ventricular rate control and regularity.

Grogan et al. studied ten patients with atrial fibrillation and functional Class III heart failure attributed to idiopathic dilated cardiomyopathy by controlling the ventricular rate with AV nodal blocking agents or by electrical cardioversion. The mean pretreatment ventricular rate at rest was 140 beats/minute. With medical therapy or cardioversion, all patients had posttreatment ventricular rates less that 80 beats/minute. Over a follow-up interval of 30 months, left ventricular ejection fraction increased from a mean of 25% to 52%. The results of this important study suggest that a chronic rapid ventricular response to

atrial fibrillation may independently result in ventricular dysfunction, which is reversible with control of the ventricular response. However, in this study, medical control of the ventricular rate response was achieved with antiarrhythmic agents, such as flecainide and encainide, known to be associated with proarrhythmia in patients with compromised ventricular function. Therefore, other investigators evaluated the role of AV node ablation and pacing to control the ventricular response.

In three separate studies Heinz et al., Twidale et al., and Brignole et al. reported on a total of 28 patients with ventricular dysfunction and atrial fibrillation and demonstrated improvements in ventricular function and exercise duration with AV node ablation and physiologic ventricular pacing. In these studies, withdrawal of medications previously used to control the ventricular response was possible, and some of the observed improvement in cardiac function may be due to withdrawal of the cardiodepressant effects of these medications.

Natale et al. performed a prospective study to evaluate the role of AV node ablation and pacing to achieve rate regularity, independent of rate control, in 14 patients with heart failure due to ischemic and dilated cardiomyopathy. All patients had a controlled ventricular response (>60 and <100 beats/minute) on 24-hour Holter recording. No patient required therapy with antiarrhythmic or AV nodal blocking medications to control the ventricular rate response. At the predetermined follow-up interval of 12 months, significant improvements in left ventricular ejection fraction, heart failure symptom severity, and quality-of-life scores were observed. This was the first chronic pacing study to document improvement in cardiac function in patients with heart failure by establishing ventricular rate regularity with pacing.

Discussion

In patients with advanced heart failure with atrial fibrillation, control of the ventricular rate response and establishment of rate regularity may result in improvement in ventricular function. A subset of patients with atrial fibrillation associated with a rapid ventricular response may have marked improvement in cardiac func-

TABLE 2. *Control of ventricular rate and regularity in advanced heart failure and atrial fibrillation*

Study	Patient no.	Left ventricular function[a]	Study design (acute/chronic)	Follow-up (mo)
Grogan et al., 1992	10	25%/52% LVEF	Chronic, uncontrolled	30
Heinz et al., 1992	5	21%/31% Fractional shortening $p = 0.02$	Acute and chronic, uncontrolled	2.5
Twidale et al., 1993	14	42%/47% LVEF	Acute and chronic, uncontrolled	1.5
Brignole et al., 1994	9[b]	23%/31% LVEF	Acute and chronic, controlled, randomized	3
Natale et al., 1996	14[b]	30%/39% LVEF $p < 0.001$	Acute and chronic, uncontrolled	12

LVEF, left ventricular ejection fraction.
[a]Percentages before and after control of ventricular rate and regularity.
[b]Number of study patients with advanced heart failure.

tion with ventricular rate control, suggesting a tachycardia-mediated cardiomyopathy.

The Dilated Cardiomyopathy and Atrial Fibrillation Trial (DCAF) is an ongoing, multicenter, randomized study designed to determine if AV node ablation and pacing is superior to standard medications used to control the ventricular rate response in chronic atrial fibrillation occurring in the setting of dilated cardiomyopathy. Study end-points include assessment of left ventricular ejection fraction, the 6-minute walk test, and quality-of-life measures. It is expected that this study will help define the optimal treatment of chronic atrial fibrillation occurring in patients with advanced heart failure.

CONCLUSIONS

The results of studies performed since the mid-1980s suggest that permanent pacemakers may benefit patients with advanced heart failure by optimizing ventricular function. The added benefit of any one of the novel pacing modalities discussed in this chapter, used alone or together in a combined device, over current medical therapy for advanced heart failure is unknown. Ongoing controlled studies will help clarify the role of pacing in heart failure and provide information on the economic and quality-of-life impact of these devices.

SELECTED REFERENCES

Bakker PF, Meijburg H, de Jonge N, et al. Beneficial effects of biventricular pacing in congestive heart failure. *Pacing Clin Electrophysiol* 1994; 17:820(abst).

Cazeau S, Ritter P, Lazarus A, et al. Multisite pacing for end-stage heart failure: early experience. *Pacing Clin Electrophysiol* 1996;19:1748–1757.

Gold M, Feliciano Z, Gottlieb S, Fisher ML. Dual-chamber pacing with a short atrioventricular delay in congestive heart failure: a randomized study. *J Am Coll Cardiol* 1995;26:967–973.

Greenberg B, Chatterjee K, Parmley WW, et al. The influence of left ventricular filling pressure on atrial contribution to cardiac output. *Am Heart J* 1979;98:742–751.

Hochleitner M, Hörtnagl H, Hörtnagl H, Fridrich L, Gschnitzer F. Long-term efficacy of physiologic dual-chamber pacing in the treatment of end-stage idiopathic dilated cardiomyopathy. *Am J Cardiol* 1992;70:1320–1325.

Kusumoto FM, Goldschlager N. Cardiac pacing. *N Engl J Med* 1996;334:89–98.

Mukharji J, Rehr RB, Hastillo A, et al. Comparison of atrial contribution to cardiac hemodynamics in patients with normal and severely compromised cardiac function. *Clin Cardiol* 1990;13:639–643.

Nishimura RA, Hayes DL, Holmes DR Jr, Tajik AJ. Mechanism of hemodynamic improvement by dual-chamber pacing for severe left ventricular dysfunction: an acute Doppler and catheterization hemodynamic study. *J Am Coll Cardiol* 1995;25:281–288.

Saxon LA. Atrial fibrillation and dilated cardiomyopathy: therapeutic strategies when sinus rhythm cannot be maintained. *Pacing Clin Electrophysiol* 1997;20:720–725.

Saxon LA, Kerwin W, Calahan MK, et al. Acute effects of multisite ventricular pacing on left ventricular function and activation/contraction sequence in patients with depressed ventricular function. *J Cardiovasc Electrophysiol* 1997;9:13–21.

Saxon LA, Natterson PD, DeLurgio DB, et al. Biventricular pacing may provide inotropic support in refractory heart failure. *Journal of Investigational Medicine* 1995;43:I-198(Abstract).

Saxon LA, Stevenson WG, Middlekauff HR, Stevenson LW. Increased risk of progressive hemodynamic deterioration in advanced heart failure patients requiring permanent pacemakers. *Am Heart J* 1993;125:1306–1310.

Shinbane J, Chu E, DeMarco T, et al. Evaluation of acute dual chamber pacing with a range of atrioventricular delays on cardiac performance in refractory heart failure. *J Am Coll Cardiol* 1997;30:1295–1300.

Stevenson WG, Stevenson LW, Middlekauff HR, et al. Improving survival for patients with advanced heart failure: a study of 737 consecutive patients. *J Am Coll Cardiol* 1995;26:1417–1423.

Management of End-Stage Heart Disease, edited by Eric A. Rose and Lynne Warner Stevenson. Lippincott–Raven Publishers, Philadelphia ©1998.

CHAPTER 9

Exercise Capacity in Heart Failure: Impairment and Improvement

Donna M. Mancini

Physical exercise involves the interaction of the respiratory, cardiac, and vascular systems to meet the increased metabolic rate of the skeletal muscles. Although each system can in theory be the limiting step to maximal physical performance, exercise capacity is primarily limited by the cardiac output response to exercise in normal humans. In patients with congestive heart failure (CHF), changes that occur in the muscles, vasculature, and lungs affect peak exercise performance in such ways that cardiac output response alone is not the sole determinant of peak exercise capacity. In this chapter, the pathophysiology of potential exercise limitations in patients with heart failure, the clinical applications of exercise testing, with particular emphasis on the use of exercise testing for risk stratification, and the types of exercise tests used in the evaluation of these patients are discussed. The impact of various therapies on exercise performance in these patients, including medical, mechanical assist devices, and, in particular, aerobic training, is reviewed.

PATHOPHYSIOLOGY OF EXERCISE PERFORMANCE IN CONGESTIVE HEART FAILURE

Decreased Cardiac Output Response

Decreased exercise capacity in heart failure has been traditionally attributed in patients with CHF to a decreased cardiac output response to exercise, which leads to skeletal muscle underperfusion and intramuscular lactic acidosis. This is based on observations that patients with heart failure exhibit reduced cardiac output responses to exercise. In 1981, Karl Weber and colleagues

performed exercise hemodynamic measurements and ventilatory gas measurements during progressive treadmill exercise in 40 patients with heart failure. This represented the first large application of the measurement of oxygen consumption in patients with heart failure as a noninvasive method for characterizing cardiac reserve and functional status in these patients. Peak oxygen consumption ($\dot{V}O_2$) provides a noninvasive assessment of the cardiac output response to exercise. Derived from the Fick equation, $\dot{V}O_2$ equals the difference between oxygen delivery and oxygen extraction. Oxygen delivery depends on cardiac output, pulmonary function, and hemoglobin content. Oxygen extraction relies primarily on the metabolic capacity of the skeletal muscle, its ability to vasodilate and extract oxygen. In subjects with a normal hemoglobin and normal lung function who maximally exercise and thus achieve near-maximal oxygen extraction, $\dot{V}O_2$ primarily reflects the ability to increase cardiac output. In Weber and colleagues' study, cardiac index response to exercise expressed as a function of percent maximum $\dot{V}O_2$ demonstrated differences between patient groups stratified by peak $\dot{V}O_2$, that is, those patients with a $\dot{V}O_2$ less than 10 mL/kg/minute, $\dot{V}O_2$ between 10 to 15 mL/kg/minute, and $\dot{V}O_2$ greater than 15 mL/kg/minute (Figure 1). Class A comprises the least limited patients, corresponding to New York Heart Association (NYHA) Class I, and Class D includes the most limited patients, corresponding to NYHA Class IV CHF. With worsening heart failure, the cardiac output response is markedly diminished. A patient with Class D heart failure may increase his cardiac output only twofold, as opposed to the normal person, who can increase his cardiac output response by approximately fivefold.

We performed a similar analysis in a larger series of 65 patients using bicycle exercise. Twenty-nine percent of patients had NYHA Class II, 65% had Class III, and 6%

Department of Medicine, Columbia-Presbyterian Medical Center, New York, New York 10032

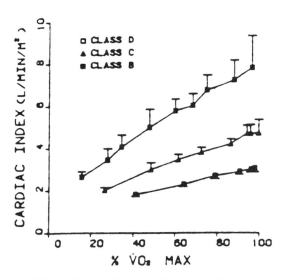 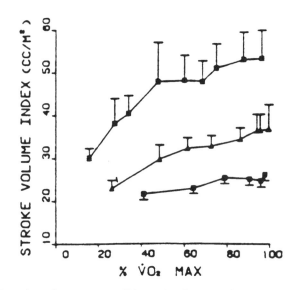

FIG. 1. Cardiac index and stroke volume index as a function of percentage $\dot{V}O_{2max}$ for Class B, C, and D patients. (From Weber K, Kinasewitz G, Janicki J, Fishman A. Oxygen utilization and ventilation during exercise in patients with chronic cardiac failure. *Circulation* 1982;65:1213–1223, with permission.)

had Class IV heart failure symptomatology. Our results are concordant with Weber and colleagues' initial observations. A series of lines are generated with a progressively lower cardiac index as a function of percent $\dot{V}O_{2max}$ as the peak $\dot{V}O_2$ declines. We also observed a highly significant correlation between peak cardiac output and peak $\dot{V}O_2$, similar to prior reports. Thus, in this and other studies, there is a significant correlation between the peak $\dot{V}O_2$ and cardiac output.

However, other investigators have emphasized that peak exercise performance in patients with heart failure is determined not only by cardiac output response, but, as is discussed later, by the vasodilator capacity of the vascular smooth muscle, metabolic capacity of skeletal muscle, and pulmonary function. Wilson et al. reported that 56% of patients with heart failure had a normal cardiac output response to exercise, and that in these patients peripheral factors were the major limitation to exercise performance. In our series, only 6% of the patients with heart failure had a normal cardiac output response. At first analysis, these results appear dramatically different. In actuality, the results are only semantically different. Although Wilson et al. concluded that more than half their population had a normal cardiac output response to exercise, the peak cardiac output of this patient cohort was only 8.5 L/minute. Of normal subjects, from whom Wilson et al. primarily derived their formula, less than 5% had a peak cardiac output in this range. Thus, in terms of absolute cardiac output, the exercise response in patients with heart failure is markedly abnormal, although it can be described by a linear equation similar to the one in normal subjects. Because oxygen consumption is the product of the cardiac output and the arteriovenous oxygen ($A\dot{V}O_2$) dif-

ference, the relationship between oxygen consumption and cardiac output should be linear, with the arteriovenous oxygen difference describing the slope. Higginbotham et al. described this relationship during bicycle exercise in 102 normal subjects. A similar relation was observed in patients with heart failure in our study. Indeed, the slopes of the two equations were the same, with the normal and heart failure groups described by different segments of the same line. Deviations from this line are likely due to differences in the arteriovenous oxygen difference, which depends primarily on muscle metabolic function.

Abnormal Peripheral Vasodilatation

Although peak oxygen consumption clearly depends on the cardiac output response to exercise, patients with similarly reduced left ventricular ejection fractions have a wide range of exercise capacity. Moreover, therapeutic interventions that acutely enhance exercise hemodynamic measurements do not increase exercise capacity. Dobutamine is a potent positive inotropic agent with combined beta1- and beta2-agonist activity. Administered at rest and during exercise, it results in significant hemodynamic benefits, with decreased pulmonary capillary wedge pressure and increased cardiac index at rest and throughout exercise. However, despite a substantial hemodynamic improvement, peak $\dot{V}O_2$ is minimally increased in these patients. Peripheral vasodilatation in the metabolically nonactive vascular beds may augment the cardiac output during exercise, with a narrowing of the $\dot{V}O_2$ difference. However, blood flow to the exercising muscles is not increased, and therefore maximal oxygen uptake remains essentially unchanged. The inability to increase exercise capacity in patients with heart failure may be due to an abnormality in arteriolar vasodilatation.

Zelis et al., in a series of elegant studies, demonstrated that fluid and sodium retention can impair arteriolar vasodilatation in humans. Rhythmic grip exercise of three different intensities was performed in 7 patients with right heart failure due to rheumatic heart disease and 22 control subjects with forearm blood flow measured using venous plethysmography. Forearm blood flow was reduced at rest and each level of exercise in patients with heart failure (Figure 2). Forearm oxygen extraction calculated from brachial venous and systemic arterial blood was also found to be consistently increased. This type of small muscle mass exercise does not require any significant increase in cardiac output, and thus the difference in forearm perfusion is not related to central hemodynamic factors.

Using a canine model of heart failure produced by rapid ventricular pacing, Zelis et al. also measured the arterial sodium content in the aorta and femoral artery in control and heart failure animals. A significant increase in the arterial sodium content in the heart failure animals was demonstrated. Zelis et al. postulated that arteriolar stiffness from increased salt and water content resulted in an abnormal vasodilatory response in heart failure. Increased sympathetic tone and an activated renin–angiotensin system are two potential mechanisms for the reduced arterial vasodilatory capacity in heart failure.

Abnormality in vasodilation may also result from changes in the vascular endothelium as well as the vascular smooth muscle. Endothelial cells produce an endothelium-derived relaxing factor (i.e., nitric oxide) that promotes local relaxation of vascular smooth muscle. Kubo et al. demonstrated that endothelium-dependent vasodilation is attenuated in patients with heart failure. Forearm blood

flow assessed by plethysmography was measured at rest and during intraarterial infusions of methacholine and nitroprusside. Metacholine releases endothelium-derived relaxing factor through stimulation of muscarinic receptors. Forearm blood flow responses to two doses of metacholine were attenuated in patients with heart failure compared with normal subjects of similar age. Forearm blood flow responses to intraarterial nitroprusside administration tended to be lower in patients with heart failure than in normal subjects. Thus, endothelial-derived vasodilation is clearly abnormal in patients with heart failure. Katz et al. confirmed these findings. Moreover, their results suggest that endothelium-independent vasodilation may also be abnormal in patients with CHF. Endothelial dysfunction of the resistance vessels impairs peripheral perfusion. Endothelial dysfunction of large conduit vessels may also have central hemodynamic effects by increasing impedance of the failing left ventricle and decreasing ejection fraction.

With chronic therapy of CHF, an improvement in leg blood flow does occur, resulting in improved exercise capacity. Using the xenon washout technique, Mancini et al. measured vastus lateralis perfusion before and after chronic treatment with captopril in eight patients with Class III to IV heart failure. Those patients who exhibited a rise in peak oxygen uptake also demonstrated a significant increase in peak skeletal muscle blood flow. Those patients who did not demonstrate an increase in peak oxygen uptake failed to experience a change in skeletal muscle blood flow. The excellent correlation between these variables supports the hypothesis that peak exercise capacity is flow limited, but the limitation is not centrally but peripherally mediated. Drexler et al. subsequently confirmed these findings in a larger, placebo-controlled trial using lisinopril. With long-term therapy, a readjust-

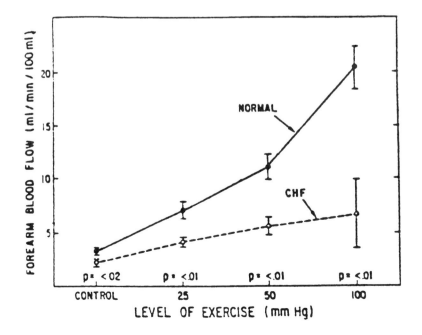

FIG. 2. Forearm blood flow at three levels of rhythmic handgrip exercise in patients with heart failure and normal subjects. (From Zelis R, et al. A comparison of regional blood flow and oxygen utilization during dynamic forearm exercise in normal subjects and patients with congestive heart failure. *Circulation* 1974;50:137–143, with permission.)

ment of the periphery mediated by interruption of the exaggerated neurohormonal function occurs. This translates into increased sodium excretion and improved aerobic capacity.

Intrinsic Skeletal Muscle Changes

A number of observations suggest that intrinsic skeletal muscle changes also contribute to exercise intolerance in heart failure. Metabolic abnormalities have been described during exercise using phosphorus-31 (^{31}P) magnetic resonance spectroscopy, which permits noninvasive monitoring of phosphocreatine, inorganic phosphate, adenosine triphosphate, and pH in working muscle. During exercise, adenosine diphosphate is a key stimulant to mitochrondrial oxidative phosphorylation. The inorganic phosphorus-to-phosphocreatine (Pi/PCr) ratio correlates closely with adenosine diphosphate concentration. By monitoring changes in the Pi/PCr ratio at different work levels, alterations in the control of oxidative phosphorylation can be detected. Exercise also activates glycolysis, producing an increase in intracellular lactate concentration and a decrease in intracellular pH. By monitoring changes in muscle pH during exercise, changes in glycolytic activity can be detected. The metabolic behavior of both the forearm and calf muscle during exercise in patients with heart failure has been examined. Patients with heart failure have a more pronounced increase in the Pi/PCr ratio and a more rapid drop in local pH than do normal subjects performing comparable workloads (Figure 3).

To determine if these metabolic abnormalities are due to skeletal muscle ischemia, plethysmographic blood flow was measured during forearm exercise in patients with heart failure and in normal subjects. There was no significant difference between forearm blood flow observed in patients and control subjects despite the presence of significant metabolic abnormalities suggesting that these abnormalities were not flow mediated. Massie and associates performed similar studies with identical results. These investigators also demonstrated persistent metabolic abnormalities compared with normal subjects even with ischemic exercise (i.e., exercise performed during arterial occlusion). Most recently, we have coupled ^{31}P magnetic resonance spectroscopy to near-infrared spectroscopy to provide simultaneous monitoring of cellular metabolism and oxygenation. Calf exercise was performed in normal subjects and patients with heart failure. This study revealed that the metabolism in the patients with heart failure was abnormal despite what appeared to be similar levels of oxygenation.

Muscle biopsy studies have also demonstrated histochemical abnormalities. A variety of histochemical changes were initially described by Lipkin et al. These included fiber atrophy and decreased oxidative enzymes. In percutaneous calf muscle biopsies obtained from 22 patients with

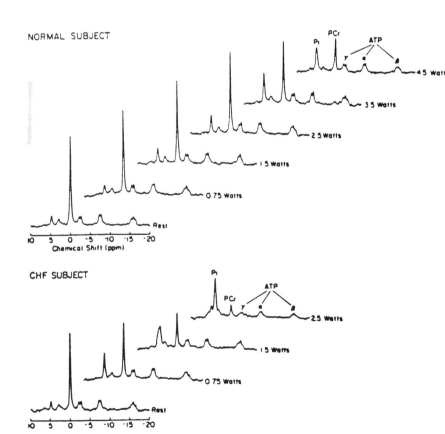

FIG. 3. Representative ^{31}P magnetic resonance spectroscopy spectra in a normal subject and a patient with congestive heart failure (CHF) at rest and during calf plantarflexion. Pi, inorganic phosphorus; PCr, phosphocreatine; ATP, adenosine triphosphate. (From Mancini DM, Wilson JR, Bolinger L, et al. *In vivo* magnetic resonance spectroscopy measurement of deoxymyoglobin during exercise in patients with heart failure: demonstration of abnormal muscle metabolism despite adequate oxygenation. *Circulation* 1994;90:500–508, with permission.)

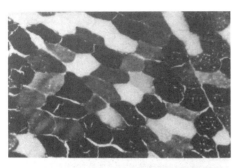
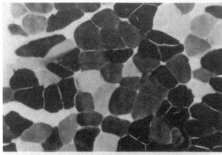
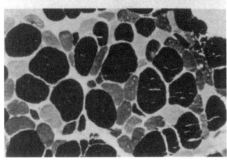

FIG. 4. Microphotographs of myofibrillar adenosine triphosphatase stain at pH 4.6 for a normal subject (*left panel*) and two representative patients with heart failure (*middle and right panels*). Black-stained fibers are Type I; gray fibers, IIb; and light fibers, IIa. In the middle panel, predominance of Type II fibers in patients with heart failure is shown. In the right panel, atrophy of Type II fibers in patients with heart failure is apparent because Type II fibers usually are equal to or larger than Type I fibers. (From Mancini DM, Coyle E, Coggan A, et al. Contribution of intrinsic skeletal muscle changes to ^{31}P NMR skeletal muscle metabolic abnormalities in patients with heart failure. *Circulation* 1989;80:1338–1346, with permission.)

heart failure, a significant increase in the percentage of Type IIb fibers (i.e., glycolytic, fast-twitch, easily fatigable fibers), Type II fiber atrophy, and a reduction in a lipolytic enzyme based in the mitochondria (i.e., beta-hydroxyl CoA dehydrogenase) were described (Figure 4). Sullivan et al. further expanded these findings and described a reduction in oxidative and glycolytic enzymes. Mitochrondrial changes, including a decrease in the volume and surface density of cristae, were described by Drexler et al.

In addition to fiber atrophy noted on muscle biopsy, patients also exhibit generalized muscle atrophy, again consistent with inactivity and deconditioning. Anthropomorphic measurements performed using Lange calipers

to measure skinfold fat thickness and arm circumference, and 24-hour urine collections for creatinine to estimate total muscle mass, were performed in 62 patients with heart failure. Patients with heart failure had adequate fat stores, but 60% had evidence of significant muscle loss. Calf muscle volume was also assessed with magnetic resonance imaging in 15 patients with heart failure and 10 control subjects. Magnetic resonance imaging studies revealed a reduced muscle volume in patients with heart failure. Significant water or fat infiltration was also noted in the muscle sections of these patients.

These intrinsic muscle changes are most likely due to deconditioning. Several studies demonstrate that aerobic training can improve maximal exercise capacity in patients with heart failure by 15% to 30%. These studies are discussed later in the section on aerobic training as a therapeutic modality for patients with heart failure. Other factors besides deconditioning may also contribute to the intrinsic skeletal muscle changes. Caloric protein malnutrition may occur; increased tissue necrosis factor, elevated serum cortisol, and chronic skeletal muscle underperfusion may also contribute to the skeletal muscle changes.

In a 1997 study, we examined the histochemical changes of the diaphragm in heart failure. If a generalized skeletal myopathy were to occur in heart failure from chronic underperfusion or cytokine activation, then similar biochemical changes would be anticipated in this muscle. As is discussed extensively in the following section, a number of pathophysiologic changes occur in the lung that lead to a markedly increased work of breathing in patients with heart failure. As a consequence of this, the diaphragm may be viewed as undergoing constant moderate-intensity exercise. Unlike in the limb musculature, the histochemical changes elicited in the diaphragm of patients with heart failure included an increase in the activity of citrate synthase, a decrease in the activity of lactate dehydrogenase, an increase in myosin heavy chain Type I isomer, and a significant decrease in myosin heavy chain Type IIB isomer. These changes were consistent with a shift from glycolytic to oxidative metabolism and imply that skeletal muscle changes are not generalized but organ specific.

Pulmonary Function Abnormalities

During exercise, patients clearly experience a greater sense of dyspnea than normal subjects at any given workload. Potential mechanisms for dyspnea in heart failure include decreased lung compliance, increased airway resistance, increased ventilatory drive from ventilation–perfusion mismatch or increased CO_2 production, and respiratory muscle dysfunction from respiratory weakness or ischemia. A pulmonary limitation to exercise performance may exist in some patients.

Airflow obstruction may contribute to reduced exercise performance. Cabanes et al. described bronchial hyperresponsiveness in patients with severely impaired left ventricular function after inhalation of the cholinergic agonist metacholine. Inhalation of the vasoconstrictive adrenergic agonist methoxamine prevented the methacholine-induced bronchial obstruction, suggesting that bronchial edema was partially etiologic for the bronchial hyperreactivity. The effect of methoxamine inhalation on exercise performance was also studied in 19 patients with heart failure. Two exercise protocols were performed: a constant maximal workload to assess the effects of inhaled methoxamine on the duration of exercise, and a graded maximal exercise with measurement of oxygen consumption. In both protocols, inhalation of methoxamine significantly improved exercise performance.

What has consistently been described in patients with heart failure is an excessive ventilatory response to exercise. With increasing severity of CHF, the ventilatory response is increased. The increase in ventilation during exercise does not appear to be related to acute increases in intrapulmonary pressure. No significant correlation is observed between the ventilatory response to exercise, expressed as ventilation normalized by CO_2 production versus peak exercise pulmonary capillary wedge pressure. Moreover, acute therapeutic interventions such as prazosin and dobutamine that acutely lower resting and exercise pulmonary capillary wedge pressures do not affect the ventilatory response to exercise.

A major factor contributing to the excess ventilatory response noted in patients with heart failure appears to be an increase in pulmonary dead space ventilation. Sullivan et al. performed exercise testing with measurement of respiratory gases in 64 patients with heart failure and 38 control subjects. Arterial blood samples were also obtained and dead space ventilation calculated using the Bohr equation. Sullivan et al. demonstrated that pulmonary dead space/breath nearly doubled during exercise in patients with heart failure, but remained unchanged in normal subjects. The etiology of this increased dead space ventilation is unclear.

The increase in exercise ventilation may partially result from metabolic changes that occur in the working skeletal muscle. Early release of lactic acid results in an increase in CO_2 production and thus stimulates ventilation. The ventilatory response to exercise can be improved with training. Aerobic training decreases submaximal exercise lactate production.

Dyspnea may be closely related to the neural drive to the respiratory muscles. Increased work of breathing or respiratory muscle weakness can cause an increased neural drive, therefore increasing dyspnea. Some studies have described an increase in diaphragmatic work with exercise in patients with heart failure. The tension time index is the product of the force of contraction and duration of contraction per breath. This value gives the work of oxygen consumption of the diaphragm per breath. In patients with heart failure, this is significantly elevated at rest and throughout exercise, with levels at peak exercise approaching the fatigue threshold.

Some investigators have demonstrated reduced maximal inspiratory and expiratory mouth pressures consistent with respiratory muscle weakness. Hammond et al. measured maximal inspiratory and expiratory mouth pressure and maximal handgrip force in 16 patients with CHF and 18 normal subjects. Maximal respiratory pressures were significantly reduced. Handgrip force was less dramatically reduced, suggesting greater respiratory muscle weakness.

Not only are these muscles weak, but during exercise they may become ischemic. Using near-infrared spectroscopy, a noninvasive technique that assesses muscle oxygenation, we have been able to demonstrate that accessory respiratory muscle oxygenation decreases more in patients with heart failure than in normal subjects at any given level of work. Progressive deoxygenation is noted throughout exercise. In normal subjects, no change in oxygenation is seen.

Respiratory muscle endurance has also been shown to be reduced in these patients. Maximal sustainable ventilatory capacity measured by progressive isocapnic hyperpnea can be used to determine endurance. This is performed by having subjects breath into a rebreathing circuit. Subjects are provided with visual feedback of their level of ventilation; essentially, they are instructed to maintain an airbag deflated. Carbon dioxide is added to the inspired air to maintain isocapnia as dictated by continuous measurements of end-tidal CO_2. Using this technique, we were able to show a significant reduction in muscle endurance. Maximal sustainable ventilatory capacity averaged 53 L/minute versus 90 L/minute in normal subjects.

The sensation of dyspnea may be exacerbated in patients with heart failure as the increased work of breathing must be performed by weak and underperfused muscles. In one study, we performed selective respiratory muscle training in a small cohort of patients with Class II to IV CHF. This study is discussed at length in the section on aerobic training. Submaximal and maximal exercise performance was increased with training. The sensation of dyspnea during activities of daily living was also ameliorated. This study demonstrates that respiratory muscle function affects the sensation of dyspnea as well as exercise performance.

Summary

In the final analysis, what is the limiting factor for maximal exercise capacity in patients with heart failure? There is no single answer. There appear to be subgroups that may be primarily limited by one factor more than another. For example, in 34 patients with heart failure and 6 normal subjects, exercise hemodynamic measurements and leg blood flow were determined. Although all

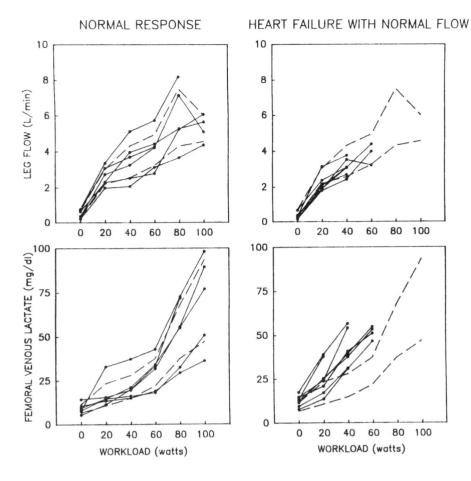

FIG. 5. Plots of leg blood flow and femoral venous lactate responses in control group and patients with heart failure and normal leg blood flow responses to exercise. (From Wilson JR, Mancini DM, Dunkman WB. Exertional fatigue due to skeletal muscle dysfunction in patients with heart failure. *Circulation* 1993;87:470–475, with permission.)

patients exhibited a reduced exercise capacity, with peak VO2 less than 18 mL/kg/minute, approximately 25% had normal leg blood flow. The plots of leg blood flow and femoral venous lactate responses in the control group and in a subgroup of nine patients with heart failure who had normal leg blood flow are shown in Figure 5. Although all these patients exhibited normal leg blood flow, lactate release was abnormal. This implies that their exercise limitation is most probably due to intrinsic skeletal muscle changes rather than limited cardiac output response. In contrast, limitation of maximal exercise capacity in other patients may primarily be related to a reduced cardiac output response; in other subgroups, pulmonary factors may be predominant. The exercise response of a patient with heart failure needs careful analysis to determine which factor may constitute the major limitation. Then, appropriate therapeutic interventions can be tailored to the patient to enhance his or her exercise performance. For example, patients who appear limited by intrinsic skeletal muscle changes will benefit more from aerobic training than from drugs that increase blood flow. Another element that has an impact on the exercise response of these patients is the chronicity of their disease. For example, in a person with severe heart failure from a recent extensive myocardial infarction, it is unlikely that exercise will be limited by vascular or skeletal muscle changes that occur only after a period of significant disability.

In summary, exercise capacity in patients with heart failure is limited not only by changes that affect the ability to increase cardiac output, but by changes that occur in the blood vessels, the muscles, and the lungs as a consequence of their disease.

Next, we review the methods for quantitating exercise capacity in patients with heart failure and the clinical usefulness of this measurement.

TYPES OF EXERCISE TESTS

Exercise capacity is best quantified by the measurement of oxygen consumption during exercise. This can be measured noninvasively by use of metabolic carts that contain rapidly responding CO_2 and O_2 analyzers. The subjects breathe through a specially constructed valve such that all the exhaled air is directed into the metabolic cart. From standard equations programmed into the computer system of the cart, a variety of ventilatory parameters are measured.

Determination of exercise capacity with measurement of oxygen consumption is usually performed with bicycle or treadmill exercise. The most commonly used exercise protocols are either constant work rate or incremental tests. Low-intensity, constant-work protocols such as the Naughton or Balke Ware are the most frequent treadmill protocols used. The Naughton protocol is particularly effective for patients with severe heart failure because the workload increment between stages equals only 1 metabolic unit (3.5 mL/kg/minute). Bicycle exercise is frequently begun with unloaded cycling and then incremented every 3 minutes by 20 to 25 watts. Bicycle exercise confers several advantages over treadmill exercise. The equipment needed is usually less expensive and much more portable, and provides a more accurate quantitation of workload. Although treadmill exercise may simulate a more familiar form of exercise, a motorized unit with variable speed and grade can be frightening to patients who have no control over the unit in the event of an immediate need to stop exercise. Besides constant–work-rate protocols, incremental exercise tests are frequently used. Continuous increase in work rate (Ramp) or 1-minute incremental workloads are used such that the test duration is approximately 10 minutes. Most investigators have found similar $\dot{V}O_{2max}$ measurements using both the continuous and discontinuous graded work rate test.

A significant improvement in $\dot{V}O_{2max}$ clearly demonstrates objective clinical improvement. Although vasodilators and positive inotropic agents can improve rest and exercise hemodynamic measurements and quality of life, in many studies peak $\dot{V}O_2$ remains unchanged despite subjective improvement. Submaximal exercise tests may therefore be a better method of assessing the benefit of interventions in patients with heart failure.

To quantitate submaximal exercise capacity, a variety of walk tests have been designed, including the 6- and 12-minute walk tests and the 9-minute self-powered walk test. These tests were initially described in the pulmonary literature, where cycle or treadmill exercise is frequently not feasible in patients with severe dyspnea from chronic pulmonary disease. In 1976, McGavin et al. introduced the 12-minute walk test, which was subsequently shortened to 6 minutes after a strong correlation between the distance walked with both tests was demonstrated. Briefly, patients are instructed to walk as much as possible in a 6-minute period. A quiet, empty corridor at least 20 m long comprises the typical course. Distance markers and chairs along the route are provided. Encouragement delivered during the test is standardized because it has been shown to improve performance. An alternative is the unencouraged walk test in which the study monitor avoids eye contact with the subject and simply informs the patient of the time remaining at 2-minute intervals. At the completion of the test, the sensations of dyspnea and fatigue are quantitated by using the Borg or visual analog scales. The 6-minute walk test has been demonstrated to provide better quantification of exercise capacity than peak $\dot{V}O_2$ in patients with severe Class III and IV CHF, but not in less ill patients. Reproducibility is optimized by performing two to three baseline studies.

Several modifications of the 6-minute walk test have been described. Distance walked on a self-powered treadmill during 9 or 12 minutes has been reported in patients with mild to severe CHF. The use of the self-powered treadmill circumvents the space limitations of the 6-minute walk test. Parameshwar et al. studied distance walked and oxygen consumption during a 12-minute self-powered treadmill test on 11 control subjects and 8 patients with heart failure. Oxygen consumption on the self-powered treadmill at a similar incline and speed as the motorized treadmill was significantly greater because of the work needed to overcome the friction of the belt. Oxygen consumption did not vary as the incline of the self-powered treadmill rose from 4% to 11%, because the energy required to overcome the friction of the belt is less with a steeper grade since body weight is more effective. In both the patients with heart failure and control subjects, measured $\dot{V}O_2$ during the self-powered treadmill test was approximately 90% of peak $\dot{V}O_2$. Oxygen consumption measurements made during 6-minute corridor walk tests were also found to be approximately 75% of peak $\dot{V}O_2$. In patients with severe Class III and IV CHF, $\dot{V}O_2$ measured during the walk test approached peak $\dot{V}O_2$, at levels of approximately 90%.

As is discussed later, we studied the submaximal exercise response of patients with left ventricular assist devices (LVAD). Sensors contained in these devices can measure the hemodynamic demands of submaximal exercise. Using a new, commercially available portable metabolic cart, the Aerosport TEEM 100 (AeroSport, Ann Arbor, Michigan), metabolic measurements were obtained during a 6-minute walk test in 6 normal subjects, 20 patients with heart failure, and 14 patients with left ventricular devices. For all subjects, distance walked was significantly correlated with oxygen consumption (r = 0.73; $p < 0.0001$). Normalization of $\dot{V}O_2$ during the walk test by peak $\dot{V}O_2$ showed that in patients with LVAD and CHF, $\dot{V}O_2$ was 90% and 85% of peak $\dot{V}O_2$, respectively, whereas in normal subjects it represented a 65% maximal effort. Peak device output was 8.2 L/minute, which represents 75% of the maximum output of the device. Thus, although the 6-minute walk test is promoted as submaximal exercise, the hemodynamic and energy requirement is near maximal $\dot{V}O_2$. Nevertheless, these tests may be valuable by providing an evaluation of endurance and thus information complementary to that obtained with maximal aerobic exercise testing.

PEAK $\dot{V}O_2$ AS A SELECTION CRITERION FOR TRANSPLANTATION CANDIDACY

Several studies have suggested that peak oxygen consumption is a good short-term predictor of mortality. In a study of 27 patients, Szlachcic et al. described a 77% 1-year mortality rate for those with a $\dot{V}O_2$ of 10 mL/kg/minute or less and a 21% mortality rate for those with $\dot{V}O_2$ of 10 to 18 mL/kg/minute. Likoff et al. described a 36% 1-year mortality rate in 201 patients with heart failure and $\dot{V}O_2$ less than 13 mL/kg/minute compared with 15% when $\dot{V}O_2$ exceeded 13 mL/kg/minute. In Veterans Administration Vasodilator in Heart Failure Trials (V-HeFT) I and II, peak $\dot{V}O_2$ was a significant independent predictor of survival. Exercise capacity as assessed from the 6-minute walk test also provides prognostic information. The Studies of Left Ventricular Dysfunction (SOLVD) investigators reported that the 6-minute walk test performed prospectively on a stratified random sample of 898 patients was an independent predictor of mortality. Patients with the lowest versus the highest performance level had a significantly higher mortality rate as well as a greater hospitalization rate for heart failure. In a logistic regression model, distance walked was comparable with the predictive value of left ventricular ejection fraction. When we compared the predictive value of peak $\dot{V}O_2$ with distance walked in patients evaluated for transplantation at Columbia, peak $\dot{V}O_2$ was found to be the more powerful predictive tool.

The use of peak exercise $\dot{V}O_2$ measurements for optimal timing of cardiac transplantation in ambulatory patients with heart failure was first described in 1991. Mancini et al. performed exercise tests on 114 ambulatory patients referred for cardiac transplantation. A peak $\dot{V}O_2$ of less than 14 mL/kg/minute was selected as a criterion for transplantation eligibility. Resting hemodynamic measurements and nuclear left ventricular ejection fractions were also obtained. Of the 114 patients, 35 were accepted for transplantation, 52 had transplantation deferred, and 27 with low $\dot{V}O_2$ were rejected for transplantation because of a significant comorbid illness. Serial exercise tests were performed at 3- to 6-month intervals, with cross-over between groups permitted. All three

groups were comparable in NYHA functional class, ejection fraction, and cardiac index. Patients with a peak $\dot{V}O_2$ greater than 14 mL/kg/minute had 1- and 2-year survival rates of 94% and 84%, respectively. In contrast, those patients accepted for transplantation had a 1-year survival rate of 70% that, when analyzed using urgent transplantation as an end-point rather than a censored observation, was reduced to 48%. Indeed, those patients who were rejected for transplantation with a reduced $\dot{V}O_2$ had 1- and 2-year survival rates of 47% and 32%, respectively (Figure 6).

Although peak $\dot{V}O_2$ is primarily determined by the cardiac output response to exercise, age, gender, muscle mass, and conditioning state also contribute to maximal exercise performance. Peak $\dot{V}O_2$ can be predicted in healthy people from standard regression equations based on age, gender, and height. We investigated whether the percentage of predicted maximal $\dot{V}O_2$ as derived from regression equations based on age, gender, and height would provide greater prognostic information than peak $\dot{V}O_2$ alone. For example, a peak $\dot{V}O_2$ of 16 mL/kg/minute may be more indicative of a poor prognosis in a muscular young man than in an elderly woman. Peak $\dot{V}O_2$ and percentage of predicted $\dot{V}O_2$ derived from the Wasserman and Astrand equations were analyzed in 272 ambulatory patients referred for transplantation evaluation. The ability of these exercise parameters to predict survival was determined by comparison of Kaplan-Meier curves, univariable proportional-hazards models, and receiver operating characteristic (ROC) curves. None of the methods of determining percentage predicted $\dot{V}O_2$ significantly improved the prediction of survival over peak $\dot{V}O_2$ alone. Peak $\dot{V}O_2$ as expressed in milliliters per minute (i.e., not normalized for body weight) and oxygen pulse (peak $\dot{V}O_2$ in mL/kg/minute/heart rate) were also not better predictive measures of survival than peak $\dot{V}O_2$ alone. A peak $\dot{V}O_2$ less than 14 mL/kg/minute remains a reliable guideline by which to time cardiac transplantation. Other

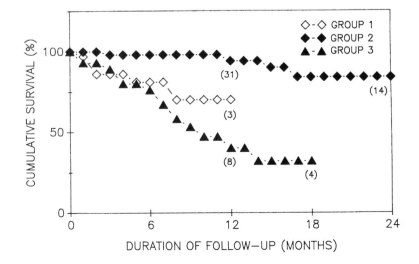

FIG. 6. Survival curves comparing patients with $\dot{V}O_2$ less than 14 mL/kg/minute accepted for transplantation (Group 1), patients with $\dot{V}O_2$ less than 14 mL/kg/minute rejected for transplantation (Group 3), and patients with $\dot{V}O_2$ greater than 14 mL/kg/minute (Group 2), in whom transplantation was deferred. (From Mancini D, Eisen H, Kussmaul W, et al. Value of peak exercise oxygen consumption for optimal timing of cardiac transplantation in ambulatory patients with heart failure. *Circulation* 1991;83:778–786, with permission.)

investigators have also examined this question, with variable conclusions.

Can the addition of exercise hemodynamic measurements to ventilatory gas parameters facilitate risk prognostication? In 65 patients with severe heart failure, we investigated this question. Oxygen consumption measurements were correlated to pulmonary artery saturation in each patient to derive a true $\dot{V}O_{2max}$. Multivariable analysis was performed using peak $\dot{V}O_2$ and all peak exercise hemodynamic variables. Using this approach, only left ventricular stroke work and left ventricular stroke work index were statistical predictors of survival. Previously, Rubin et al. had examined the prognostic significance of exercise hemodynamic variables in 49 patients. Multiple logistic regression analysis in that study identified peak exercise stroke work index as the only exercise-derived hemodynamic predictor of mortality. The results of these studies are similar. However, many of the patients with heart failure have significant mitral valve regurgitation; thus, the formula used to calculate left ventricular stroke work is frequently inaccurate in this population. Without simultaneous quantitation of the extent of mitral valve regurgitation, it is difficult to advocate the widespread application of this particular hemodynamic variable.

Although peak $\dot{V}O_2$ is a powerful short-term predictor, no single variable should be the exclusive criterion by which to time cardiac transplantation. Aaronson et al. developed an objective pretransplantation risk stratification system from multivariable analyses performed on 268 ambulatory patients referred for transplantation from July, 1986, to December, 1991, at the Hospital of the University of Pennsylvania. Eighty clinical variables were collected prospectively, including items derived from the history and physical examination, cardiac catheterization, exercise, and electrocardiographic data. Patients were prospectively followed to death or to urgent or elective transplantation. Using proportional hazards modeling, a model was developed that included seven variables most predictive of survival: etiology of heart failure, resting heart rate, left ventricular ejection fraction, mean arterial blood pressure, left ventricular conduction defect, peak $\dot{V}O_2$, and serum sodium. The ability of this model to predict survival was subsequently validated in an independent sample of 199 ambulatory patients followed at Columbia-Presbyterian Medical Center. Model discrimination was evaluated by constructing receiver operating characteristic curves. The areas under the curve were 0.81 and 0.88 for the Penn and Columbia data sets, respectively; model discrimination was therefore excellent. An equation consisting of the seven clinical variables and their model coefficients was derived to yield a prognostic score. Stratum-specific likelihood ratios were then used to determine accurate threshold values for the prognostic scores. Three distinct strata were observed: low risk (i.e., prognostic score >8.1); medium risk (score 7.2–8.09); and high risk (score <7.19). Event-free survival rates for the low-, medium-, and high-risk strata were 93%, 72%, and 43%, respectively, in the University of Pennsylvania derivation sample and 88%, 60%, and 35% in the Columbia validation sample. Thus, in both groups the model identified patients with an anticipated good prognosis in whom transplantation could be safely deferred. Medium- and high-risk patients would proceed for transplantation. Analysis as to whether any single parameter in the model similarly predicted survival revealed that no single variable approached the discriminatory power of the model in the derivation cohort. However, in the validation subset, peak $\dot{V}O_2$ alone was nearly equal to the total model. Importantly, in the derivation sample, $\dot{V}O_2$ was one of the weakest variables. It can be justifiably concluded that by incorporating multiple, partially correlated variables, the multivariable model is more likely to be a better predictor of survival than any single variable when tested in new samples.

Stevenson et al. have used serial assessment of peak $\dot{V}O_2$ to identify patients who could be safely deactivated from the transplantation list. These investigators have demonstrated that improvement of peak $\dot{V}O_2$ to greater than 14 mL/kg/minute after treatment with high-dose diuretic and vasodilator therapy tailored to near-normal filling pressure and systemic vascular resistance, identifies transplantation candidates who can safely defer cardiac transplantation.

AEROBIC TRAINING

Exercise training has long been advocated as a means to delay aging and decrease cardiovascular mortality in normal subjects. The evidence to support either of these outcomes in normal or disease states is lacking. However, aerobic training can confer a multitude of significant hemodynamic, morphologic, and metabolic changes in humans. In this section, the benefits of aerobic training in both normal subjects and patients with heart failure are reviewed.

What is exercise training? It can be defined as maintaining a habit of exercise above that usually performed. We train to achieve physical fitness. The President's Council on Fitness defines a physically fit person as one who can perform vigorous work without undue fatigue and with sufficient remaining energy to enjoy recreational activities and meet emergencies—or, more simply, in the words of the great former Dallas Cowboy coach Tom Landry, "the ability of a man to do what a man has to do." Objectively, physical fitness is quantitated by measurements of muscle strength, endurance, and cardiovascular capacity ($\dot{V}O_{2max}$). Key features of a training program include the mode of exercise, duration of exercise, intensity (i.e., percentage of peak $\dot{V}O_2$ or maximum heart rate), and frequency of exercise sessions. The mode

TABLE 1. *Benefits of aerobic training*

Morphologic
↑Myocardial mass
↑LVEDV
↑Diameter of coronary arteries
↑Myocardial and skeletal muscle capillary-to-fiber ratio
Skeletal muscle
↑Capillary density
↑Mitochondrial volume and cristae
↑Enzymes of citric acid cycle and electron transport chain
±↑Myoglobin
↑Use of free fatty acids
↑Potential to store glycogen
↑Local arterial-venous O_2 difference
↑Maximal flow rate through muscle
Hemodynamic
↓Resting heart rate
↓Double product at submaximal workloads
↑Stroke volume
↑Maximum cardiac output
↑Maximum $\dot{V}O_2$
Metabolic
↑Skeletal muscle mitochondrial and enzymatic changes
↑HDL
↓Triglycerides
↓Fasting glucose
↓Catecholamines
↑Lipoprotein lipase (acts on VLDL, TG →FFA + glycerol)
↓hepatic lipase (converts HDL2 →HDL3)
↑LCAT (esterifies cholesterol with FFA, enhancing
   cholesterol transport)
↑Beta-hydroxyacyl Co dehydrogenase (↑beta oxidation of
   FFA)

↑, increase; ↓, decrease; HDL, high-density lipoprotein; VLDL, very–low-density lipoprotein; FFA, free fatty acid; LVEDV, left ventricular end-diastolic volume; LCAT, lecithin-cholesterol acyltransferas

of exercise is most commonly continuous submaximal exercise involving large muscle groups, such as bicycling, running, and swimming. Dash and interval exercise training are frequently used and involve brief periods of near-maximal or supramaximal exercise alternating with low-level activity. This form of training enhances aerobic as well as anaerobic metabolism.

Table 1 summarizes the hemodynamic, morphologic, and metabolic benefits of training.

Hemodynamic Changes

The classic study on the hemodynamic effects of chronic exercise was performed by Saltin et al. Using a longitudinal design, five young subjects, 19 to 21 years of age, underwent an initial assessment followed by 3 weeks of bed rest and 2 months of intense training. Measurements of cardiac output during supine and upright exercise, heart rate, blood pressure, $\dot{V}O_2$, pH, and lactate were performed, and skeletal muscle biopsies were taken. With deconditioning, there was a rapid decline in $\dot{V}O_2$, a 15% decrease in cardiac output, a

widening of the $A\dot{V}O_2$ difference, and an increase in lactate production. With training, all of these changes were reversed, with significant increases in $\dot{V}O_2$, cardiac output, and stroke volume, a widening of the $A\dot{V}O_2$ difference, and a decrease in lactate production. In the sedentary people, the improvement in $\dot{V}O_2$ was derived equally from a widening of the $A\dot{V}O_2$ difference and the increase in cardiac output. A general axiom of training derived from this classic study is that the greater the intensity and frequency of exercise, the greater the gain in $\dot{V}O_2$.

Morphologic Changes

Much of the information on the morphologic consequences of training are derived from animal studies. Myocardial hypertrophy is a well described result of prolonged vigorous exercise in both human and animal studies. Physiologic hypertrophy is usually concentric, with occasional disproportional increases in septal thickness. The increased left ventricular mass is associated with a constant myocardial fiber diameter such that the diffusion distance from surrounding capillaries to central myofibrils is unchanged. In human echocardiographic studies, left ventricular mass may increase by as much as 45%.

A variety of myocardial microcirculatory changes may also be observed with training. An increase in capillarization can result from the mechanical stimulus for growth (i.e., a chronic increase in blood flow) or a metabolic stimulus (i.e., hypoxia). The physiologic significance of this lies in the decrease in the diffusion distance. This enhances the delivery of oxygen and substrates as well as the removal of metabolites.

Morphologic changes are also evidenced in the epicardial vessels. Coronary luminal diameter is increased. This increase is in general proportional to the increase in left ventricular mass. These changes are well documented in animal studies, where casts of the coronary trees are examined in trained and untrained animals. Epicardial morphologic changes in humans are best illustrated by the case of Clarence DelMar, nicknamed by the public "Mr. Marathon." One of the first advocates of physical fitness, he was instrumental in raising public awareness on the importance of exercise. Mr. Marathon participated in more than 1,000 long-distance races up to age 69 years, authored the book *Marathon*, and was the study subject in an article in the *Journal of Applied Physiology* that was the initial description of lower lactate levels in well-trained subjects. When he died, autopsy showed coronary arteries with a luminal diameter two to three times normal. A left main coronary artery lesion was observed that was not significant only because of the luminal enlargement.

The obvious clinical question that follows these observations is whether the changes in the myocardial circulation as a consequence of exercise will decrease angina or limit infarct size. There have been a series of elegant animal studies by several investigators examining this question. The constraints of this review preclude a detailed examination of these studies. The results of these studies have been conflicting, and there is no consensus as to whether exercise superimposed on severe stenosis increases collateral formation and limits angina or infarct size.

Studies on the effect of exercise on contractility are also conflicting. In normal humans and animals, exercise does not appear to decrease contractility. Most studies demonstrate no change in isometric tension development or isotonic shortening velocity of myocardial papillary muscle and trabeculae in trained animals with or without hypertrophy. Scheuer has studied isolated perfused working hearts in rat exercise models and has described increased myocardial contractile performance, left ventricular compliance, and relaxation. Studies in open-chested rats have also shown a shift of the end-diastolic pressure–volume relationship to the right with training. Whether similar changes can be observed in diseased states such as heart failure is unclear. Echocardiographic studies in patients after myocardial infarction suggest that aerobic training results in left ventricular dilation with a deterioration of function. This remains a very active area of clinical research.

Metabolic Changes

The changes that occur in the skeletal muscle with training are well described. Briefly, with training there is an increase in capillarization, an increased mitochondrial volume and number of cristae, an increase in the concentration of oxidative enzymes of the Krebs and electron transport chains, and an increase in beta oxidation of free fatty acids.

Skeletal muscle perfusion has been described to be reduced in some studies during submaximal exercise with training at the same absolute workload, but unchanged at a relative workload. An increase in skeletal muscle blood flow at maximal exercise has also been reported.

The changes that occur in lipid metabolism have important clinical implications with regard to the development or progression of atherosclerosis. Lipoprotein lipase is located on the luminal surface of capillaries. With training and subsequent capillarization, lipoprotein lipase activity increases. This results in the increased degradation of very low-density lipoprotein to free fatty acids and glycerol. Hepatic lipase activity is also decreased with training. This enzyme converts high-density lipoprotein (HDL)-2 to HDL-3. Accordingly, HDL-2, which is cardioprotective, is increased. Apolipoprotein I also increases with training. Thus, aerobic training improves the lipid profile.

Aerobic Training in Heart Failure

There are multiple central and peripheral changes induced by aerobic training in healthy subjects (see Table 1). Potential advantages of training in heart failure include central hemodynamic changes such as an increase in stroke volume, a potential increase in contractility, alteration of autonomic tone with a decrease in sympathetic stimulation, an improvement in endothelial and vascular function with a decrease in peripheral vascular resistance, muscle enzymatic changes with an increased oxidative capacity, and a decrease in lactate production.

There is a growing literature on the benefits of aerobic training in these patients. However, many questions remain, such as which mode of training is optional for these patients and what is the effect of training on long-term morbidity and mortality.

Table 2 summarizes the clinical studies investigating aerobic training in patients with heart failure. Initial studies by Letac et al., Lee et al., Williams et al., and Cohn et al. established the safety of training in this population. They also showed that patients with reduced left ventricular function can demonstrate the hallmarks of training (i.e., improvement in work capacity with a concomitant decline in heart rate). These studies did not investigate the physiologic mechanisms underlying the improved work state.

Using an ischemic rat model of heart failure, Musch et al. studied the effects of endurance training. Fifty rats underwent thoracotomy. A sham procedure was performed in 25 animals. In the remaining 25 rats, the left anterior descending artery was ligated. These groups were then randomized to a sedentary versus trained protocol. The training protocol consisted of 60-minute sessions of treadmill exercise 5 days a week for 10 to 12 weeks. Parameters studied included infarct size, $\dot{V}O_2$, heart rate and blood pressure response, rest and exercise hemodynamic measurements, succinate dehydrogenase activity in the soleus and plantaris muscles, lactate levels, and regional perfusion of the skeletal muscle and renal and splanchnic beds. After the training program in the rats with heart failure, $\dot{V}O_2$ was higher, succinate dehydrogenase activity increased, and lactate levels were lower during submaximal exercise. No differences were observed in regional perfusion or in hemodynamic measurements. In this rat model of heart failure, all derived benefits were from peripheral mechanisms.

Studies by Sullivan et al., Coats et al., Hambrecht et al., and Drexler et al. have attempted to characterize the physiologic mechanisms behind the clinical improvement in patients with heart failure. Sullivan et al. studied 12 patients with heart failure with a mean $\dot{V}O_2$ of 16.3 mL/kg/minute and an ejection fraction of 21%. Aerobic training was performed 3 to 5 hours a week for 6 months. Hemodynamic measurements, skeletal muscle perfusion, oxygen consumption, and left ventricular ejection frac-

TABLE 2. *Whole-body aerobic training in heart failure*

Investigator	No. of patients (CAD)	EF (%)	Duration of training (mo)	Training effects
Letac et al., 1977	8	<45	2	↑Work capacity ↓HR; ↓BP
Lee et al., 1979	18	35	12–42	↑Work capacity, ↓HR ↔CO or EF
Williams et al., 1984	6	<55	6	↔EF, ↓HR
Cohn et al., 1982	10	27	12	↑VO₂
Sullivan et al., 1988	12	21	6	↑VO₂, ↑peak CO, ↑arterial-venous O₂ difference ↓lactate
Coats et al.,	17	20	2	↑VO₂, ↑CO, ↓VE, ↓SVR, ↑vagal tone
Hambrecht	22	26	6	↑VO₂, ↑peak CO, ↑Mitochondria volume density
Belardinelli	27	30	2	↑VO₂, ↑Mitochondria volume density
Adamopoulos et al., 1991	12	24	2	↓PCr deletion, ↓PCr recovery time

↑, increase; ↓, decrease; ↔, no change; CAD, coronary artery disease; HR, heart rate; BP, blood pressure; $\dot{V}O_2$, peak oxygen consumption; CO, cardiac output; VE, minute ventilation; SVR, systemic vascular resistance, PCr, phosphocreatine; EF, ejection fraction.

tion were measured before and after training. With training, peak $\dot{V}O_2$ rose 23%, from 16.8 to 20.6 mL/kg/minute. Peak cardiac output, peak $A\dot{V}O_2$ difference, and peak leg blood flow also significantly increased. Ejection fraction was unchanged. Training decreased leg lactate production. Leg blood flow during submaximal exercise did not increase, suggesting that the major benefit derived from training was through increased oxygen extraction by the skeletal muscles. The largest proportion of the increase in $\dot{V}O_2$ was derived from peripheral adaptation, with a possible small central contribution.

Coats et al. performed a controlled, cross-over, home-based trial of 8 weeks of exercise training in 17 patients with stable, moderate to severe CHF. Peak $\dot{V}O_2$ increased from 13.2 to 15.6 mL/kg/minute. They also studied the effect of training on autonomic tone by measuring heart rate variability and radiolabeled norepinephrine spillover. After training, these measurements demonstrated a shift from sympathetic to enhanced vagal activity. Other investigators have demonstrated a decrease in serum catecholamine levels both at rest and during submaximal exercise in these patients after aerobic training.

Two studies using selective arm training and another study using aerobic exercise have demonstrated an improvement in but not normalization of the metabolic abnormalities observed with exercise in patients with heart failure. Percutaneous muscle biopsies of the vastus lateralis were obtained before and after 6 months of aerobic training in 22 patients. Aerobic training increased the volume density of mitochondria. Staining for cytochrome oxidase-positive mitochondria was used as a qualitative index of oxidative enzyme activity in skeletal muscle. This measurement was also significantly increased with training. Thus, aerobic training in patients with heart failure results in improved skeletal muscle oxidative function.

The effect of aerobic training on endothelial function has also been studied in this patient population. Isolated forearm training using handgrip exercise was performed for 4 weeks in 12 patients with chronic heart failure. Flow-dependent dilatation of the radial artery was assessed using a high-resolution ultrasound system. Measurements were performed at rest; during reactive hyperemia; during an intraarterial infusion of sodium nitroprusside, an endothelial-independent vasodilator; and after an intraarterial infusion of N-monomethyl-L-arginine (L-NMMA), an inhibitor of endothelial synthesis and nitric oxide release. The impaired flow-dependent dilatation observed in the patients with heart failure was improved by training. L-NMMA attenuated this improvement, implying that the normalization of flow-dependent dilatation with training resulted from enhanced endothelial release of nitric oxide. This is an important finding in that it may indicate that training improves skeletal muscle perfusion. Improvement in the endothelial function of large-conduit vessels may also decrease impedance to the failing left ventricle and thus improve left ventricular ejection fraction. Other investigators have demonstrated increases in skeletal muscle leg perfusion and cardiac output at maximal but not submaximal activity.

Many questions remain regarding the value of exercise training in these patients. Indeed, even what mode of training would be most advantageous is not clear. A study by Jugdutt et al. suggests that a 12-week exercise training program in patients after extensive anterior infarctions can further distort left ventricular shape, increase infarct expansion, reduce scar thickness, and reduce ejection fraction. Endurance training in rats after large myocardial infarctions resulted in reduced survival and left ventricular dilatation. The Exercise in Anterior Myocardial Infarction (EAMI) trial by Italian investigators randomized 93 patients within 2 months of their anterior wall myocardial infarction to 6 months of exercise training versus a sedentary protocol. Echocardiographic indices of ventricular size and function were obtained before and at the completion of the study. In this study, where most of the patients had ejection fractions greater than 40%, exercise training did not produce greater ventricular dilatation or reduction in ejection fraction compared with the control group. In a subgroup analysis including 30 patients with ejection fractions below 40%, no echocardiographic evidence of deterioration of left ventricular function was observed. However, in this group the mean left ventricular ejection fraction was still quite high, averaging 35%, and only a small percentage of patients were maintained on angiotensin-converting enzyme inhibitors. The question as to the effect of prolonged exercise training on cardiac remodeling in this subcategory of patients deserves further investigation.

To circumvent the potential deleterious effects of high-intensity aerobic training, a few studies have focused on either low-intensity or specific-muscle training. Studies that focus on small muscle mass training that does not stress the cardiovascular system may have the added advantage of inducing peripheral skeletal muscle changes without adverse cardiac effects.

Belardinelli et al. investigated the value of low-intensity exercise training in 27 patients with chronic heart failure randomized to training versus control groups. The exercise prescription in this study called for 3 weekly training sessions of bicycle exercise at 40% of peak $\dot{V}O_2$ for 8 weeks. Measurements of peak $\dot{V}O_2$, serum catecholamines, and lactate were taken, and vastus lateralis skeletal muscle biopsies were obtained before and after training. Peak $\dot{V}O_2$ increased as serum lactate and catecholamine levels declined during submaximal exercise, and the volume density of mitochondria was enhanced at the conclusion of the study only in the trained group.

We performed selective respiratory muscle training in 14 patients with Class II to IV CHF. Six patients dropped out early in the training period and formed a comparison group. Respiratory muscle strength, respiratory muscle endurance, and submaximal and maximal exercise capacity were measured before and after 3 months of training. The training protocol combined both endurance and strength training. As discussed previously, submaximal and maximal exercise performance was increased in the trained but not the comparison group.

Future studies investigating the clinical benefit of low-intensity exercise training or regional muscle group training in patients with heart failure appear warranted.

IMPACT OF LEFT VENTRICULAR ASSIST DEVICES ON EXERCISE PERFORMANCE

Left ventricular assist devices are increasingly used as a bridge to cardiac transplantation and may represent a permanent alternative therapy for the management of end-stage heart failure. After insertion of an LVAD, patients frequently become ambulatory. Reports have described peak exercise performance with measurement of oxygen consumption in small numbers of patients. Jaski et al. were the first to report on the maximum exercise capacity in patients with Thermocardiosystems (TCI) devices. In that report, peak $\dot{V}O_2$ measured in two patients was 14.3 and 16.7 mL/kg/minute. Murali et al. described a similar peak $\dot{V}O_2$ in a small cohort of patients with the Novacor system. Peak $\dot{V}O_2$ was dramatically better than the preoperative exercise capacity of these patients. We reported on the maximal and submaximal exercise capacity of 14 patients with the TCI device. Mean peak $\dot{V}O_2$ for this group averaged 17 mL/kg/minute, consistent with the earlier reports of Jaski et al. and Murali et al. Interestingly, this value is considerably lower than what would be predicted from the maximal device output. Assuming a peak $A\dot{V}O_2$ difference of 18 and a maximum device output of approximately 11 L/minute, the calculated peak $\dot{V}O_2$ for a 70-kg man should be roughly 25 mL/kg/minute. The mechanisms precluding achievement of this level of exercise warrant future investigation.

Submaximal capacity of LVAD patients was also measured and compared with that of patients with dobutamine-dependent, chronic CHF and normal subjects. Distance walked during a 6-minute walk test was comparable with that in patients with stable Class II to III CHF, and markedly better than that in dobutamine-dependent patients. Inotropic therapy and devices are both used as bridges to cardiac transplantation. Functional capacity is an integral component of a person's overall sense of well-being, satisfaction, and quality of life. These findings suggest that the quality of life is better in LVAD recipients than in the dobutamine-dependent patients who are bridged to transplant. Because the submaximal and maximal exercise capacity of LVAD patients is similar to that of patients with moderate CHF, this study suggests that permanent placement of LVADs represents effective alternative therapy for patients with end-stage refractory heart failure.

Sequential measurements of submaximal exercise capacity of LVAD patients demonstrated an increase in endurance over time without an alteration of the device output. Peripheral mechanisms such as muscle conditioning or reversal of neurohormonal activation, rather than central mechanisms, may underlie this observed improvement. All our LVAD patients participated in a progressive physical therapy program. A preliminary report by Katz et al. describes a delayed and incomplete reversal of impaired metabolic vasodilatation in patients with heart failure after device implantation. Whether the improvement we observed in the submaximal exercise capacity of LVAD patients is due to continued reversal of the abnormal metabolic vasodilatation, reversal of intrinsic skeletal muscle abnormalities, or recovery of the native heart, cannot be determined from this study but requires further investigation.

CONCLUSION

This chapter reviews the potential limitations of exercise performance in patients with heart failure, the value of exercise capacity for risk stratification, and, finally, the potential benefit of exercise as a therapeutic intervention. Exercise physiology in these patients and in patients after device implantation or transplantation remains an active area of clinical research.

SELECTED REFERENCES

Aaronson K, Goin J, Wong K, Schwartz S, Mancini D. Clinical index to predict survival in patients with heart failure. *Circulation* 1997;95:2660-2667.

Adamopoulos S, Coats A, Arnolda L, et al. Effects of physical training on skeletal muscle metabolism in chronic heart failure: ^{31}P NMR spectroscopy study. *J Am Coll Cardiol* 1993;21(5):1101–1106.

Belardinelli R, Georgiou D, Scocco V, Barstow TJ, Purcaro A. Low intensity exercise training in patients with chronic heart failure. *J Am Coll Cardiol* 1995;26:975–982.

Cabanes L, Costes F, Weber S, et al. Improvement in exercise performance by inhalation of methoxamine in patients with impaired left ventricular function. *N Engl J Med* 1992;326:1661–1665.

Coats A, Adamopoulos S, Radaelli A, et al. Controlled trial of physical training in chronic heart failure. *Circulation* 1992;85:2119–2131.

Cohn E, Williams R, Wallace A. Exercise responses before and after physical conditioning in patients with severely depressed left ventricular ejection fraction. *Am J Cardiol* 1982;49:296–300.

Froelicher VF. The hemodynamic effects of physical-conditioning in healthy, young, and middle-aged individuals, and in coronary heart disease patients. In: Naughton J, Hellerstein H, Mahler I, eds. *Exercise testing and exercise training in coronary heart disease.* New York: Academic Press, 1973: 341–385.

Hambrecht R, Niebauer J, Fiehn E, et al. Physical training in patients with stable chronic heart failure: effects on cardiorespiratory fitness and ultrastructural abnormalities of leg muscles. *J Am Coll Cardiol* 1995; 25:1239–1249.

Katz S, Biasucci L, Sabba C, et al. Impaired endothelium-mediated vasodilation in the peripheral vasculature of patients with congestive heart failure. *J Am Coll Cardiol* 1992;19:918–925.

Kubo S, Rector T, Bank A, Williams R, Heifetz S. Endothelium-dependent vasodilation is attenuated in patients with heart failure. *Circulation* 1991;84:1589–1596.

Lee AP, Ice R, Blessey R, et al. Long-term effects of physical training on coronary patients with impaired ventricular function. *Circulation* 1979; 60:1519–1526.

Letac B, Cribier A, Desplances JF. A study of LV function in coronary patients before and after physical training. *Circulation* 1977;56:375–378.

Mancini D, Eisen H, Kussmaul W, Mull R, Edmunds LH, Wilson JR. Value of peak exercise oxygen consumption for optimal timing of cardiac transplantation in ambulatory patients with heart failure. *Circulation* 1991;83:778–786.

Mancini D, Walter G, Reichek N, et al. Contribution of skeletal muscle atrophy to exercise intolerance and altered muscle metabolism in heart failure. *Circulation* 1992;85:1364–1373.

Mancini DM, Coyle E, Coggan A, et al. Contribution of intrinsic skeletal muscle changes to ^{31}P NMR skeletal muscle metabolic abnormalities in patients with heart failure. *Circulation* 1989;80:1338–1346.

Mancini DM, Henson D, La Manca J, et al. Benefit of selective respiratory muscle training on exercise capacity in patients with chronic congestive heart failure. *Circulation* 1995;91:320–329.

Mancini DM, Henson D, La Manca J, Levine S. Respiratory muscle function and dyspnea in patients with chronic congestive heart failure. *Circulation* 1992;86:909–918.

Musch T, Moore R, Leathers D, Bruno A, Zelis R. Endurance training in rats with chronic heart failure induced by myocardial infarction. *Circulation* 1986;74:431–441.

Saltin B, Hartley LH, Kilbom A, et al. Physical training in sedentary middle-aged and older men. *Scand J Clin Lab Invest* 1969;24:323–344.

Scheuer J. Effects of physical training on myocardial vascularity and perfusion. *Circulation* 1982;66:491–495.

Sullivan M, Higginbotham M, Cobb F. Exercise training in patients with severe left ventricular dysfunction: hemodynamic and metabolic effects. *Circulation* 1988;78:506–515.

Wasserman K, Hansen J, Sue D, Whipp B. *Principles of exercise testing and interpretation.* Philadelphia: Lea and Febiger, 1987:1–45.

Weber K, Janicki J. *Cardiopulmonary exercise testing: physiologic principles and clinical applications.* Philadelphia: WB Saunders, 1986.

Weber K, Kinasewitz G, Janicki J, Fishman A. Oxygen utilization and ventilation during exercise in patients with chronic cardiac failure. *Circulation* 1982;65:1213–1223.

Williams R, McKinnis R, Cobb F, et al. Effects of physical conditioning on left ventricular ejection fraction in patients with coronary artery disease. *Circulation* 1984;70:69–75.

Wilson JR, Mancini DM, Dunkman WB. Exertional fatigue due to skeletal muscle dysfunction in patients with heart failure. *Circulation* 1993;87: 470–475.

Zelis R, Mason D, Braunwald E, Winterhalter M, King C. A comparison of the effects of vasodilator stimuli on peripheral resistance vessels in normal subjects and in patients with congestive heart failure. *J Clin Invest* 1968;47:960–970.

Management of End-Stage Heart Disease, edited by Eric A. Rose and Lynne Warner Stevenson. Lippincott–Raven Publishers, Philadelphia ©1998.

CHAPTER 10

When Is Heart Failure a Surgical Disease?

Lynne Warner Stevenson

THE CHANGING SPECTRUM OF HEART FAILURE

Heart failure has become a leading diagnosis for mortality, morbidity, and dollar costs throughout developed countries. In the United States, it accounts for over 40,000 deaths, 2.3 million hospitalizations as primary or secondary diagnosis, and 1% to 3% of the entire health care budget annually. The term "heart failure" encompasses a wide spectrum of disease severity, and the definition continues to evolve. Increasing recognition of early heart failure because of surveillance of postinfarction patients and greater availability of echocardiography has expanded the population and led to demonstration that intervention is beneficial even before the onset of symptoms. At the other end of the spectrum, the lure of transplantation has attracted patients with severe symptoms of advanced heart failure to centers where alternative therapies have now been developed by unified medical/surgical programs specializing in heart failure. Without these options, many such patients were previously relegated to suffer in bed under the assumption that there was no way to relieve their congestion.

The distribution of heart failure etiologies is also evolving. Aggressive therapy of hypertension has rendered this a less common cause of heart failure than coronary artery disease and nonischemic cardiomyopathy. The most common cause of heart failure is now coronary artery disease, but this may be affected by the growing use of lipid reduction therapies, which decrease the incidence and recurrence of infarction as well as the progression to heart failure after myocardial infarction. Earlier detection and therapy of left ventricular dysfunction with therapies such as angiotensin-converting enzyme (ACE) inhibitors and adrenergic blocking agents may further change the spectrum of heart failure within the next 10 years. At the same time, the aging population contributes an increasing proportion of patients in whom the syndrome of congestive heart failure presents with relatively preserved systolic function. Many of the principles for medical heart failure therapy apply to this population as well, in whom congestive symptoms can be as severe as in patients with low ejection fractions. Such patients are less likely to have hypoperfusion, however, and the better overall prognosis with preserved left ventricular ejection fraction renders these patients less likely to benefit from the surgical interventions considered here for advanced heart failure.

HOW MANY "END-STAGE" HEART FAILURE PATIENTS ARE THERE?

This chapter describes the population currently considered to have "end-stage" heart disease with low ejection fractions. It is difficult to determine the target population for which end-stage options may be indicated. Calculations from the prevalence and hospitalization rates for heart failure in the United States, combined with an estimate that approximately 20% of patients with New York Heart Association (NYHA) functional Class III to IV symptoms are truly refractory to optimal medical therapy, yield somewhere between 100,000 and 200,000 patients with end-stage heart failure. This estimate is compatible with those of Drs. Robbins and O'Connell in Chapter 1 and Dr. Evans in Chapter 2, as well as with the Institute of Medicine estimates from 1991 that the number of patients younger than 75 years of age potentially eligible for mechanical cardiac support devices ranges from 35,000 to 200,000, depending on the clinical severity included.

WHEN IS HEART FAILURE A SURGICAL DISEASE?

When surgery offers a better outcome than available medical therapies, heart failure is a surgical disease. Major benefits of any procedure can be measured in

Department of Medicine, Cardiovascular Division, Brigham and Women's Hospital, Boston, Massachusetts 02115 terms of either survival or quality of life, with multiple intermediate end-points as discussed in Chapter 3. For advanced heart failure, however, in which the clinical status remains the most robust predictor of survival, almost all interventions that produce a *substantial* and *sustained* improvement in quality of life provide either a positive or at worst neutral impact on length of life.

Surgical procedures for heart failure can be repairs of underlying structural causes of heart failure, or primary therapy for the heart failure condition itself. Coronary artery disease and structurally abnormal valves are examples of anatomic abnormalities leading to heart failure, which can be to some degree reversible with revascularization or valve repair/replacement, as discussed in Chapters 11 and 13, respectively. Congenital heart disease and hypertrophic cardiomyopathy are other examples of potential indications for surgical approaches in the setting of symptoms of heart failure. This chapter, however, addresses the identification of patients for whom surgery is designed primarily to improve or remodel the dilated failing heart directly, regardless of the underlying etiology.

There are three major principles in evaluating patients and techniques for primary heart failure surgery:

1. Most patients initially evaluated for such procedures can enjoy a quality and length of life superior to that provided by current surgical techniques, if available medical therapies are used effectively in conjunction with the other components of a dedicated heart failure program, even after referral on ACE inhibitors, digoxin, and diuretics as initially prescribed. The "natural history" of such patients is best predicted not by baseline profiles but by their responses after optimal medical therapy.
2. The evolution of surgical therapies, in contrast to development of most new drugs for heart failure, has been characterized by initial experimentation in moribund patients, followed by extension to less compromised and eventually relatively compensated patients, in whom both perioperative risks and potential benefits are less dramatic. This pattern of downshifting risks mandates frequent reevaluation of all surgical therapies for heart failure.
3. Patients undergoing newer surgical therapies must be compared with similar patients receiving concurrent medical therapy, not with historical control subjects from an era when neither the current surgical nor medical options were used.

OPTIMAL MEDICAL THERAPY

All patients referred with severe symptoms of heart failure should undergo careful evaluation for reversible causes of heart failure and superimposed reversible factors that may have led to decompensation of established heart failure, as described in Table 3, Chapter 4. Specific considerations apply to the increasing number of patients being referred for primary surgical therapy of cardiogenic shock early after myocardial infarction or cardiac surgery. Cardiac replacement or other irreversible procedures should, if possible, be avoided during the first 3 to 5 days after an acute injury, during which there is often substantial clinical improvement that allows these procedures to be deferred indefinitely, or at least until they can be performed electively in more favorable circumstances. This is particularly important for the previously healthy patient who needs time to accept the commitment to chronic reliance on medications and the medical system.

A separate group comprises the patients with recent onset of cardiomyopathy in the absence of structural heart disease. In general, almost half of patients with less than 3 months of symptoms or other evidence of disease demonstrate substantial improvement over the next 3 months. Even after patients are sufficiently compromised to be referred for cardiac transplantation, one study demonstrated 27% to have major subsequent improvement in left ventricular function, which was associated almost uniformly with survival. Those patients who did not improve after referral with recent-onset symptoms, however, had a worse prognosis than patients referred in the chronic stage of their disease. A specific subset of patients in previous normal health, presenting usually with only a few days of symptoms progressing to cardiogenic shock, are considered to have "fulminant" myocarditis, often preceded by a febrile viral illness. Such patients may require massive intravenous inotropic agents or urgent mechanical support, but at least 50% improve within 7 to 14 days to near-normal left ventricular ejection fractions. Therapies during this time should thus be planned according to the potential for cardiac recovery.

Patients with chronic heart failure present many different profiles of symptoms and hemodynamic derangements, which require individualized therapy, as discussed in Chapter 4. The current status of medical interventions specifically for advanced heart failure is shown in Table 1. Approximately 75% to 80% of patients are referred already on ACE inhibitors, digoxin, and diuretics, but improve after further adjustments and combinations. Drug efficacy and dose responses vary widely among this population, some of whom may benefit from high doses of both ACE inhibitors and angiotensin II (AII) receptor antagonists, whereas others tolerate only low doses of ACE inhibitors and require supplementation with nitrates or hydralazine to achieve adequate vasodilation. Some patients need relatively little diuretic to maintain fluid balance, whereas others require up to 400 mg of furosemide daily plus frequent metolazone. The strategy is more aptly termed "optimal" therapy rather than "maximal" therapy.

In addition to development of specific drugs for heart failure, a major difference from the heart failure therapy of the early transplantation era is the strategy emphasizing reduction of the elevated filling pressures of heart failure rather than direct increase of cardiac output, as

TABLE 1. *Outpatient therapies for advanced heart failure*

Routine use	Selected use	Detrimental	Under clinical investigation
Angiotensin-converting enzyme inhibitors	β-blockers	Amrinone, milrinone	Carvedilol
Digoxin	Amiodarone	Flosequinan	Amlodipine
Diuretics	Anticoagulation	Ibopamine	All receptor antagonists
Nitrates	Hydralazine	Vesnarinone	
Potassium replacement	Magnesium	Home prostacyclin infusion	Home dobutamine infusion
Exercise	Automatic implantable defibrillator		Ubiquitin (coenzyme Q_{10})
For CAD coronary artery disease	Ultrafiltration	Diltiazem, nifedipine	L-Carnitine
Acetylsalicylic acid	Nocturnal oxygen	Type I antiarrhythmic agents	CPAP
Lipid-lowering agents	CPAP		
		Nonsteroidal antiinflammatory agents	

CPAP, continuous positive airway pressure.

discussed in Chapter 4. This emphasis is also evident in the recently developed algorithm for advanced heart failure, with the first branch point of therapy defined by the distinction between "wet" and "dry" heart failure, as shown in Figure 1. Whereas earlier strategies aimed merely to reduce filling pressures by some percentage, the current goal, regardless of initial congestion, is to establish near-normal filling pressures, at which cardiac output in the chronically dilated heart with low ejection fraction is in general not only maintained but maximal. Even in populations with initial pulmonary capillary wedge pressures over 30 mm Hg, the reduction of these pressures into the range of 15 mm Hg correlates with freedom from congestion and with survival.

Therapy of elevated filling pressures requires optimization of volume status and venous and arterial vasodilation. In mild to moderate heart failure, and frequently in advanced heart failure without marked hypoperfusion, optimal therapy can be designed according to clinical goals (Table 2). When success of therapy is limited by poor perfusion, renal dysfunction, or other factors, hemodynamic monitoring can often help to guide initial stabilization and design of an effective oral regimen to maintain stability after discharge. Although there remains controversy regarding the exact indications for hemodynamic monitoring to tailor therapy for heart failure, there is general consensus that patients in whom aggressive surgical approaches might be appropriate should not be considered "refractory" until medical therapy has been tailored to optimize loading conditions (Table 3). This has previously been emphasized for cardiac transplantation at the Bethesda Conference.

What happens to the medical regimen after referral to a heart failure/transplantation program? In the current era, most patients are referred already on ACE inhibitors, and it is rare to initiate therapy after referral, although doses are often increased. Patients unable to tolerate the longer-acting ACE inhibitors often can be slowly titrated onto increasing doses of captopril. The most universal change after referral for expert management is establishment of optimal fluid balance, which in some experiences

averages over 4 L of net diuresis, often 15 to 20 L in a patient with anasarca or ascites. Identification of a regimen to maintain that balance after discharge is equally important, usually requiring extensive patient education regarding the flexible diuretic regimen. Oral nitrates are frequently added in combination with ACE inhibitors. Hydralazine, usually with nitrates, may be added to supplement the vasodilation with less reduction of blood pressure in patients whose blood pressures hover at 80 mm Hg or less. Some patients who do not tolerate any dose of ACE inhibitor nonetheless can be stabilized on hydralazine and nitrates, sometimes allowing later outpatient initiation of ACE inhibitor therapy. In some patients with persistent resting heart rates over 90 beats/minute, the cautious initiation of amiodarone, as discussed in Chapter 6, may lead to clinical improvement over the next 4 to 6 weeks. The coronary vasodilating and negative chronotropic actions of amiodarone also make it a reasonable drug to consider in patients with heart failure and frequent ischemic episodes without potential for revascularization. Patients with recent decompensation or with persistent difficulty maintaining fluid balance are not appropriate candidates for initiation or increase of beta-adrenergic blocking agents.

In the current experiences, congestion cannot be relieved in approximately 20% to 25% of the patients with advanced heart failure referred to heart failure programs for consideration of further therapies. (As increasing heart failure sophistication moves into the community, this proportion would be expected to grow.) These patients are often limited by renal dysfunction due to intrinsic renal disease or maladaptive renal responses to chronic fluid retention and loss. Such patients represent the majority of those dependent on intravenous inotropic infusions, although, as discussed in Chapter 5, such true dependence is rare. After initial relief, the most common reason for congestion to recur in ambulatory patients is poor compliance with sodium and fluid restriction and with the flexible diuretic regimen guided by daily weights. For most of the patients currently being referred, however, freedom from congestion can be maintained

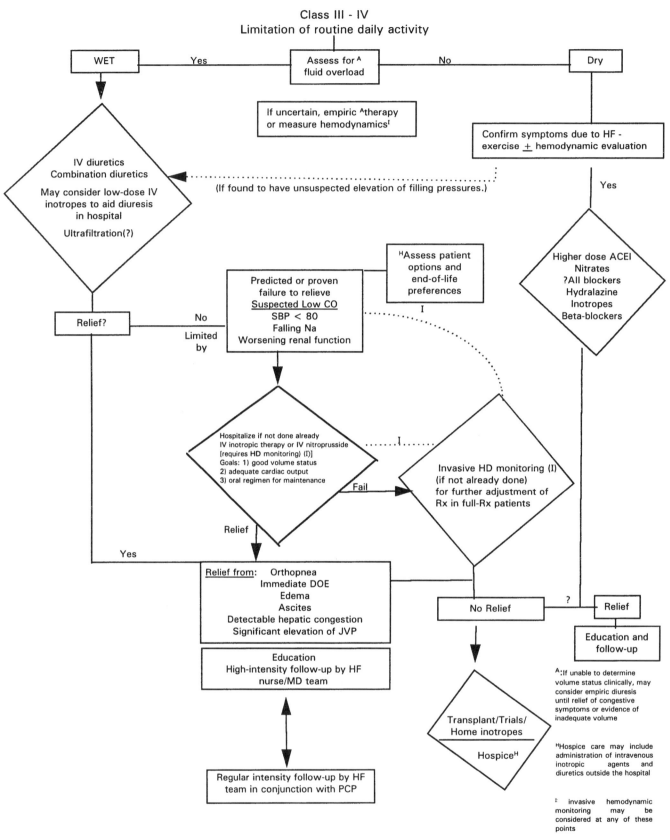

FIG. 1. Algorithm for management of heart failure with persistent severe symptoms after initiation of therapy with angiotensin-converting enzyme inhibitors, digoxin, and diuretics. Developed by the Advanced Heart Failure Task Force. (Modified from Stevenson LW, Massie BM, Francis GS. Optimizing therapy for complex or refractory heart failure: report of the Task Force on Complex Heart Failure. *Am Heart J* 1998 [*in press*], with permission.)

TABLE 2. *Hemodynamic goals for therapy of advanced heart failure*

Assessed clinically	Measured directly
Absence of orthopnea	Pulmonary capillary wedge
No peripheral edema	pressure ≤15 mm Hg
No hepatomegaly/ascites	Right atrial pressure ≤8 mm Hg
Valsalva square wave absent	
Jugular venous pressure ≤8 cm	
Warm extremities	Systemic vascular resistance
	1000–1200 dynes-sec-cm^{-5}
SBP ≥80 mm Hg	SBP >80 mm Hg
$\dfrac{\text{SBP} - \text{DBP}}{\text{SBP}}$ ≥25%	

DBP, diastolic blood pressure; SBP, systolic blood pressure.
Adapted from Stevenson LW. Therapy tailored for symptomatic heart failure. *Heart Failure* 1995;11:87–107.

TABLE 3. *Principles of tailored therapy*

0.5. Reduce obvious volume reservoir, if present
1. Measure baseline hemodynamics
2. Tailor intravenous nitrodilators and diuretics to hemodynamic goals:
  Pulmonary capillary wedge pressure ≤15 mm Hg
  Systemic vascular resistance ≤1000–1200 dynes-sec-cm^{-5}
  Right atrial pressure ≤8 mm Hg
  Systolic blood pressure ≥80 mm Hg
3. Define optimal hemodynamics by 24–48 hr
4. Titrate oral vasodilators as nitroprusside weaned:
  Captopril, isosorbide dinitrate,
  hydralazine, if necessary
5. Monitor ambulation and diuretic adjustment for 24–48 hr
6. Maintain digoxin levels 0.7–1.2 ng/dL if no contraindication
7. Provide detailed patient education
8. Provide flexible outpatient diuretic regimen
9. Institute progressive walking program
10. Vigilant follow-up

when supported by a heart failure program that provides extensive patient education, consistent phone contact, and high-intensity clinic follow-up from a dedicated multidisciplinary team, as shown by Fonarow et al.

Ambulatory patients who are relieved of congestion but then become limited instead by "dry" heart failure demonstrate less clinical compromise because of the absence of the resting congestive symptoms that usually characterize Class IV heart failure (Table 4). Because this contemporary population of dry heart failure has only recently been recognized, principles of therapy are less well developed than for classic "wet" heart failure. The greater stability of these patients with dry heart failure may permit more potential interventions, but the relative benefit of interventions may be harder to demonstrate.

TABLE 4. *The two profiles of advanced heart failure optimized on current therapy*

	Congestive ("wet")	Low-output only ("dry")
Frequency	Less common after optimal therapy	Underrecognized
New York Heart Association Class	III–IV	Usually III
Objective diagnosis	Examination, resting HD	Exercise (peak $\dot{V}O_2$, hemodynamics)
Further medical therapy	Intravenous inotropes	Beta blockers
	Ultrafiltration	Amiodarone, training
Transplantation	Indicated if eligible	Sometimes indicated
	Oral inotropes	Oral inotropes if no excess risk
Investigational therapies	Specific agents for renal perfusion	Assist devices; cardiomyoplasty considered
	Assist devices	Mitral valve modification
	Nonreplacement surgery carries high	Left ventricular reduction in
	operative risk from multiorgan failure	dilated nonischemic disease

HD = hemodynamics

ASSESSMENT BEFORE AND AFTER OPTIMAL MEDICAL THERAPY

The First Look

Most of the prognostic factors and models have focused on patients at the time of presentation, although it is well recognized that most patients improve after referral to a heart failure center. For instance, many such patients are considered "dependent" on intravenous inotropic infusions merely because they have received them and then deteriorated when the infusions are discontinued without optimization of fluid status and oral vasodilators. Most of these patients on infusions can be stabilized on oral regimens of vasodilators and diuretics, as discussed earlier. Earlier experiences suggested that up to 80% of these patients can be discharged home without nonglycosidic inotropic support, with reasonable short-term outcome. This proportion is likely to diminish with increasing community expertise in the management of heart failure before referral, but all such patients continue to merit careful evaluation, with repeated documentation of deterioration of symptoms or renal function, before being declared "inotrope dependent" or "refractory to oral therapy."

The major challenge is to select from the larger group of ambulatory patients those who remain at high risk for early adverse outcome despite hospital discharge without intravenous inotropic support. The practical utility of prognostic factors for advanced heart failure is to separate ambulatory patients at high risk from patients at low risk who superficially appear similar (Table 5). A prognostic factor that is usually worse in hospitalized patients than in out-patients thus may not add much practical prognostic value, although it may provide interesting pathophysiologic information. The most relevant analyses for defining the need for newer therapies may be those that consider ambulatory and intensive care unit patients separately.

The estimation of prognosis in advanced heart failure differs from the estimation for other heart failure populations. Many of the adverse prognostic factors from healthier and more heterogeneous populations are routinely present in patients with advanced heart failure. In a

---

TABLE 5. *Risk for mortality in advanced heart failure*

Etiology: Valvular
   Coronary artery disease
Large left ventricular end-diastolic dimension (>SD)
Left ventricular ejection fraction <10
Picture of congestion
   Class IV
   High PCW/(RA) persistent
   MR/TR
   Right ventricular function
   Natriuretic peptides high
Systolic blood pressure
Heart rate (untreated)
Arrhythmia substrate (>SD)
   History of syncope
   Nonsustained ventricular tachycardia/premature ventricular contraction
   Abnormal sinoatrial electrocardiogram
Systemic integration/response
   Neuroendocrine (e.g., low Na)
   Exercise (e.g., peak $\dot{V}O_2$)

>SD, greater likelihood of sudden death
Multiple investigators have contributed to this list, including the following:
Mancini DM, Eisen H, Kussmaul W, et al. *Circulation* 1991;83:778–783.
Cintron G, Johnson G, Francis G, et al. *Circulation* 1993;[Suppl VI]:VI17–VI23.
Conti JB, Mills RM. *Am J Cardiol* 1993;71:617–618.
Gottleib SS, Kukin ML, Ahern D, Packer M. *J Am Coll Cardiol* 1989;13:1534–1539.
DiSalvo TG, Mathier M, Semigran MJ, Dec DW. *J Am Coll Cardiol* 1995;25:1143–1153.
Moriguchi J, Kirklin J, Stevenson LW, et al. *J Heart Lung Transplant* 1997;16(abst).
Lee WH, Packer M. *Circulation* 1986;73:257–267.
Lee TH, Hamilton MA, Stevenson LW. *Am J Cardiol* 1003;72:672–676.
Aaronson KD, Schwartz JS, Chen T-M, et al. *Circulation* 1997;95:2660–2667.
Kubo SH, Ormaza SM, Francis GS, et al. *J Am Coll Cardiol* 1993;21:975–981.
Rickenbacher PR, Trinidad PT, Haywood GA, et al. *J Am Coll Cardiol* 1996;27:1192–1197.
Anguita M, Arizon JM, Bueno G, et al. *Am J Cardiol* 1990;66:413–417.
Keogh AM, Freund J, Baron DW. *Am J Cardiol* 1988;61:418–422.
Morley D, Brozena SC. Assessing risk by hemodynamic profile in patients awaiting cardiac transplantation. *Am J Cardiol* 1994;73:379–383.
Campana C, Gavazzi A, Berzuini C. Predictors of prognosis in patients awaiting heart transplantation. *J Heart Lung Transplant* 1993;12:756–765.

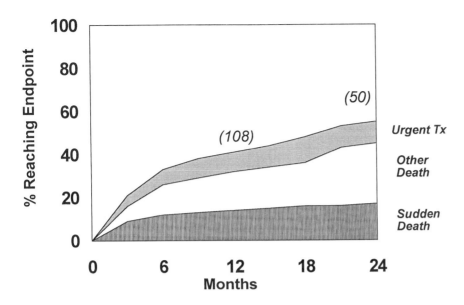

FIG. 2. Outcomes for 265 patients discharged after referral with Class IV symptoms and left ventricular ejection fraction of 25% or less. At 2 years, actuarial survival was 55%. Considering urgent transplantation as an end-point, 45% were alive without urgent transplantation. This population at the time of referral is typical of the transplantation population: 70% male, age 52 ± 13 years, left ventricular ejection fraction 18% ± 5%, left ventricular diastolic diameter 75 ± 10 mm, mitral regurgitation 2 ± 0.8 and tricuspid regurgitation 1.7 ± 0.9 on a 0- to 3-point scale, and serum sodium 134 ± 5 meq/L. (Data derived from Stevenson LW, Couper G, Natterson BJ, et al. Target heart failure populations for newer therapies. *Circulation* 1995;92[Suppl I]:II-174–II-181, with permission.)

milder population with relatively good prognosis, change is slow and event rates are low. In advanced heart failure, improvement, deterioration, and death frequently occur during the short interval after initial referral, after which the subsequent estimates of prognosis can be refined. Another difference is the application of the prognosis, which for patients with mild heart failure is assessed primarily to provide general information to the patient and family or to support pharmaceutical claims. In advanced heart failure, the estimated survival is frequently used to influence a specific therapeutic decision for an individual patient, a practice at odds with the wide variability of individual parameters and outcomes. A population may have a 50% mortality rate at 1 year, but each individual patient is 100% alive or 100% dead.

Most models are derived from large series that have focused largely on the snapshot of the patient at the time of referral. NYHA Class IV symptoms at referral confer a poor prognosis. In large heart failure series, the 1-year survival rate is estimated to be approximately 50%. In patients discharged after referral for transplantation with Class IV symptoms and left ventricular ejection fractions of 25% or less, 50% were without either death or urgent transplantation at 2 years (Figure 2). As discussed previously, the difference between Class IV symptoms and Class III symptoms is largely the presence of congestive symptoms, correlated with elevated intracardiac filling pressures. Thus, the correlates of these elevated filling pressures are also predictors of mortality in advanced heart failure (see Table 5). The predictive value of natriuretic peptides, both in asymptomatic left ventricular dysfunction and in advanced heart failure, likely derives from their reflection of intracardiac filling pressures. Preservation of right ventricular function is a more recently recognized predictor of favorable outcome that is at least partly determined by the duration and intensity of pulmonary hypertension due to elevated left-sided filling pressures.

Left ventricular ejection fraction is a valuable prognostic factor in broad populations such as the postinfarct survivors, but is less useful once heart failure has progressed to Class III or IV symptoms. In this setting, an ejection fraction over 30% is associated with better survival, but once below 30%, there is little additional prognostic information (Figure 3). Some series have shown that a left ventricular ejection fraction below 10% to 15% is associated with a particularly poor outcome, but there are few patients and significant technical problems of measurement in this range.

The degree of left ventricular dilatation from echocardiography is a consistent predictor of poor outcome in studies in which it was measured. A left ventricular diastolic dimension index greater than 4.0 cm/m² predicted twofold higher mortality, even when hemodynamic and clinical status were equivalent. The contribution is more obvious when the analysis separates patients with coronary artery disease from those with nonischemic cardiomyopathy, which tends to be more dilated. In the population discharged after referral with Class IV symptoms and left ventricular ejection fraction 25% or less, a left ventricular diastolic dimension less than 72 mm correlated with a 2-year survival rate of 58%, compared with 36% in the population with the larger dimension (Figure 4). As with other continuous variables, expected survival is a continuous function, such that much information is lost when a specific threshold value is used to separate high from low risk.

Low serum sodium predicts mortality, largely from heart failure death rather than sudden death. Patients with hyponatremia are less likely to tolerate standard doses of ACE inhibitors, although these agents, when tolerated, may be particularly beneficial in this group. Unlike some parameters, the serum sodium has its greatest predictive value in the first 12 months, after which many of the survivors after an initial low sodium have a better sodium. A serum

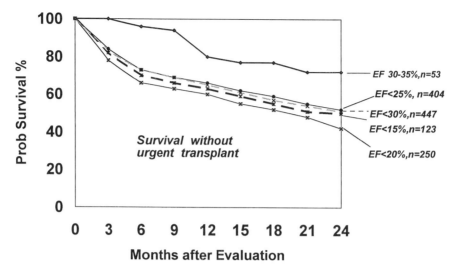

FIG. 3. Actuarial survival for 500 patients discharged after referral to transplantation with Class III or IV symptoms, demonstrating the limited prognostic significance of left ventricular ejection fraction in a population already selected by severe symptoms. Death and urgent transplantation are both considered end-points of medical therapy. The patients are divided into progressively smaller groups by lower threshold left ventricular ejection fractions. Although patients with left ventricular ejection fractions above 30% had a better prognosis, there was no further useful division in this population. (Data derived from Stevenson LW, Couper G, Natterson BJ, et al. Target heart failure populations for newer therapies. *Circulation* 1995;92[Suppl I]:II-174–II-181, with permission.)

sodium over 136 mEq/L defines a group with an almost 70% 1-year survival rate, compared with only 40% if the sodium is less than 130 mEq/L (Figure 5). Like other continuous functions, there is no single threshold value, but a progressively worse prognosis with more abnormal values.

Initial hemodynamic parameters, although useful for guiding therapy in advanced heart failure, are of less utility for assessing prognosis. In advanced heart failure causing resting symptoms, the filling pressures are usu-

ally elevated, with the degree of elevation often more a reflection of inadequate therapy than of the underlying cardiac dysfunction. More important for prognosis is the early response of these filling pressures to therapy designed to normalize them. When therapy is adjusted in the hospital during hemodynamic guidance, patients have a better prognosis if they are able to achieve pulmonary capillary wedge pressures ≤16 mm Hg. In one study of 152 patients with left ventricular ejection fractions of

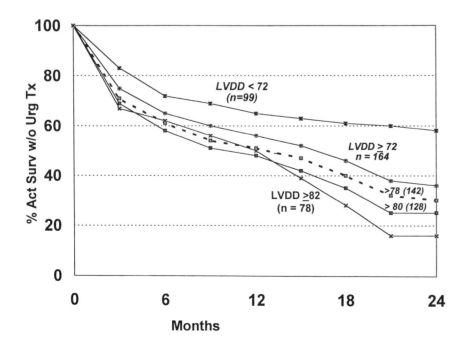

FIG. 4. Actuarial survival for 263 patients discharged after referral with Class IV symptoms and left ventricular ejection fraction of 25% or less, demonstrating the progressive impact of greater left ventricular diastolic dimension (not available in 2 patients) on prognosis. Population is as described in Fig. 2. Death and urgent transplantation are both considered end-points of medical therapy. As in Fig. 3, patients are divided into progressively smaller groups by left ventricular diastolic dimension in millimeters.

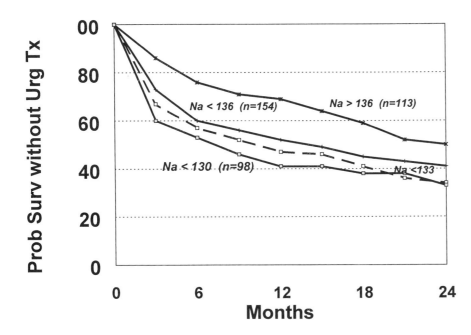

FIG. 5. Actuarial survival for 265 patients discharged after referral with Class IV symptoms and left ventricular ejection fraction of 25% or less, demonstrating the relationship of hyponatremia to poor outcome. Population is as described in Fig. 2. Death and urgent transplantation are both considered end-points of medical therapy. As in Fig. 3, patients are divided into progressively smaller groups by the risk factor, in this case lower serum sodium. The impact of the lowest sodium on mortality is most evident during the first year after referral, during which sodium often improves in survivors.

20% or less, those achieving pulmonary capillary wedge pressures ≤16 mm Hg had a 1-year survival rate of 83%, compared with 38% in those with higher filling pressures. Cardiac index and related parameters are less predictive and in some series not predictive of subsequent survival in this population. In broader populations, however, preservation of cardiac index does predict better outcome than severely compromised cardiac output. In advanced heart failure populations for which detailed clinical assessment is available, clinical findings in combination with noninvasive measurements are almost as good for predicting outcome as when hemodynamic information is added.

Multiple circulating factors have been reported to correlate with worse symptoms and worse survival. The ability of these factors to distinguish between Class I to II heart failure and worse heart failure does not render them very useful for this population of patients. Serum norepinephrine, for example, does not appear to provide significant prognostic information once the level is above 800 ng/ml, as it commonly is in patients with severe heart failure.

Peak oxygen consumption during exercise provides information about prognosis in every clinical class, and is even more valuable because it also provides a measure of functional capacity that can be compared with that expected with procedures such as transplantation or implantation of assist devices. This is discussed in detail in Chapters 3 and 9. The most consistent threshold value is a peak oxygen consumption of no more than 10 mL/kg/minute, which in general seems to predict a 1-year survival rate of less than 50%. Peak oxygen consumption of over 16 to 18 mL/kg/minute identifies patients with 1-year survival rates of over 80% in the

absence of other limitations such as severe angina or ventricular arrhythmias. The worst prognosis, however, is in patients unable to perform exercise tests during evaluation. This test helps to identify high- and low-risk patients from among the ambulatory population, not to confirm compromise in a patient virtually bedridden from resting symptoms.

Time Offers Wisdom

We remain limited in our ability to correctly identify patients at high risk for early deterioration or death. Many patients have already outlived their odds by the time of referral and continue to do so after referral. The event rates are highest in the first 6 months after referral. In one study, ambulatory patients who survived the first 6 months after listing for transplantation had a subsequent 12-month survival rate almost equivalent to that after transplantation. Rather than condemning patients to a prognosis based on presenting profiles, assessment of risk can be continually revised as time passes. This has become standard in the guidelines for transplantation candidacy, which now require reevaluation at 3- to 6-month intervals to determine whether transplantation remains indicated in ambulatory candidates.

What changes suggest improved prognosis? Improvement of five points in left ventricular ejection fraction correlated with better prognosis in the mild to moderate heart failure population of the Veterans Administration Vasodilator in Heart Failure Trials (V-HeFT). Such improvement occurs occasionally in patients with advanced heart failure, but is most often seen in recent-onset cardiomyopathy or after heavy alcohol consumption has been discontinued.

Improvement in peak oxygen consumption occurs frequently after adjustment of medical therapy that allows exercise rehabilitation, whether as a result of enhanced daily activity after resolution of dyspnea or as a result of formal exercise training. An increase of 15% to 20% is common during training programs. The ability to improve exercise capacity may be a particularly favorable sign of overall compensation and circulatory reserve. One study followed 107 ambulatory candidates listed for transplantation with an average initial peak VO_2 of 11 mL/kg/minute (Table 6). At an average of 6 months after listing, 39 could not be reexercised on medical therapy because of transplantation, death, angina, or deterioration, whereas 38 of the 68 patients undergoing repeat exercise testing (28% of all the ambulatory candidates) had a peak VO_2 improved by at least 2 mL/kg/minute to a value of at least 12 mL/kg/minute (average, 15 mL/kg/minute). To be removed from the active transplantation list, patients with improved peak VO_2 also had to meet criteria for clinical stability, based largely on absence of clinical congestion, angina, or symptomatic arrhythmias (see Table 6). The 31 patients who were thus "delisted" had a 100% survival rate at 2 years, with only five patients undergoing relisting for transplantation.

Although these criteria for delayed reevaluation concentrate the transplantation waiting list on those most likely to benefit from transplantation, it is difficult to postpone other aggressive interventions for 3 to 6 months. The highest interval risk occurs during this early period. Beyond transplantation, therapies not limited by donor supply would best be performed as soon as it is clear that the outcome without such intervention is dis-mal. From among the ambulatory patients initially referred as Class IV patients, it remains critical to be able to select as early as possible the patients who remain at high risk *after* provision of optimal therapy.

Because Class IV symptoms, which are associated with the highest mortality, primarily reflect the presence of resting congestion, subsequent freedom from congestion should portend the best prognosis, whereas persistent or recurrent congestion should portend the worst outcome. This was tested in a group of 146 patients discharged after initial referral for transplantation with Class IV symptoms of heart failure. After intensive education and clinic follow-up on the flexible diuretic regimen, sodium and fluid restriction, and the oral medications tailored to hemodynamic goals, all patients were reevaluated at 4 to 6 weeks for evidence of congestion (i.e., orthopnea, jugular venous distention ≥ 8 cm, peripheral edema, increasing weight, or increasing baseline diuretic requirement). Those who had no evidence of congestion had a subsequent 2-year survival rate of over 80%, similar to those returning for follow-up after initial referral with Class III symptoms (Figure 6). Of those with multiple persistent criteria for congestion, over 60% died or required urgent transplantation by 2 years. Interestingly, the most predictive single component on assessment was the persistence of orthopnea despite all attempts to maintain relief. For these measures of successful therapy, there is no easy way to discern whether persistent congestion reflected poor patient compliance or true refractory heart failure, but compliance may be at least as important a predictor of outcome in heart failure as it is with other chronic illnesses. Thus, the presence or absence of congestion, par-

---

TABLE 6. *Reassessment for clinical stability in advanced heart failure*

Clinical criteria
1. Stable fluid balance without evidence of congestion
   (determined after ≥ 1 mo of regular heart failure clinic visits after hospital discharge)
   Congestion defined as any of the following:
   Orthopnea
   Jugular venous pressure ≥ 8 cm above right atrium
   Peripheral edema or ascites
   Increasing weight over past week
   Need for increasing baseline daily diuretics
2. Stable blood pressure with systolic blood pressure ≥ 80 mm Hg
   (except occasional decreases into the 70s after medication doses)
3. Stable serum sodium levels (usually ≥ 132 mEq/L) and renal function
   (usually creatinine ≤ 2.0 and blood urea nitrogen ≤ 60)
4. Absence of frequent symptomatic ventricular arrhythmias
   (or automatic implantable cardiac defibrillator firings)
5. Absence of frequent or progressive angina
6. Absence of severe drug side effects (inability to tolerate angiotensin-converting
   enzyme inhibitors due to hypotension may suggest tenuous compensation)
7. Stable or improving activity level without dyspnea during self-care or exertion for one block
Exercise criteria
1. Peak oxygen consumption ≥ 12–14 mL/kg/min *and* $\geq 50\%$ predicted for gender, age, and height
2. If initially lower, improvement in peak oxygen consumption by ≥ 2 mL/kg/min by 3–6 mo

Adapted from Stevenson LW, Steimle AE, Fonarow G, et al. Improvement in exercise capacity of candidates awaiting heart transplantation. *J Am Coll Cardiol* 1995;25:163–170.

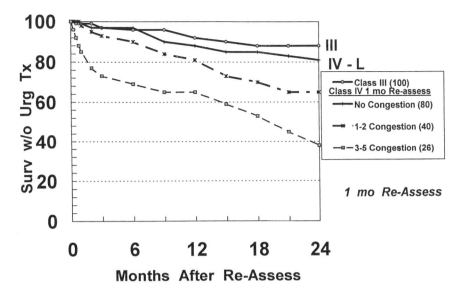

FIG. 6. Actuarial survival in relation to persistence of congestion for 146 patients who were initially referred with Class IV symptoms and survived to be reevaluated 1 month after discharge. Survival with urgent transplantation for 100 patients seen after initial referral with Class III symptoms was the same as for the patients who were Class IV initially, but at 1 month had no evidence of congestion on medical therapy tailored to maintain near-normal filling pressures (Class IV L = lightened). The five components of congestion evaluated were presence of orthopnea, edema, jugular venous pressure at least 8 cm, weight gain during the past week, or new need to increase baseline diuretic dose. (Data derived from Lucas C, Johnson W, Flavell C, et al. Freedom from congestion at one month predicts good two-year survival after hospitalization for class IV heart failure. *Circulation* 1996;94:I-93, *abstract,* with permission.)

ticularly orthopnea, after a medical regimen designed to relieve congestion may be one of the most powerful as well as one of the simplest ways to update prognosis for an individual patient with end-stage heart failure.

Patients referred with end-stage heart failure merit detailed initial assessment and revision of medical therapy before reassessment of clinical status and risk of future deterioration or death. There is sufficient time for this process in most patients with chronic heart failure. Unfortunately, some health care plans allow only one referral visit, no ongoing specialty care, and no opportunity for reassessment. If we are to make optimal use of the health care resources for advanced disease, however, the element of time and continuity is critical to the selection of the most appropriate therapy for each patient.

THE END OF THE ROAD IS MOVING ON

Downshifting Risks after Introduction of New Procedures

The evolution of new procedures for advanced disease often follows a progressive pattern of improving results and expanding populations. This differs from the development of pharmacologic and exercise therapies for heart failure, which have usually been tested and developed first in patients with relatively mild disease, validated in large trials of moderate disease, and ultimately extended to patients with severe disease, although such patients

would usually have been excluded from the trials that demonstrated benefit. Surgical therapies for heart failure are associated with considerable front-loaded risk that is initially easier to accept for patients expected to have a high early mortality from the natural history of their disease. As survival and improved function are demonstrated in these desperate patients, the procedure may then be sought for patients with less initial compromise. As better operative candidates, these patients have better survival rates than the earlier population. With downshifting risks, however, the actual benefit, calculated as the outcome with the procedure minus the outcome without the procedure, may become less significant (Figure 7).

Cardiac transplantation presents the best-known example of the downshifting risks (Figure 8). Transplantation candidates were originally considered to have "less than 6 months to live." At that time, survival rate after transplantation was only 60% to 70% at 1 year. Now, the 1-year survival rate after transplantation is 80% to 85%, with a 10-year survival rate of up to 40%. The survival *without* transplantation, however, has also improved. For the total population of patients listed for transplantation in the Pre-Transplant Research Database (1992–1994), the 1-year survival rate without transplantation was over 80%. The current benefit of transplantation can be more clearly shown if the different groups are considered (see Figure 8B). Those patients who were initially listed for urgent transplantation had a survival rate of less than 60% at 6 months, by which time most were dead or trans-

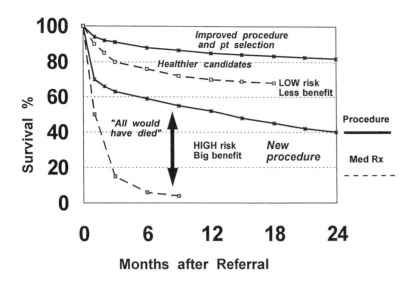

FIG. 7. Downshifting risk concept for evolution of surgical therapies for "end-stage" heart failure. Initially tried only in patients facing imminent death, procedures found to be successful are then performed in less desperate patients. The outcome of the surgery is better in these patients, who are better operative candidates, but the benefit is less dramatic because the natural history of the disease is also more favorable.

planted. For patients requiring frequent hospitalization or out-patient intravenous inotropic therapy, the rate of death or urgent transplantation was almost 50% at 6 months. The largest group of patients were those waiting at home without intravenous infusions for whom the actuarial survival rate without death or urgent transplantation was 64% at 1 year. For all patients listed nonurgently for transplantation, the single most likely actual outcome at the end of 1 year was to be still alive at home without a transplant (Figure 9), as shown by the Pre-Transplant Research Database Centers. This good survival without transplantation is in part possible because the patients were followed closely at the heart failure/transplantation centers where they could be hospitalized for urgent transplantation, which took place in 18% of patients initially listed as Status II.

Cardiomyoplasty is a more recent example of downshifting risks. The early results yielded poor perioperative outcomes in patients with Class IV symptoms, who were then largely excluded from subsequent experience (Figure 10). Other indicators of advanced disease such as significant mitral regurgitation were also considered exclusion criteria. On the other hand, severe symptoms of heart failure are rare in patients without significant mitral regurgitation. The most recent data indicate that patients with left peak oxygen consumption over 16 mL/kg/minute have the best outcome after cardiomyoplasty. As discussed in Chapter 9, these patients have a good outcome in general. Current 1-year survival rates after cardiomyoplasty in patients with Class III symptoms are approximately 70%, similar to those seen with medical therapy in Class III patients, for whom 1-year survival rates are in general 70% to 80% when followed in heart failure programs.

Left ventricular assist devices represent the most current example of a therapy originally introduced for salvage of the dying patient. Most early recipients were in cardiogenic shock with incipient organ failure, not expected to survive 24 to 48 hours. A cohort population study showed over 50% mortality before 3 months for these patients unsupported, compared with 25% to 40% early mortality on implantable left ventricular assist devices. The gratifying results in this population have led to earlier implantation of devices and pretransplantation rehabilitation in patients waiting in hospital for transplantation. As this therapy is extended to ambulatory patients, however, the front-loaded risk of device support will take longer to be exceeded by the natural history of unsupported heart failure (Figure 11). These studies will require more precise definition of a high-risk ambulatory population and longer trial duration to show benefit. Once ambulatory patients are enrolled, it will be more important to consider functional capacity as well. The current functional capacity supported by the device is in the range of 13 to 16 mL/kg/minute peak oxygen consumption, which corresponds with Class III heart failure and potentially with the results achievable in some Class IV patients by exercise training or after improvement on medical therapy alone.

Changing Profiles of "End-Stage" Heart Failure

The evolution of medical therapies continues concomitantly with the evolution in surgical therapies. Not only are the selection criteria changing for surgical intervention, as described previously, but the population from which patients are selected is undergoing fundamental changes. The outlook for patients referred for transplantation has improved as the application of therapies such as ACE inhibitors and the avoidance of detrimental therapies such as Type I antiarrhythmic therapies extend into advanced heart failure, in combination with integrated

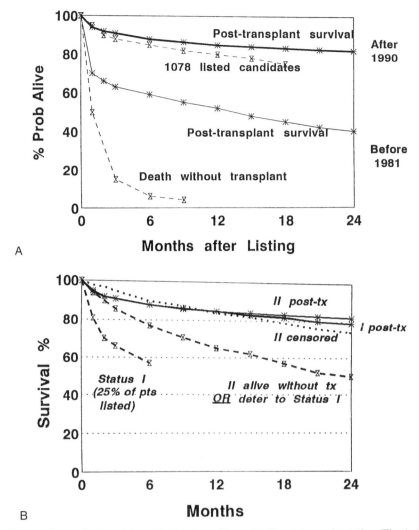

FIG. 8. A: Comparison of actuarial survival rates with and without transplantation. The lower curves are based on the pioneering Stanford experience before 1981. The posttransplantation survival rate is based on the current International Registry. The risk of the procedure has diminished greatly, but the mortality of candidates without transplantation has also decreased markedly. The interpretation is misleading, however, because the survival curves without transplantation censor a patient at the time of transplantation, which may have averted death that would otherwise have occurred on medical therapy. (From Jamieson SW, Oyer PE, Reitz BA, et al. Cardiac transplantation at Stanford. *Journal of Heart Transplantation* 1981;1:86–95; and Hosenpud JD, Novick RJ, Bennett LE, et al. The Registry of the International Society for Heart and Lung Transplant 1996. *J Heart Lung Transplant* 1996;15:655–674, with permission.) **B:** More accurate representation of benefits of transplantation for candidates, in relation to priority at the time of listing. Patients listed as Status I have a high mortality without transplantation, but a virtually equivalent survival rate after transplantation as in patients transplanted electively as Status II. The benefit for Status II patients is more evident if deterioration to a requirement for urgent transplantation (Status I) is displayed *(dashed lines)* instead of censoring all patients at the time of transplant *(dotted line)*. Presumably, most deterioration events would have been deaths if transplantation had not been expeditious. (Data derived from Stevenson LW, Bourge RC, Naftel DC, and the Cardiac Transplant Research Database Group. Deterioration and death on the current waiting list: a multicenter study of patients awaiting heart transplantation. *Circulation* 1995;92:I-702, *abstract;* and Rodeheffer RJ, Naftel DC, Stevenson LW, et al. Secular trends in cardiac transplant recipient and donor management in the United States, 1990–1994: a multiinstitutional study. *Circulation* 1996;94:2883–2889, with permission.)

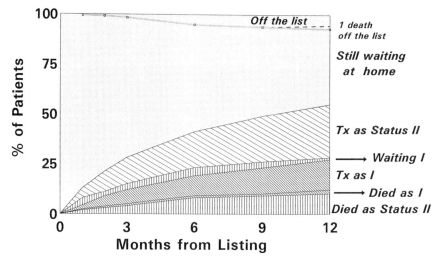

FIG. 9. Actual (not actuarial) outcome for 516 patients with complete 1-year follow-up after listing (1992–1994) among the 12 centers of the Pre-Transplant Research Database for transplantation as Status II. Note that the *actual* mortality rate is only 13%, because many patients underwent transplantation. The *actuarial* mortality rate would be higher, expressed as a percentage of the decreasing number of patients remaining without transplantation. The single most likely outcome at the end of a year for a patient originally listed as a Status II candidate is to be still alive and waiting at home. (From Stevenson LW, Bourge RC, Naftel DC, and the Cardiac Transplant Research Database Group. Deterioration and death on the current waiting list: a multicenter study of patients awaiting heart transplantation. *Circulation* 1995;92:I-702, *abstract,* with permission.)

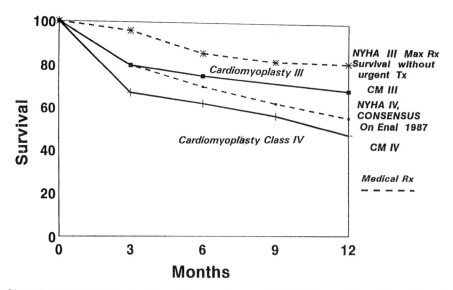

FIG. 10. Changing populations considered for cardiomyoplasty. Initial results in Class IV patients indicated less than a 50% 1-year survival rate when perioperative mortality was added to mortality after hospital discharge, as described in Furnary et al. This was comparable to the mortality from the CONSENSUS Trial Study Group. The more recent experience of Grandjean et al. indicates low operative mortality rates and an overall 1-year survival rate of approximately 70% for Class III patients. This survival rate is comparable to that observed by Stevenson et al. and Lucas et al. for Class III patients receiving medical therapy through heart failure programs. (From Furnary AP, Jessup M, Moreira LFP. Multicenter trial of dynamic cardiomyoplasty for chronic heart failure. *J Am Coll Cardiol* 1996;28:1175–1180; CONSENSUS Trial Study Group. Effects of enalapril on mortality in severe congestive heart failure. *N Engl J Med* 1987;316:1429–1435; Grandjean PA, Austin L, Chan S, et al. Dynamic cardiomyoplasty: clinical follow-up results. *J Card Surg* 1991;6:80–88; Stevenson LW, Couper G, Natterson BJ, et al. Target heart failure populations for newer therapies. *Circulation* 1995;92[Suppl I]:II-174–II-181; and Lucas C, Johnson W, Flavell C, et al. Freedom from congestion at one month predicts good two-year survival after hospitalization for class IV heart failure. *Circulation* 1996;94:I-93, *abstract,* with permission.)

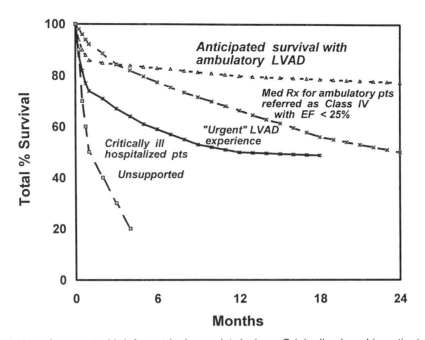

FIG. 11. Evolution of support with left ventricular assist devices. Originally placed in patients critically ill with cardiogenic shock, they allowed rehabilitation and survival to transplantation. As the indications are broadened to include ambulatory patients with heart failure, perioperative risk should decrease. Many patients referred with Class IV heart failure subsequently improve on optimal medical therapy, such that the overall mortality after referral with Class IV symptoms for ambulatory patients does not approach 50% until into the second year. For ambulatory patients with advanced heart failure, the risks and benefits of permanent left ventricular support devices have not been determined. (From Frazier OH, Rose EA, McCarthy P, et al. Improved mortality and rehabilitation of transplant candidates treated with a long-term implantable left ventricular assist system. *Ann Surg* 1995;222:327–336; and Stevenson LW, Hamilton MA, Tillisch JH. Decreasing survival benefit from cardiac transplantation for outpatients as the waiting list lengthens. *J Am Coll Cardiol* 1991;18;919–925, with permission.)

programs of education and management. Presenting with similar baseline clinical and hemodynamic parameters, such patients treated after 1990 have only a 16% 1-year mortality rate, compared with 33% for patients referred in 1986, with reductions in both heart failure death and sudden death (Figure 12). For trials of new therapy, it is no longer easy to identify a target population with a 50% early mortality rate (Table 7).

The changing population considered for "end-stage" therapies is indicated by the current transplant candidates. In the Pre-Transplant Research Database from 1992 to 1994, only 562, or 42% of the 1,344 candidates listed among the 12 major transplantation centers participating were described as Class IV at the time of listing. Using the more specific descriptors of hospitalized or ambulatory "wet" or "dry," the experience at the Brigham and Women's Hospital from 1995 to 1997 includes refractory congestion in only 38% of the ambulatory patients listed, the remainder being primarily limited by low cardiac output reserve during modest exercise, or, less commonly, by refractory angina or arrhythmias (Figure 13). Among the hospitalized candidates, only 31% had a chronic history of heart failure, the remainder being newly diagnosed disease, frequently in the setting of recent infarction.

The emphasis on relief of congestion has allowed definition of the wet and dry heart failure populations (see Table 4). The classic picture of end-stage heart failure was the patient with wet heart failure, of whom there are relatively fewer now. The reciprocal increase in the prevalence of patients with dry heart failure has created a population whose disability may be underappreciated by the average practitioner, because edema and resting dyspnea are absent. Peak oxygen consumption is often required to confirm the limited cardiac reserve in these patients. Invasively measured exercise hemodynamics may occasionally be useful to determine which patients are limited because of central cardiac reserve and which are limited more because of peripheral factors in the face of adequate cardiac response to exertion. More precise definition of the cardiovascular limitations in terms of congestion and perfusion may replace previous approximations of Class III and IV, and determine the further therapeutic options after standard medical therapy has failed.

A major development whose impact has not yet been appreciated is the growing use of the automatic implantable defibrillator, as discussed in Chapter 7. It has long been recognized that there are multiple causes for sudden death in heart failure, among which primary ventricular arrhythmias are only one. The availability of both

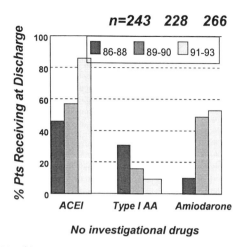

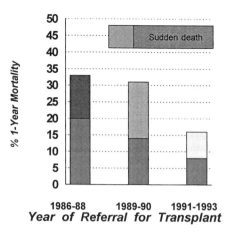

FIG. 12. Changing therapies and improving outcomes for patients discharged after evaluation for cardiac transplantation. The actuarial mortality rate at 1 year decreased from 33% for the 243 patients referred between 1986 and 1988 to 16% for the 266 patients referred between 1991 and 1993. In the Cox proportional hazards model, the improved survival for the more recent cohort was largely explained by an increased use of angiotensin-converting enzyme inhibitors and preference of amiodarone over Type I antiarrhythmic agents. The decrease in mortality resulted both from a decrease in sudden death (*lower bars*) and a decrease in heart failure death. (From Stevenson WG, Stevenson LW, Middlekauff HR, et al. Improving survival for patients with advanced heart failure: a study of 737 consecutive patients. *J Am Coll Cardiol* 1995;26:1417–1423, with permission.)

defibrillation and back-up bradycardia pacing, however, may allow rescue from multiple potential causes of sudden death, including tachyarrhythmias related to ischemic events and primary bradyarrhythmias related to autonomic abnormalities.

The availability of mechanical assist devices further decreases the need to anticipate clinical deterioration with a long lead time. Previously, there was concern that patients might become "too sick" to undergo transplantation or another definitive procedure if the natural history

TABLE 7. *Hierarchy of "end-stages" of heart failure*

Stage	50% Expected mortality[a]
Intensive care unit—critical	<3 mo
Ambulatory on intravenous inotropic support	<6 mo
Ambulatory with history of Class IV symptoms	
Persistent "wet" heart failure despite optimal therapy	<1 yr
Stable "dry" heart failure with very limited cardiac reserve (peak oxygen consumption ≤12–14 mL/kg/min)	<2 yr

[a]This is based on data in patients with left ventricular ejection fractions ≤25%. The mortality for similar severity of symptoms in ambulatory patients would be different when symptoms result from abnormalities of relaxation and circulating volume in patients with relatively preserved left ventricular ejection fraction. In addition, the available survival data reflect primarily the population referred for transplantation, with a median age of 52 years, and no other obvious comorbidity. The mortality would be expected to be worse for patients unsuitable for cardiac transplantation.

of heart failure was followed too long. Current therapies continue to modify this natural history, providing long periods of stability in what was previously thought to be a rapid and inexorable deterioration to death. Even when deterioration occurs unexpectedly, the improving technology and experience with assist devices can often provide adequate stabilization for other therapies to be undertaken electively.

Both the sudden death and unanticipated hemodynamic deterioration can thus be addressed more effectively than in previous eras. There is then decreasing need to act on projected future risks during a period of clinical stability. The more obvious predictors of imminent outcome such as current clinical symptoms and stability will assume greater weight. As the weight of future risk is lessened, there will be less incentive to perform heart transplantations or other procedures to prevent sudden or rapid deterioration in the setting of an otherwise acceptable quality of life.

With reduction of daily uncertainty regarding survival, the assessment of quality of life with different therapies will become relatively more important. This is particularly true for therapies that themselves necessitate substantial adaptation to a different daily routine. Cardiac transplantation provides a good example of a therapy that improves survival and improves measured left ventricular function, but may not always improve functional capacity or global quality of life above that enjoyed by patients with stable heart failure (Figure 14). Patients will need more information and guidance to participate in the decisions regarding choices among different therapies. There

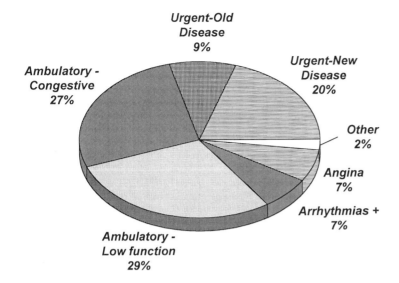

FIG. 13. Distribution of indications for transplantation in the last 100 patients accepted at Brigham and Women's Hospital. Increasing numbers are being listed with newly diagnosed heart failure, usually due to recent myocardial infarction. On therapy to relieve congestion, there are relatively fewer ambulatory patients being listed primarily for congestive symptoms. For patients without symptomatic congestion, the indication of low functional capacity must be confirmed by measurement of peak oxygen consumption (<12–14 mL/kg/minute). Some patients are listed primarily for arrhythmias or angina in the setting of very low left ventricular ejection fraction.

will often be no globally "right" choice, but only a decision that fits an individual patient. When considering options associated with significant morbidity and mortality, patient preference should become a more explicit factor in evaluation and decision making. Preferences may involve a trade-off of time versus quality of life, or a choice between different morbidity burdens.

CONCLUSION

Increasing experience with advanced heart failure demonstrates that very few patients truly have "end-stage" heart disease that is refractory to currently available medical therapies. Prognosis is more accurately estimated not by baseline profiles at referral but by responses to optimal therapy, particularly as guided by the goal of relieving congestion. Evaluation of new surgical therapies is complicated by the downshifting risks of procedures as they become more widely applied to better surgical candidates, and by the simultaneous evolution of contemporary medical therapies. Although these rapid changes will soon render obsolete the survival data provided in this chapter, it is hoped that the principles developed will continue to define the challenges. Heart failure is and will be a surgical disease in those patients for whom surgery offers greater benefits than medical therapy for quality and length of life.

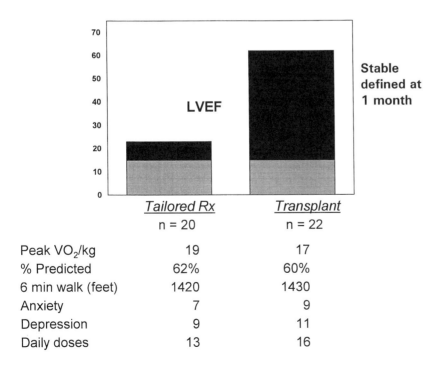

	Tailored Rx	Transplant
	n = 20	n = 22
Peak VO$_2$/kg	19	17
% Predicted	62%	60%
6 min walk (feet)	1420	1430
Anxiety	7	9
Depression	9	11
Daily doses	13	16

Stable defined at 1 month

FIG. 14. Similarity between measured functional capacity at 1 year in patients stable at 1 month after evaluation for cardiac transplantation, regardless of subsequent transplantation. Both groups had an initial average left ventricular ejection fraction of 15%. Patients remaining on tailored therapy had contraindications to transplantation. Peak oxygen consumption, the 6-minute walk distance as a measure of capacity for routine daily activity, and assessment of mood were similar between the two groups of patients despite return to normal left ventricular ejection fraction in the posttransplantation patients. (Data derived from Stevenson LW, Sietsema K, Tillisch JH, et al. Exercise capacity for survivors of cardiac transplantation or sustained medical therapy for stable heart failure. *Circulation* 1990;81:78–85, with permission.)

SELECTED REFERENCES

Aaronson KD, Schwartz JS, Chen T-M, et al. Development and prospective validation of a clinical index to predict survival in ambulatory patients referred for cardiac transplant evaluation. *Circulation* 1997;95:2660–2667.

Coats AJ, Adamopoulos S, Radaelli A, et al. Controlled trial of physical training in chronic heart failure. *Circulation* 1992;85:2119–2131.

DiSalvo TG, Mathier M, Semigran MJ, Dec DW. Preserved right ventricular ejection fraction predicts exercise capacity and survival in advanced heart failure. *J Am Coll Cardiol* 1995;25:1143–1153.

Fonarow GC, Stevenson LW, Walden JA, et al. Impact of comprehensive heart failure management program on rehospitalization and functional status for patients with advanced heart failure. *J Am Coll Cardiol* 1997; 30:725–732.

Hamilton MA, Stevenson LW, Child JS, et al. Sustained reduction in valvular regurgitation and atrial volumes with tailored vasodilator therapy in advanced congestive heart failure secondary to dilated cardiomyopathy. *Am J Cardiol* 1991;67:259–263.

Keogh AM, Freund J, Baron DW. Timing of cardiac transplantation in dilated cardiomyopathy. *Am J Cardiol* 1988;61:418–422.

Kubo SH, Ormaza SM, Francis GS, et al. Trends in patient selection for heart transplantation. *J Am Coll Cardiol* 1993;21:975–981.

Mancini DM, Eisen H, Kussmaul W, et al. Value of peak oxygen consumption for optimal timing of cardiac transplantation in ambulatory patients with heart failure. *Circulation* 1991;83:778–783.

Rickenbacher PR, Trindad PT, Haywood GA, et al. Transplant candidates with severe left ventricular dysfunction managed with medical treatment: characteristics and survival. *J Am Coll Cardiol* 1996;27:1192–1197.

Steimle AE, Stevenson LW, Chelimsky-Fallick, et al. Sustained hemodynamic efficacy of therapy tailored to reduce filling pressures in survivors with advanced heart failure. *Circulation* 1997;96:1165–1172.

Stevenson LW, Couper G, Natterson BJ, et al. Target heart failure populations for newer therapies. *Circulation* 1995;92[Suppl I]:II-174–II-181.

Stevenson LW, Hamilton MA, Tillisch JH, et al. Decreasing survival benefit from cardiac transplantation for outpatients as the waiting list lengthens. *J Am Coll Cardiol* 1991;18;919–925.

Stevenson LW, Massie BM, Francis GS. Optimizing therapy for complex or refractory heart failure: report of the Task Force on Complex Heart Failure. *Am Heart J* 1998 (*in press*).

Stevenson LW, Steimle AE, Fonarow G, et al. Improvement in exercise capacity of candidates awaiting heart transplantation. *J Am Coll Cardiol* 1995;25:163–170.

Stevenson LW, Tillisch JH. Maintenance of cardiac output with normal filling pressures in dilated heart failure. *Circulation* 1986;74:1303–1308.

Conventional Surgical Options

Management of End-Stage Heart Disease, edited by Eric A. Rose and Lynne Warner Stevenson. Lippincott–Raven Publishers, Philadelphia ©1998.

CHAPTER 11

High-Risk Myocardial Revascularization

John A. Kern and Irving L. Kron

Patients with coronary artery disease and severe left ventricular dysfunction often receive standard medical therapy, which may result in poor long-term survival. Despite improvements in vascularization techniques and the evaluation of myocardial viability, many patients who could benefit from surgical revascularization do not receive this treatment. Patients with severe ischemic left ventricular dysfunction, for example, are often not referred for coronary bypass surgery, partly because many surgeons are not willing to perform such high-risk revascularization. One of the major problems with surgical revascularization of these patients is the inability to predict postoperative outcome for any particular patient. Historically, patients whose dominant symptoms were low ejection fraction and angina often did better after revascularization than patients with congestive heart failure (CHF) without angina. Current studies continue to document this phenomenon, showing a higher operative risk and lower 5-year survival rate for patients with CHF without angina. Patients with angina may have a higher survival rate because angina is a marker for jeopardized, but still viable, myocardium. Unfortunately, the lessons learned from these retrospective studies are often difficult to apply to individual patients.

BACKGROUND

Ejection fraction alone is not an adequate predictor of postoperative outcome for any particular patient. Although patients with low ejection fraction clearly have an abnormal ventricle, the clinician must understand what is happening at the cellular level to stratify these high-risk patients accurately. No longer is an ejection fraction of less than 40% (or 30%, or 20%) acceptable (with or without angina or heart failure) as the sole criterion for a "bad" ventricle. We need to identify and examine other predictors of ventricular performance as well, such as measures of ventricular compliance and oxygen consumption. In a recent study by Chan et al., a subgroup of patients with low ejection fraction experienced symptomatic improvement in heart failure with no measurable increase in ejection fraction after surgical revascularization. Patients who show areas of redistribution on preoperative stress thallium-201 scintigraphy, however, usually experience improved ejection fraction after revascularization. This improvement may be caused by the recruitment of poorly perfused "hibernating" myocardium. Subjective improvements in patients' conditions without corresponding improvements in measurable indices of ventricular performance could be explained by the maintenance of the present level of functioning myocardium. Such patients are more likely to show no evidence of reversible ischemia on preoperative thallium studies, and are likely to have replacement of functioning or hibernating myocardium by fibrous tissue and scar.

Each year, approximately 300,000 people in the United States are diagnosed with ischemic heart failure. Also each year, 80,000 people die of this condition, usually because of progressive CHF or ventricular arrhythmias. Most of these patients have been treated medically, but many have received revascularization. Determining which patients should be treated medically and which should be treated surgically can be a difficult task. It may also be difficult to decide when to operate. Patients with ischemic cardiomyopathy and who have undergone high-risk revascularization may be candidates for cardiac transplantation. Prior coronary artery bypass surgery does not appear to increase the risks of cardiac transplantation. Unfortunately, because the number of donor organs are limited, only about 2,100 Americans can undergo cardiac transplantation each year.

The question may then be not who to revascularize, but when should someone be revascularized. The medical management of ischemic heart failure is improving. In the past, patients treated medically had 5-year survival

Department of Surgery, University of Virginia Health System, Charlottesville, Virginia 22908 rates of 20% to 30%. Today, patients with ischemic heart failure who are referred for transplantation can usually live 3 to 4 years while awaiting transplantation. Evaluating and weighing the potential risks and benefits of coronary bypass in these patients is very difficult. Studies have shown acceptable operative mortality, but existing data analyzing predictors of long-term performance are difficult to apply clinically. Most studies are retrospective reviews, and the definition of poor ventricular function is too varied. In addition, some studies have included patients with recent acute myocardial infarction, and the revascularization of these patients may falsely enhance long-term results.

More data are needed to determine when to revascularize patients with ischemic cardiomyopathy. Some authors have reported a series of patients who were referred for heart transplantation but instead underwent high-risk cardiac surgical procedures, mainly revascularization. In all series, acceptable functional status and survival were noted. A retrospective, nonrandomized review of 143 patients was reported by Luciani and colleagues. Medically treated patients had a 5-year survival rate of 28%. Surgically revascularized patients had a 5-year survival rate of 80%, but an operative mortality rate of 20%. Patients undergoing transplantation had a 5-year survival rate of 82% and an operative mortality rate of 11.6%. Medically treated patients deteriorated despite treatment, whereas revascularized patients improved.

Another question then arises: which patients with advanced left ventricular ischemic dysfunction should not undergo surgical revascularization? Obvious factors come to mind. Patients with life-limiting noncardiac diseases, for example, should not undergo an operation. In addition, good target vessels are needed to which to sew. Repeat cardiac revascularization surgery should also be carefully considered before being undertaken. Until further prospective studies are undertaken to identify risk factors that predict poor outcomes, the decision whether to perform high-risk revascularization will often be made based on the individual surgeon's experience. The remainder of this chapter reviews preoperative, intraoperative, and postoperative issues that may help the surgeon to make a decision.

FACTORS INFLUENCING SURVIVAL IN HIGH-RISK REVASCULARIZATION

Preoperative Assessment

Some of the earliest reports of high-risk revascularization appeared in the early 1970s. Reported results were variable. Operative and early postoperative mortality rates were high, and the long-term survival of patients treated surgically was often not better than that of the patients treated medically. Surgeons noted, however, that patients with angina pectoris had a lower operative risk.

In addition, patients with a greater severity of congestive heart failure had a greater chance for poor outcome. By the late 1970s, the operative mortality rates for patients with low ejection fraction who underwent high-risk revascularization had decreased to between 4% and 10%, and long-term survival was often better in patients treated surgically than in patients treated medically. Around this time, a study from Stanford reported that the actual 5-year survival rate for medically treated patients was only 18%, whereas the 5-year survival rate for surgically treated patients was 66%. This study also found that patients with angina fared better with surgical treatment than with medical treatment. Patients with severe CHF and no angina, however, had a poor prognosis when treated medically or surgically. In fact, the severity of heart failure was the strongest determinant of death. The enhanced postoperative life expectancy in patients with poor ventricular function and angina pectoris was due to the reduction in time-related incidence of myocardial infarction.

Since these early reports, many authors have reported improved survival of patients undergoing high-risk revascularization who present with minimal angina and severe heart failure. The introduction of more sophisticated preoperative imaging techniques, such as thallium-201 scintigraphy, single-photon emission computed tomography, and positron emission tomography, has helped surgeons determine more precisely which patients might benefit most from revascularization. Two studies have attempted to define more accurately the predictors of surgical outcome. Chan et al. performed a prospective study in an attempt to define the preoperative variables that best predict a favorable outcome in patients with poor ventricular function who are undergoing surgical revascularization. This study included 57 consecutive patients with stable coronary artery disease with a mean ejection fraction of 28%. Patients with acute myocardial infarction or ischemic events within 4 weeks of surgery, as well as patients with unstable angina or significant left main disease, and patients requiring repeat coronary surgery, were excluded from the study. Thirty-seven of the 57 patients underwent thallium-201 scintigraphy before operation; 31 of these 37 patients had some degree of reversibility, with 18 patients showing large areas of redistribution. In this study, a favorable outcome was defined as survival at 12 months and postoperative improvement in left ventricular ejection fraction of 0.05% or more. The only clinical variable found to predict a good surgical outcome was the presence of a large reversible defect on preoperative thallium-201 imagery. In addition, 16 of the 18 patients with a large reversible defect noted subjective improvement in heart failure symptoms 1 year after surgery. Patients with fixed, small or moderate-sized reversible defects did not fare so well. Four patients died within 1 year, mean ejection fraction did not change, and only seven patients had improvement in heart failure symptoms. In general, the authors concluded that most patients demonstrated an improvement in angina and heart failure symptoms after surgical revascularization, independent of objective improvement in left ventricular ejection fraction. Perhaps there was a "placebo effect" of surgery, or perhaps the revascularization procedure provided an improvement in coronary flow reserve that was clinically evident only as improved postoperative exercise tolerance. Other studies have corroborated these results by showing that successful revascularization can improve subjective symptoms of heart failure without improvements in objective measures of cardiac function. Objective improvements in left ventricular ejection fraction can be expected most in patients with large reversible defects suggestive of significant viable myocardium on preoperative thallium-201 scanning.

Another retrospective study attempted to quantify survival in patients undergoing high-risk revascularization and to characterize the patients most likely to benefit from surgery. Ejection fraction in all study patients was less than 20%. Reasons for revascularization included unstable angina, recurrent angina after previous revascularization, CHF symptoms, or ventricular arrhythmias. All patients with CHF had reversible ischemia on preoperative imaging. Patients with dilated cardiomyopathy, left ventricular aneurysm, or severe segmental dysfunction were not included in the study. Preoperative predictors of increased perioperative mortality included advanced age, female gender, and increasing severity of coronary artery disease. Patients with preoperative ventricular arrhythmias and patients with renal failure also had an increased risk of death early after operation. Others have noted similar findings.

A retrospective study by Milan et al. from Duke University identified four variables associated with higher perioperative mortality: other vascular disease, female gender, hypertension, and elevated left ventricular end-diastolic pressure. Marginally significant preoperative variables predictive of increased mortality included older age, sustained ventricular tachyarrhythmias, the need for preoperative intraaortic balloon counterpulsation, and low preoperative cardiac index.

Intraoperative Factors

There exists no standardized surgical technique used by all surgeons for coronary artery bypass surgery. Reports of successful high-risk coronary revascularization have found that patients with advanced ischemic left ventricular dysfunction can be safely revascularized with operative mortality rates as low as 2% to 3%. Although outstanding results have been achieved using a variety of surgical techniques, we believe the improved results are largely due to improved myocardial management techniques. We also believe the best operation for any patient is the use of techniques most familiar to the operating surgeon.

The most commonly used technique for myocardial management during coronary revascularization may not be known, but most surgeons probably use a single cross-clamp technique with mild to moderate systemic hypothermia and blood-based cardioplegia. Having said this, early reports of successful high-risk revascularization documenting low operative mortality rates, including our own series from the University of Virginia, include patients managed with cold crystalloid cardioplegia. We have since changed to cold blood cardioplegia and believe this change enhances myocardial protection during aortic cross-clamping. Because studies are ongoing and various reports continue to appear, we will not comment as to the potential advantages of warm versus cold cardioplegia, or on the potential roles for warm induction cardioplegia and warm substrate-enhanced reperfusates (the so-called "hot-shot"). Recent studies are indicating, however, that blood cardioplegia is superior to crystalloid cardioplegia during the revascularization of these high-risk patients.

The use of retrograde cardioplegia through a coronary sinus cannula has been identified in one retrospective study as a predictor of improved early postoperative survival in high-risk revascularization. In a report in patients with an ejection fraction of less than 20%, those who did not receive retrograde coronary sinus cardioplegia had an increased risk of death early after surgery compared with patients receiving combined antegrade and retrograde cardioplegia. These patients were not randomized into different treatment groups, however, and other factors could have been responsible for the survival difference. In theory, retrograde perfusion may improve delivery of cardioplegic solution to the ischemic myocyte, particularly in patients with severe multivessel coronary artery disease, and may result in improved cardiac function in the early postoperative period. Uniform myocardial cooling may not be an adequate explanation because studies have appeared documenting the efficacy of warm blood cardioplegia. In general, we believe optimal myocardial management and protection are crucial to successful high-risk revascularization. Electrical silence with minimal myocardial oxygen requirements coupled with either continuous or, at the least, intermittent delivery of oxygenated-blood cardioplegic solution is the optimal situation for these patients.

Although complete revascularization is an important goal when performing high-risk coronary bypass surgery, one study reported that when the number of distal anastomoses performed increased, survival decreased. The possible reason for this decrease was not clear, but perhaps it may have been related to longer bypass or operative times. In the study by Milano et al., a longer cardiopulmonary bypass time was predictive of an increased length of hospital stay after surgery, but had no impact on early or late survival.

Langenburg et al. from our institution reported that the quality of the distal coronary vasculature may have a profound effect on survival after revascularization of patients with low ejection fractions. Ninety-six patients with heart failure and ejection fractions of 25% or less underwent coronary bypass. The operative mortality rate was 8%. The catheterization films were examined retrospectively by a blinded, nonbiased cardiac surgeon who was not involved in the management of any of the patients. Target vessels were graded as poor, fair, or good. The results of this retrospective study indicated that increasing age and poor vessel quality were the only two predictors of poor surgical outcome. The presence of angina and the number of bypass grafts had no significant bearing on perioperative outcome (Table 1). The conclusion was made that even in the presence of angina, coronary bypass grafting is contraindicated in older patients with poor vessel quality.

Finally, the use of the internal mammary artery should not be denied to patients with severe left ventricular dysfunction undergoing surgical revascularization. Long-term survival benefits may result from internal mammary artery grafts, and problems with low early flow rates and susceptibility to inotropic agents have not been significant problems in our hands. We and others have reported series in which the internal mammary artery was routinely used in high-risk revascularization with little or no difficulty. We therefore strongly recommend the use of the internal mammary artery in high-risk revascularization.

Postoperative Considerations

We use pharmacologic inotropic support in every patient coming off cardiopulmonary bypass. We do not routinely use an intraaortic balloon pump in high-risk revascularization patients, but if difficulty is encountered weaning a patient from bypass on inotropic support alone, a balloon pump is inserted. Some authors, however, believe that unsuccessful attempts at weaning from cardiopulmonary bypass can cause irrevocable harm to already jeopardized myocardium, and that prophylactic use of intraaortic balloon counterpulsation should be routinely considered for the poorest of ventricles or the most tenuous coronary supply. A report by Dietl et al. stated that the preoperative prophylactic insertion of an intraaortic balloon pump should be strongly considered in most patients with low ejection fraction. In particular, patients with an ejection fraction of less than 25% and with New York Heart Association heart failure Class III or IV, or patients undergoing reoperation, are likely to have improved survival and shorter hospital stays if a balloon pump is inserted before surgery. The authors believe that an intraaortic balloon pump is the most predictable method of myocardial protection during induction of anesthesia and the prebypass period, and that perhaps this leads to improved postoperative myocardial function.

If we are still unable to wean from cardiopulmonary bypass, a ventricular assist device or extracorporeal membrane oxygenation circuit, depending on the situation, should be considered. Prolonged mechanical support of the failing postcardiotomy ventricle is not often successful in high-risk revascularization, but recovery of acceptable cardiac function is occasionally achieved, and if indicated, the patient can be considered for cardiac transplantation.

RESULTS AND CONCLUSIONS

Surgical vascularization should be considered as a treatment option in the management of patients with ischemic left ventricular dysfunction and CHF. Operative mortality rates have been reduced to the range of 5%. No longer does the presence of CHF without angina contraindicate successful coronary bypass surgery. In a review of treatment options for the failing left ventricle, two clinical studies were summarized, one by Elefteriades from Yale, the other by Kron from the University of Virginia. Independent series of patients with severe left ventricular dysfunction undergoing vascularization yielded remarkably similar results.

In the Yale series, 83 consecutive patients with a mean ejection fraction of 24.2% underwent coronary bypass surgery by a single surgeon over a 6-year period. The Virginia series included 39 patients with an ejection fraction lower than 20% (mean ejection fraction, 18.3%). Both series excluded patients with associated cardiac surgical procedures (e.g., valve replacement or aneurysm resection), and the Virginia series excluded patients with acute coronary events in order to evaluate only patients with chronic ischemic cardiomyopathy. These studies independently documented the safety of the revascularization, as reflected by low mortality rates, excellent long-term survival (>80% at 3 years), improved ventricular dysfunction, and improved quality of life (relief of angina and reduction in CHF symptoms). The authors concluded that surgical revascularization in this high-risk patient population protects already normal myocardium, recruiting hibernating viable muscle and improving ejection fraction exercise tolerance and subjective symptoms of heart failure.

TABLE 1. *Possible predictors of postoperative outcome*

Predictor	Hospital survivors (n = 88)	Hospital deaths (n = 8)
Age (yr)	62.6±0.9	68.8±2.0[a]
Angina		
Stable	80% (70)	75% (6)
Unstable	11% (10)	12.5% (1)
None	9% (8)	12.5% (1)
Ejection fraction	0.2±0.00	0.20±0.02
Number of bypass grafts	3±0.1	3±0.3
Cross-clamp time	49.8±2.8	40.3±8.4

[a]$p < 0.05$.

When not to perform revascularization on a patient with ischemic left ventricular dysfunction may be difficult to determine. We believe that in the absence of fatal, noncardiac disease, any high-risk patient with evidence of ischemia and good-quality, graftable target vessels should be considered for coronary bypass surgery. Most can be expected to show postoperative improvement. If symptoms persist or recur, improvements in medical management may provide temporary relief while other therapeutic options, such as transplantation, are considered.

SELECTED REFERENCES

Baker DW, Jones R, Hodges J, et al. Management of heart failure: III. the role of revascularization in the treatment of patients with moderate or severe left ventricular systolic dysfunction. *JAMA* 1994;272:1528–1534.

Chan RKM, Raman J, Lee KG, et al. Prediction of outcome after revascularization in patients with poor left ventricular function. *Ann Thorac Surg* 1996;61:1428–1434.

Dreyfus GC, Duboc D, Blasco A, et al. Myocardial viability assessment in ischemic cardiomyopathy: benefits of coronary revascularization. *Ann Thorac Surg* 1994;57:1402–1408.

Elefteriades JA, Kron IL. CABG in advanced left ventricular dysfunction. *Cardiol Clin* 1995;1:35–42.

Langenburg SE, Buchanan SA, Blackbourne LH, et al. Predicting survival after coronary revascularization for ischemic cardiomyopathy. *Ann Thorac Surg* 1995;60:1193–1197.

Lansman SL, Cohen M, Galla JD, et al. Coronary bypass with ejection fraction of 0.20 or less using centigrade cardioplegia: long-term follow-up. *Ann Thorac Surg* 1993;56:480–486.

Luciani GB, Faggian G, Razzolini R, et al. Severe ischemic left ventricular failure: coronary operation or heart transplantation. *Ann Thorac Surg* 1993;55:719–723.

Magovern JA, Magovern GJ, Maher TD, et al. Operation for congestive heart failure: transplantation, coronary artery bypass, and cardiomyoplasty. *Ann Thorac Surg* 1993;56:418–425.

Mickleborough LL, Maruyama H, Takagi Y, et al. Results of revascularization in patients with severe left ventricular dysfunction. *Circulation* 1995;92[Suppl II]:73–79.

Milano CA, White WD, Smith LR, et al. Coronary artery bypass in patients with severely depressed ventricular function. *Ann Thorac Surg* 1993;56:487–493.

Miller DC, Stinson EB, Alderman EL. Surgical treatment of ischemic cardiomyopathy: is it ever too late? *Am J Surg* 1981;141:688–693.

Tyras DH, Kaiser GC, Barnes HB, et al. Global left ventricular impairment and myocardial revascularization: determinants of survival. *Ann Thorac Surg* 1984;37:47–51.

Management of End-Stage Heart Disease, edited
by Eric A. Rose and Lynne Warner Stevenson.
Lippincott–Raven Publishers, Philadelphia ©1998.

CHAPTER 12

Ventricular Aneurysmectomy and Surgical Ablative Approaches for Malignant Arrhythmias

Lynda L. Mickleborough

A surgical approach that combines revascularization with surgical remodeling of the ventricle should be considered in patients with coronary artery disease when myocardial infarction has occurred and resulted in a significant decrease in left ventricular function and a wall motion abnormality or potential aneurysm. Such procedures can be accomplished with low risk to the patient and may offer several benefits, including prolonged survival and control of symptoms due to ischemia or congestive heart failure. In patients with ventricular arrhythmias, an ablation procedure can be performed at the time of surgery to reduce the risk of recurrent ventricular tachycardia or sudden death.

DIAGNOSTIC CONSIDERATIONS FOR ANEURYSM REPAIR

To understand the role of surgery in the treatment of patients with a ventricular aneurysm, the clinician must first consider the criteria used to define the presence or absence of an aneurysm. Angiographically, an aneurysm is an area of the ventricle that is clearly demarcated from the surrounding tissue by hypokinesis, akinesis, or dyskinesis. Anatomically, however, an aneurysm may manifest as an obvious sac of thinned scar tissue (classic pathologic definition of an aneurysm) or as a region composed of scar and viable muscle of variable thickness.

Based on the angiogram, it may be difficult to determine whether a patient may benefit from revascularization (with the hope of recruiting hibernating myocardium and improving regional wall motion), or from resection with ventricular reconstruction. Thus, preoperative perfu-

sion scans, positron emission tomography, and dobutamine echocardiography have been used to try to separate scar from viable nonfunctioning myocardium. In our experience, however, the final decision whether to perform revascularization or resection can best be made at the time of surgery.

When operating on patients with a suspected aneurysm, the degree of thinning in the affected area may not be apparent even when the patient is placed on cardiopulmonary bypass. Because thrombotic material may exist inside the cavity, insertion of a vent to decompress the ventricle further is associated with risk of embolism. Therefore, we prefer to assess the degree of thinning of the infarcted wall by simple needle aspiration. If the area that appears aneurysmal on the angiogram corresponds to a thick region of myocardium mixed with scar, then revascularization is performed. If the area appears thin, an aneurysm is present and the area is resected regardless of whether myocardium has been completely replaced by transmural scar. Throughout this chapter, the word "aneurysm" has been used with this surgical definition in mind.

HEMODYNAMIC CONSEQUENCES OF A LEFT VENTRICULAR ANEURYSM

Almost all ventricular aneurysms result from myocardial infarction due to coronary artery disease. After infarction, the affected region experiences a loss of contractile function and distention of the ventricular chamber. Thus, wall stress increases, systolic shortening decreases, and oxygen consumption increases in areas that are removed from the original infarct. Expansion and thinning of the infarcted area may produce additional work because of paradoxic motion of the thinned segment. Infarct expansion may also cause muscle fibers in

Department of Surgery, University of Toronto, The Toronto General Hospital, Toronto, Ontario, M5G 2C4 Canada the surrounding contractile segments to realign, further decreasing the efficiency of contraction. At the same time, extensive scarring and calcification may cause decreased compliance of the left ventricle. These changes in ventricular function may precipitate or aggravate symptoms related to ongoing ischemia in noninfarcted areas, or may lead to symptoms of congestive heart failure (CHF). Finally, mitral regurgitation may occur if papillary muscles were involved in the original infarct or if changes in ventricular geometry secondary to the formation of the aneurysm interfere with function of the subvalvular mitral apparatus.

NATURAL HISTORY OF LEFT VENTRICULAR ANEURYSMS

Patients whose angiograms suggest the presence of an aneurysm after extensive transmural myocardial infarction often have a high early mortality rate. Patients with this condition may require urgent surgery because of ongoing ischemia or complications from infarction. Surgery often reveals that the dyskinetic area of the ventricular wall is an area that has still not undergone significant fibrosis and thinning (nonaneurysmal by surgical definition). In these instances, revascularization of the stunned myocardium may significantly improve regional wall motion.

If an associated anatomic defect (such as a ventricular septal defect or free wall rupture) is present, incision into the nonthinned infarcted area is required. In such cases, a special repair called "endoaneurysmorrhaphy," which avoids suturing to necrotic muscle, may be used if it can be accomplished without compromising the size of the residual ventricular cavity. Alternatively, an onlay patch repair of the septum or a patch exclusion of an apical rupture can be combined with linear closure of the ventriculotomy.

Late chronic ventricular aneurysms may develop in patients who survive acute infarction. In these patients, fibrous tissue slowly replaces necrotic muscle in the expanded infarct area. This process is often associated with thinning of the walls (compatible with the surgical definition of aneurysm). Despite this thinning, however, a significant amount of viable myocardium may remain in the infarct zone or aneurysm.

INDICATIONS FOR ANEURYSM REPAIR

In patients with a chronic left ventricular aneurysm, large aneurysms, low global ejection fractions, and extensive coronary artery disease are associated with poor prognosis. In these patients, modern medical therapy, including angiotensin-converting enzyme inhibitors, may effectively control symptoms, often delaying hemodynamic decompensation for years. Once decompensation occurs, however, deterioration may be rapid. Patients may

die before surgery can be properly considered. For these reasons, patients in whom an aneurysm develops after myocardial infarction should be followed closely and considered for operation when signs of decompensation first occur. These signs include symptoms of increasing angina or CHF, the occurrence of ventricular arrhythmias, or recurrent embolic events.

In addition, ventricular aneurysm resection should be considered in asymptomatic patients who have critical coronary anatomy (left main stem stenosis or triple-vessel disease) and vessels that can be bypassed. We also advocate aneurysm resection in asymptomatic patients who show evidence of deteriorating left ventricular function (increasing diastolic dimensions, decreasing ejection fraction, or increasing mitral regurgitation). We believe that, in these cases, surgery should be performed before the patient becomes so ill that cardiac transplantation is the only reasonable alternative.

Patients with a ventricular aneurysm often have some degree of mitral regurgitation. This combination has been associated with increased operative risk. Angiograms often do not detect mitral regurgitation because dye may be diluted in the enlarged ventricle, making it difficult to see the regurgitant jet. In our experience, Doppler echocardiographic studies taken before surgery may detect 2+ mitral regurgitation not found by the angiogram.

The degree of mitral regurgitation depends on loading conditions and left ventricular geometry. Repair of the aneurysm with or without revascularization may significantly improve valve function because of (a) decreased annular dilatation secondary to decreased left ventricular size; (b) improved function of the valvular apparatus due to realignment of the papillary muscles secondary to aneurysm repair; or (c) improved function of ischemic papillary muscles secondary to revascularization. If the patient has a fairly discrete aneurysm, the degree of improvement in mitral regurgitation following repair will increase with aneurysm size and its proximity to the mitral valve.

FALSE ANEURYSMS

Both angiographic and pathologic criteria can be used to differentiate true and false aneurysms. The classic definition states that true aneurysms arise when transmural infarcts expand and thin, whereas false aneurysms develop when pericardial adhesions contain a rupture of the free wall (Figure 1). Pathologically, however, distinguishing between true and false aneurysm is often difficult. In fact, Davies has suggested that differentiation may have no clinical relevance. We believe that when the aneurysm is chronic (and not discovered after acute infarction), "false aneurysms" are no more likely to rupture than "true aneurysms," and thus are not surgical emergencies.

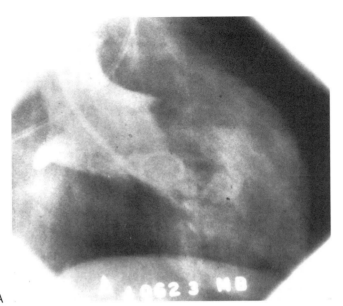
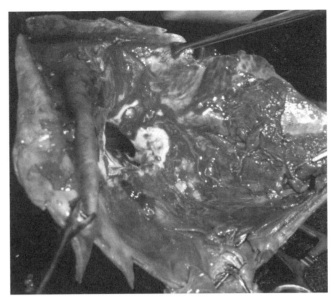

A

B

FIG. 1. A: Ventriculogram showing large apical aneurysm superimposed on left ventricular cavity of normal size and shape. **B:** Intraoperative photograph after removal of clot from large aneurysm sac. A relatively small defect in the ventricular wall is seen. (Reproduced with permission from Mickleborough LL, Takagi Y, Ohashi M. Ischemic heart disease: left ventricular aneurysm: linear closure. In: *Mastery of cardiothoracic surgery.* Boston: Little, Brown and Company [*in press*].)

ANATOMIC CONSIDERATIONS

Most aneurysms are anteroapical and follow the distribution of the left anterior descending artery. Such aneurysms often extend over the apex; to what extent depends on the relative distribution of the vessel. In these cases, the diagonal branch and anterior papillary muscle are displaced laterally after infarct expansion and thinning.

In posterior aneurysms, the posterior interventricular artery is the occluded vessel. The posterior papillary muscle is often located close to the lateral margin of the thinned myocardium. Therefore, great care must be taken to avoid compromising this structure during the repair. In anterior and posterior aneurysms, the interventricular septum may be involved in the scarring and thinning process. In such cases, a patch should be used to exclude the aneurysmal septum.

Occasionally, an aneurysm may occur in the distribution of an obtuse marginal or diagonal branch. In all of the aforementioned variations, the principles of repair are the same.

Extensive calcification occurs in 10% to 15% of aneurysms. Often, this calcification primarily involves the endocardial and mid-myocardial layers and is covered epicardially by scar mixed with surviving muscle. In rare cases, the calcification extends through all layers of the ventricular wall. To help excise the scar tissue adequately and to allow safe myocardial repair, all of the calcification must be removed before any attempt at closure.

RECOMMENDED SURGICAL TECHNIQUE

Tailored Scar Excision and Primary Closure

While the patient is supported on cardiopulmonary bypass, the heart is carefully examined. If there is any doubt that the infarct area is significantly thinned, aspiration with an 18-gauge needle can be used to determine wall thickness. The aneurysm is opened and all of the clot carefully removed. A vent is then inserted through the right superior pulmonary vein. With the heart open and beating, all obviously thinned transmural scar is excised. The surrounding edges are palpated and assessed for contractility. Whenever possible, areas capable of significant contraction or thickening in the unloaded state are not resected, but revascularized. Areas that do not contract should be considered for excision, even when they are 4 to 5 mm thick. To determine the extent of excision, the size and shape of the remaining ventricular cavity is evaluated. When the residual chamber has a relatively normal size and shape, linear closure can be easily accomplished. In patients with marked chamber dilatation, diffuse hypokinesis, and distortion of ventricular shape (spherical vs. conical), however, restoring the left ventricular cavity toward normal size or shape is not possible (Figure 2). In such patients, some of the nonfunctioning wall may have to be left behind so that linear closure can be performed without distorting ventricular geometry (specifically, the relationship between papillary muscles and the septum).

In patients with an obvious septal aneurysm, a patch septoplasty should be performed using bovine preserved

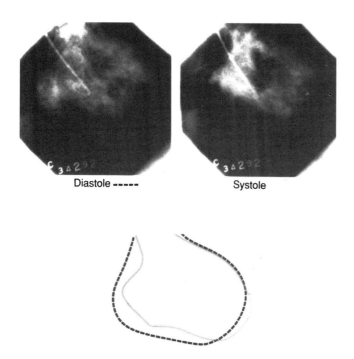

FIG. 2. Representative diastolic and systolic frames from ventriculogram of patient in aneurysm series. Ventricular wall is diffusely hypokinetic. Chamber is markedly dilated and distorted. (Reproduced with permission from Mickleborough LL, Maruyama H, Liu P, Mohamed S. Results of left ventricular aneurysmectomy with a tailored scar excision and primary closure technique. *J Thorac Cardiovasc Surg* 1994;107: 690–698.)

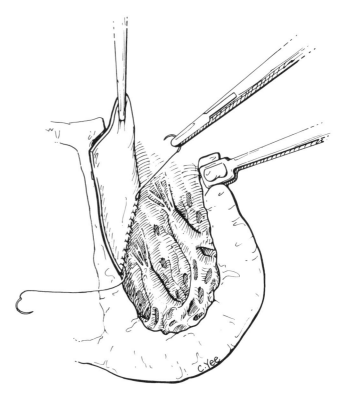

FIG. 3. Diagram showing coronal section of the heart with bovine epicardial patch used to reinforce thinned septum. The patch is attached to the septum with a 4-0 prolene suture. (Reproduced with permission from Mickleborough LL. Operative techniques in cardiac and thoracic surgery: a comparative atlas. JL Cox and TM Sundt III, editors. W. B. Saunders, 1997;2(2):118–131.

pericardium. The patch is applied to the left ventricular aspect of the septum and is sewn to the surrounding myocardium with 4-0 prolene (Figure 3). Deep stitches are avoided because they may compromise collateral flow through the septum. Anteriorly, the patch is incorporated into the ventriculotomy repair. Such patches can be safely sewn in place without inducing cardioplegic arrest.

In patients with calcified aneurysms, the epicardium over the calcium is incised and calcified tissue is removed *en bloc* by carefully dissecting the calcified layer from the surrounding tissue (Figure 4). Often, calcification extends on the endocardial surface well beyond the planned area of resection. Complete excision of the calcified layer helps in approximating the walls during the repair, reducing the risk of excessive bleeding.

In many patients, the aneurysm consists of a mixture of viable muscle and scar. It is rarely possible to leave behind a rim of fibrous tissue, as mentioned in the classic description of aneurysm repair. Often, closing sutures have to be placed through fairly thick areas of myocardium. Closure is performed using interrupted prolene sutures buttressed with two felt strips (Figure 5).

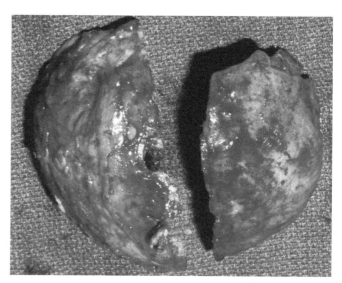

FIG. 4. Resected specimen from patient with calcified aneurysm. The defect was closed with modified linear closure technique. (Reproduced with permission from Mickleborough LL. Surgical management of left ventricular ventricular aneurysms. *Semin Thorac Cardiovasc Surg* 1995;7: 233–239.)

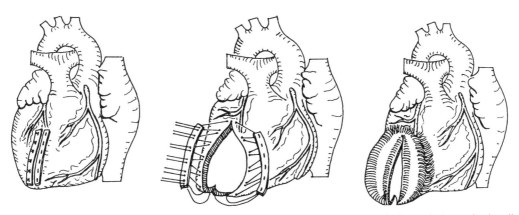

FIG. 5. Diagram showing preoperative appearance and suture closure technique that results in plication of the repair to restore more normal shape to the ventricle. Each mattress suture incorporates a wider distance on edge of left ventricular resection than it does in felt strips. When sutures are tied, resection margins are plicated in a longitudinal direction, which restores left ventricular size and shape toward normal. Additional continuous sutures are later added to obtain hemostasis. (Reproduced with permission from Mickleborough LL, Maruyama H, Liu P, Mohamed S. Results of left ventricular aneurysmectomy with a tailored scar excision and primary closure technique. *J Thorac Cardiovasc Surg* 1994; 107:690–698.)

Sutures are placed further apart in the tissue than on the felt, plicating the length of the incision in the closure. This helps restore the shape of the ventricle toward normal. After deairing, the sutures are tied and cut. The closure is then reinforced with a continuous, over-and-over suture technique to ensure hemostasis. By performing the entire repair without cross-clamping, ischemic time is kept to a minimum. Minimizing ischemic time may decrease perioperative morbidity and mortality, especially in patients with severe triple-vessel disease.

After completing the ventricular repair, the aorta is cross-clamped and cardioplegia is given so that aorto-coronary bypass grafting may be performed. Myocardial protection is essential to achieve optimal results. We originally used temperature mapping to ensure adequate cardioplegia delivery. More recently, we switched to retrograde cardioplegia to protect the left ventricle, where adequate temperature mapping may be difficult because of diffuse scarring. The right ventricle is cooled by antegrade cardioplegia through the root or through a graft to the right coronary artery when indicated.

We revascularize the proximal portion of the left anterior descending artery whenever possible, even if the distal vessel has been amputated in the repair. We believe that revascularization of even a small portion of the septum may be important in improving short- and long-term results.

The basic principles of tissue resection and repair apply to most patients with an inferior aneurysm. In some patients, however, a thin scar extends up to the level of the mitral valve annulus, making it impossible to excise the entire thinned area and reapproximate the edges without plication or distortion of the valve ring. In such cases, a portion of the thinned posterior wall adjacent to the atrioventricular groove is retained. Satisfactory repair is accomplished in this region using a triangular patch of pericardium to reinforce the closure (Figure 6). This patch is incorporated into the posterior linear repair, which has been previously described.

In a few patients with inferior aneurysms, there is thinning of the entire posterior wall between the septum and the base of the papillary muscle. In such patients, primary closure of the defect would result in gross distortion of the subvalvular apparatus. Instead of primary closure, a free wall patch must be inserted to obtain satisfactory results.

Alternate Repair Techniques

Likoff and Bailey first reported successful surgical repair of an aneurysm in 1955. Cooley et al. reported the first resection using cardiopulmonary bypass in 1958. Their technique involved removing the aneurysm and leaving a rim of scar, followed by linear repair. This approach remained the standard technique until Jatene questioned whether such a closure deformed the geometry of the ventricle and led to a decreased efficiency of contraction. He advocated resection of the scar tissue followed by use of a circumferential suture to decrease the size of the defect before performing linear or patch closure. More recently, a more complex internal patch repair technique called "endoaneurysmorrhaphy" has been advocated. This technique is indicated for repair of acute ventricular septal defects or free wall rupture. It has also been advocated for use in repairing chronic aneurysms. Some believe using this technique can avoid causing ven-

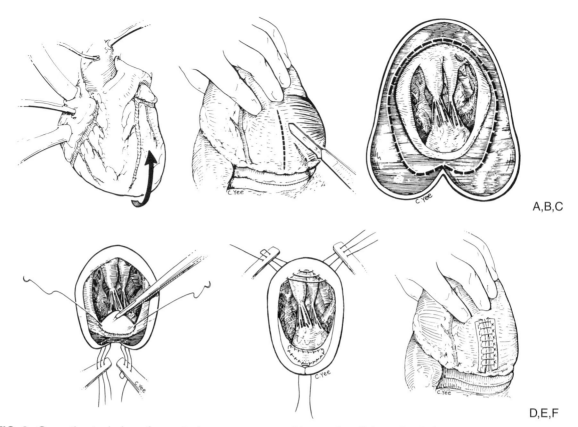

A,B,C

D,E,F

FIG. 6. Operative technique for posterior aneurysm requiring pericardial patch reinforcement along the mitral valve annulus. **A:** The apex of the heart is elevated. **B:** The proposed incision in the posterior aneurysm is indicated. **C:** Close-up of opened aneurysm. The edges are retracted and the thinned portion of the posterior wall is indicated (*shaded area*). The proposed resection margin is outlined by the dashed line. **D:** Most of the thinned area has been resected. The remaining edge to be closed is shown in cross-section. To accomplish the repair without distortion of the mitral valve annulus, and to reinforce the closure close to the valve posteriorly, a pericardial patch is used. It is attached first along the mitral valve annulus. In this diagram, the patch is elevated to show sutures in the remaining thinned scar tissue (*shaded area*), which is closed posteriorly as a separate layer. **E:** After tying the sutures in the thinned posterior layer, the pericardial patch is reflected posteriorly to cover and reinforce the repair. The patch is then attached laterally and medially to relatively normal myocardium. The apex of the patch is incorporated into the posterior linear repair, which is performed with interrupted sutures and felt strips. **F:** The diagram shows plicated posterior repair. An over-and-over continuous suture is used to complete the closure and ensure hemostasis. (Reproduced with permission from Mickleborough LL. Operative techniques in cardiac and thoracic surgery: a comparative atlas. JL Cox and TM Sundt III, editors. W. B. Saunders, 1997;2(2):118–131.)

tricular distortion and improves results. Dor and colleagues have described a modification of this technique that they call "endoventricular circuloplasty," which involves insertion of a patch where endocardial scar and viable muscle meet to exclude the noncontracting portion of the ventricle. Attempts to compare results achieved with linear and more complex repair techniques have thus far been inconclusive because of lack of randomization and failure to control for important variables such as infarct size, function of the nonaneurysmal segment, and the effect of concomitant revascularization on ventricular function. We believe that modified linear closure, the technique outlined in this chapter, is relatively simple,

easily reproducible, and can be used successfully in the vast majority of cases.

SURGICAL ABLATIVE APPROACHES FOR MALIGNANT ARRHYTHMIAS

In most patients with coronary artery disease and a ventricular aneurysm who present with clinical ventricular tachycardia, the arrhythmia is due to reentry in a fixed anatomic substrate and can be induced by programmed stimulation. In these patients, chamber dilatation, increased wall tension, and subendocardial ischemia may also play a role in causing the arrhythmia. Results of extensive intraoperative mapping studies have shown that the ventricular tachycardia substrate consists of sheets of surviving muscle fibers mixed with areas of fibrosis, and is usually located in the border zone between viable myocardium and scar. In most cases, at least part of the reentry circuit has been found to be subendocardial. The target area for ablation almost always lies outside the area of aneurysm resection and is most often located in the fibrosed septum.

Intraoperative mapping and ventricular tachycardia ablation should be considered in patients who have a history of clinical ventricular tachycardia or who have inducible ventricular tachycardia at electrophysiologic study, unless contraindicated by advanced age or other factors associated with prohibitive operative risk.

Intraoperative Mapping

Mapping techniques include preoperative catheter mapping, intraoperative exploration of the epicardium and endocardium using a single-point, hand-held probe, and use of sophisticated, online, computer-aided systems that acquire data simultaneously from multiple electrode arrays. Single-point mapping is still used at some centers, but this technique is time consuming and useful only if a stable, monoform ventricular tachycardia can be induced. To use this technique to perform endocardial mapping, an incision is made in the left ventricle to introduce the

probe and guide its positioning. A major drawback of this approach is that after the ventriculotomy incision has been made, it is often difficult or impossible to reinduce the arrhythmia.

In 1984, we introduced a transatrial balloon approach to mapping that, when used in combination with an epicardial sock array, allows data to be acquired simultaneously from a large number of endocardial and epicardial sites. With the patient on cardiopulmonary bypass, the balloon is introduced by a left atriotomy incision and passed across the mitral valve into the intact left ventricle (Figure 7). Using computer-aided techniques, it is possible to generate an online display of activation maps on a beat-to-beat basis. A different system for data analysis developed by Cox and his group allows rapid generation of serial potential distribution maps. Whether the information derived is displayed as a series of color-coded isochron maps, a real-time video light display of the activation sequence, or a dynamic, color-coded potential map display, is largely a matter of preference and availability.

Three basic patterns of activation have been observed with intraoperative mapping (Figure 8). Based on our understanding of these patterns, we have modified ablation efforts to target not only the earliest site of activation, but critical areas of the presumed reentry circuit (indicated by the dynamic flashing light display). Once mapping has been completed, the ventricle is opened through the area of scarring, the balloon orientation is noted, and

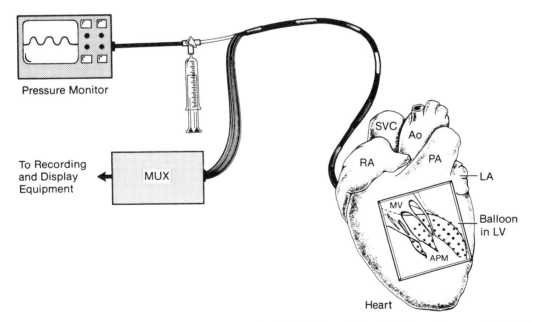

FIG. 7. Diagram of transatrial approach to mapping. The balloon is inserted through a small left atrial incision and passed across the mitral valve. When positioned in the left ventricle, it is inflated to achieve good electrical contact with the endocardium. Intraballoon pressure is monitored to prevent overinflation and possible subendocardial ischemia. (Reproduced with permission from Mickleborough LL. Surgery for ventricular arrhythmias following myocardial infarction. In: David T, ed. *Mechanical complications of myocardial infarction.* Austin, TX: RG Landers Co., 1993:211–231.)

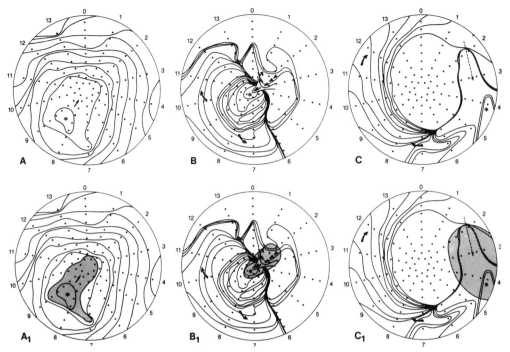

FIG. 8. Patterns of endocardial activation observed with transatrial balloon mapping technique. **A:** Monoregional endocardial activation radiates from a well-defined focus (*asterisks*). Shaded area **(A₁)** corresponds to target area identified from video display. Surgical ablation techniques encompass this region of interest. **B:** Figure-of-eight pattern. Earliest site of endocardial activation (*asterisks*) lies close to one side of two areas of block. Endocardial activity radiates in two directions around areas of block in a figure-of-eight pattern. An area of slow conduction can be identified between two areas of block that appears to lead up to the site of earliest endocardial activation. We believe that this narrow corridor between areas of block represents the reentry pathway. The target area, as indicated by shading **(B₁)**, was chosen to include both the presumed reentry pathway and the earliest site of endocardial activity observed. **C:** Circle (complete or incomplete). A large portion of the myocardium is involved in a sweeping circular front of activation. Earliest site of activity is identified by an asterisk. There is a spatial and temporal gap in the upper right-hand quadrant of the circle, and the presumed pathway of reentry in this area is indicated by broken arrow. The shaded area **(C₁)**, which includes both the presumed reentry circuit and the earliest site of endocardial activation, is the target area chosen for surgical ablation. (Reproduced with permission from Mickleborough LL, Harris L, Downar E, Parson I, Gray G. A new intraoperative approach for endocardial mapping of ventricular tachycardia. *J Thorac Cardiovasc Surg* 1988;95: 271–280.)

the location of specific electrodes is used to identify target areas on the endocardial surface. As mentioned previously, areas for ablation most often occur on the scarred septum. Any visible subendocardial scar in the target areas is excised (2–3 mm thick). After removal of the scar, a 15-mm cryoprobe is used to apply overlapping cryolesions (–60°C for 2 minutes) along the perimeter of the target area to isolate possible deep septal foci (Figure 9). If the septum is markedly thinned after ventricular tachycardia ablation, a septoplasty patch is inserted as previously described. Ventricular repair is then accomplished using methods previously outlined.

In these patients, a postoperative electrophysiologic study is performed in 7 to 10 days. If there are any inducible arrhythmias, the patient is discharged home on amiodarone or considered for implantable defibrillator insertion.

Visually Directed Ventricular Tachycardia Ablation

In centers where mapping is not available, visually directed approaches have been advocated. These procedures involve extensive resection of all visible subendocardial scar (which may include three fourths of the endocardial surface of the left ventricle) with or without cryoablation around the perimeter of the excision. Such extensive ablation procedures often necessitate resection and reimplantation of the posterior papillary muscle or mitral valve replacement, and may decrease ventricular function. Jatene et al. reported excellent results with another visually directed approach involving a U-stitch septoplasty and routine aneurysm repair.

Woelfel et al. demonstrated that ventricular tachycardia is often inducible during preoperative electrophysiologic testing in patients with an aneurysm and no clini-

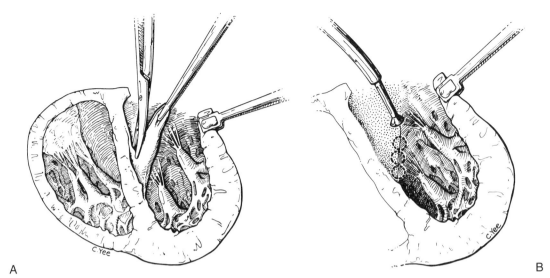

FIG. 9. A: Coronal section of the heart in a patient with ventricular tachycardia. Diagram shows the edge of free-wall resection (retracted with Babcocks) and profile of the papillary muscle. Scissors are being used to establish a plane for resection of a sheet of endocardial scar from the septum. **B:** After endocardial excision, overlapping cryolesions are applied at the perimeter of the target area to isolate potential deep septal ventricular tachycardia foci. (Reproduced with permission from Mickleborough LL, Takagi Y, Ohashi M. Ischemic heart disease: left ventricular aneurysm: linear closure. In: *Mastery of cardiothoracic surgery.* LR Kaiser, IL Kron, TL Spray, editors. Philadelphia: Lippincott–Raven Publishers, 1998:438–445.)

cal history of ventricular arrhythmia. Because of this result, Dor et al. have advocated visually directed "endoventricular circuloplasty" in all patients with aneurysms, asserting that if the arrhythmia substrate is not modified by the aneurysm repair, the potential for arrhythmias during follow-up is significant. Whether this approach is justified in all patients with an aneurysm requires further study.

RESULTS ACHIEVED WITH ANEURYSM REPAIR AND SURGICAL ABLATION OF VENTRICULAR TACHYCARDIA FOCI

Since the mid-1980s, mortality associated with aneurysm repair has decreased significantly. Using the principles of patient selection and operative technique outlined in this chapter, ventricular surgical remodeling can be accomplished with a low surgical morbidity and mortality. We reported a consecutive series of 92 patients in whom the surgical mortality was 3%, despite a high proportion of patients with diffuse coronary artery disease, advanced left ventricular dysfunction, and ventricular arrhythmia. This mortality rate compares favorably with others reported in the literature using linear or more complex repair techniques.

In our series, only 18% of patients required intraaortic balloon support. Few perioperative complications occurred, including one perioperative stroke.

Using multiple-gated acquisition data, we provided objective evidence that postoperative left ventricular function improves; ejection fraction increased an average of 7%. In addition, echocardiographic data available in a limited number of patients showed a significant decrease in left ventricular dimensions and mitral regurgitation after surgery. Interestingly, there was no correlation between postoperative ejection fraction or postoperative end-diastolic dimension and functional class. Possible reasons for this discrepancy have been previously discussed.

In our series, there were 15 late deaths as a result of CHF after a 10-year follow-up. The actuarial survival rate, including hospital deaths, was 88% at 1 year, 86% at 2 years, and 80% at 5 years. There was no difference in survival between patients with a preoperative ejection fraction greater than 20% and those with an ejection fraction less than 20%. Global ejection fraction, usually an important predictor of operative risk for cardiac surgery, was not helpful in these patients. Risk was better assessed by the contractility of the nonaneurysmal segment. Patients who had symptoms of CHF on presentation had poorer survival rates than those who did not.

Our results were comparable to those reported in other series, where operative mortality ranged from 3 to 7% and the long-term survival rate was 80% at 5 years, even in patients with diffuse coronary artery disease and left ventricular dysfunction. As would be expected, surgical risk did appear to increase with advancing age, increasing severity of coronary artery disease, decreasing preoperative functional class, and the presence of significant associated diseases.

Patients with ventricular arrhythmias had a surgical mortality rate of 7%. Seventy-four percent of these patients had a completely negative postoperative electrophysiologic study. All patients with positive tests were discharged on amiodarone. In this subgroup, only one sudden death occurred during follow-up (1–10 years). The overall survival rate was 80% at 5 and 8 years.

These results in patients with ventricular tachycardia and a poor ejection fraction compare favorably with those obtained using other approaches, including revascularization and defibrillator insertion (mortality rate of 30–40% at 2–4 years). Furthermore, quality of life in patients cured of ventricular tachycardia with a surgical ablation approach is greatly improved, with no need for antiarrhythmic medications and no fear of defibrillator discharge.

SUMMARY

With proper patient selection and surgical techniques, ventricular aneurysm resection and surgical remodeling can be performed with good results, even in patients with severe coronary artery disease and poor ventricular function, including those with ventricular arrhythmias. We believe these results support more liberal indications for surgical repair. We recommend performing surgical aneurysm excision and left ventricular remodeling even in patients with critical coronary anatomy who are asymptomatic, and in those with deteriorating left ventricular function (increasing diastolic dimensions, increasing mitral regurgitation or decreasing ejection fraction). We believe that earlier surgical intervention in these patients should be considered before decompensation progresses to the point that cardiac transplantation or an implantable assist device become the only reasonable options for treatment.

SELECTED REFERENCES

Cooley DA. Ventricular endoaneurysmorrhaphy: a simplified repair for extensive postinfarction aneurysm. *J Cardiac Surg* 1989;4:200–205.

Cooley DA, Collins HA, Morris GC, Chapman DW. Ventricular aneurysm after myocardial infarction: surgical excision with use of temporary cardiopulmonary bypass. *JAMA* 1958;167:557–560.

Davies MJ. Ischaemic ventricular aneurysms: true of false? *Br Heart J* 1988;60:95–97.

Dor V, Saab M, Coste P, Kornaszewska M, Montiglio F. Left ventricular aneurysm: a new surgical approach. *J Thorac Cardiovasc Surg* 1989;37:11–19.

Elefteriades JA, Solomon LW, Salazar AM, et al. Linear left ventricular aneurysmectomy: modern imaging studies reveal improved morphology and function. *Ann Thorac Surg* 1993;56:242–252.

Jatene AD. Left ventricular aneurysmectomy: resection or reconstruction. *J Thorac Cardiovasc Surg* 1985;89:321–331.

Komeda M, David TE, Malik A, Ivanov J, Sun Z. Operative risks and long-term results of operation for left ventricular aneurysm. *Ann Thorac Surg* 1992;53:22–28.

Likoff W, Bailey CP. Ventriculoplasty: excision of myocardial aneurysm. Report of a successful case. *JAMA* 1955;158:915–920

Mickleborough LL. Surgical management of left ventricular ventricular aneurysms. *Semin Thorac Cardiovasc Surg* 1995;7:233–239.

Mickleborough LL, Harris L, Downar E, Parson I, Gray G. A new intraoperative approach for endocardial mapping of ventricular tachycardia. *J Thorac Cardiovasc Surg* 1988;95:271–280.

Mickleborough LL, Maruyama H, Liu P, Mohamed S. Results of left ventricular aneurysmectomy with a tailored scar excision and primary closure technique. *J Thorac Cardiovasc Surg* 1994;107:690–698.

Mickleborough LL, Takagi Y, Ohashi M. Ischemic heart disease: left ventricular aneurysm: linear closure. In: *Mastery of cardiothoracic surgery*. Boston: Little, Brown and Company (*in press*).

Rokkas CK, Nitta T, Schuessler RB, et al. Human ventricular tachycardia: precise intraoperative localization with potential distribution mapping. *Ann Thorac Surg* 1994;57:1628–1635.

Management of End-Stage Heart Disease, edited by Eric A. Rose and Lynne Warner Stevenson. Lippincott–Raven Publishers, Philadelphia ©1998.

CHAPTER 13

Valve Surgery in Patients with Severe Left Ventricular Dysfunction

Francis D. Pagani and Steven F. Bolling

Because of the donor shortage, many patients who could benefit from cardiac transplantation die on the waiting list. Thus, surgical strategies to manage patients with severe end-stage heart disease have evolved to cope with the donor shortage in heart transplantation, including high-risk coronary artery revascularization, cardiomyoplasty, and high-risk valvular repair or replacement. This chapter discusses the efficacy of performing valve surgery in certain patients with severe left ventricular dysfunction.

MITRAL REGURGITATION

Mitral regurgitation is a significant complication of dilated cardiomyopathy and end-stage heart disease. The incidence of mitral regurgitation complicating dilated cardiomyopathy is variable, but has been reported to occur in as many as 60% of patients. It occurs as a consequence of (a) dilation of the mitral annular–ventricular apparatus with altered ventricular geometry; (b) ischemic papillary muscle dysfunction; or (c) a combination of both mechanisms. Mitral regurgitation leads to a cycle of continuing volume overload of the dilated left ventricle, with progressive annular dilation, increasing degrees of mitral regurgitation, and congestive heart failure (CHF). Finally, patients with uncontrollable, severe mitral regurgitation refractory to medical therapy have a poor survival rate.

Mitral regurgitation is frequently observed in patients with either idiopathic or ischemic dilated cardiomyopathy, and can be caused by many different factors. In patients with nonischemic dilated cardiomyopathy who do not have organic disease of the mitral valve (i.e., myxomatous degeneration, or calcific or rheumatic disease),

mitral regurgitation is thought to occur predominantly because of progressive dilation of the mitral valve annulus with subsequent loss of coaptation of the valve leaflets. In comparisons of patients with dilated cardiomyopathy (with or without mitral regurgitation), patients with dilated cardiomyopathy and mitral regurgitation had significantly greater mitral leaflet areas (i.e., surface area of the mitral valve orifice) and significantly larger dimensions of the mitral valve annulus. As the mitral valve annulus increases in size, an increasing amount of redundant mitral leaflet tissue covers the surface area of the mitral valve orifice. A relatively large amount of leaflet area is required for coaptation to seal effectively the mitral valve; the area of the mitral valve leaflet is 2.5 times greater than the area of the mitral valve orifice. The mitral leaflet tissue available for coaptation is reduced to the point that coaptation of the mitral leaflets becomes "ineffective," and a central regurgitant jet of insufficiency develops. This pathologic process has been referred to as "functional" mitral regurgitation. The most significant determinant of mitral valve leaflet orifice area is the dimensions of the mitral valve annulus. Left ventricular dimensions, although clearly related to annulus size, are not as important a factor in the etiology of functional mitral regurgitation. Chordal length and angulation and papillary muscle length are not significantly different in patients with idiopathic cardiomyopathy, with or without mitral regurgitation.

In patients with ischemic heart disease and dilated cardiomyopathy, the mechanisms that contribute to mitral regurgitation are more complex and controversial; they may include a component of functional mitral regurgitation through dilation of the mitral valve annulus as well as papillary muscle dysfunction. Normal function of the mitral valve depends on the structural and functional integrity of the subvalvular apparatus. Papillary muscle

Department of Surgery, Section of Thoracic Surgery, University of Michigan Hospitals, Ann Arbor, Michigan 48109-0344 dysfunction, also called "papillary–annular dysfunction," is related to an unsuccessful coordination of the mitral valve apparatus, which includes the annulus, leaflets, chordae tendineae, papillary muscles, and the left ventricular wall, and is not simply a disorder of the papillary muscle. In experimental studies by Tsakiris et al., isolated injection of both papillary muscles in dogs, which induced fibrosis of the papillary muscle, did not by itself induce mitral regurgitation; however, if the left ventricular free wall beneath the papillary muscles is injected and made fibrotic at the same time—so that regional asynergy develops—mitral regurgitation may result because of restriction of the mitral leaflet motion.

Experimental acute myocardial infarction involving approximately 33% of the left ventricular posterior wall causes significant acute and chronic mitral regurgitation in sheep. Using sonomicrometer array localization after acute myocardial infarction in sheep, Gorman et al. reported that mitral regurgitation appeared to involve asymmetric enlargement of the posterior annulus, lengthening of the posterior papillary muscle, failure of the posterior papillary muscle to contract, and movement of the papillary muscle tip toward the posterior mitral valve commissure during systole. These changes occurred in addition to asymmetric enlargement of the left ventricle and development of rotational abnormalities in left ventricular contraction, resulting in significant abnormalities in the mitral valve annulus.

In a study by Izumi et al. investigating the anatomic and functional bases of mitral regurgitation in the setting of ischemic heart disease, a correlation was observed between the site of mitral regurgitation and the region of myocardial infarction (left ventricular wall asynergy) in patients with eccentric mitral regurgitation (i.e., regurgitation from either the posteromedial or anterolateral commissural areas). Patients with eccentric mitral regurgitation through the anterolateral mitral commissure had corresponding anterior wall myocardial infarctions, whereas patients with eccentric mitral regurgitation through the posteromedial commissure had associated inferior myocardial infarctions. Eccentric mitral valve regurgitation occurred independent of direct involvement of the papillary muscles by infarction. Thus, asynergy (i.e., hypokinesis, dyskinesis, or akinesis) caused by myocardial infarction or ischemia in the papillary muscle influences the orientation of the papillary muscles on contraction, resulting in an insufficient area of coaptation of the mitral leaflet. The incidence of eccentric mitral regurgitation was not influenced by the site of the myocardial infarction. Furthermore, in patients with central regurgitant jets, the degree of central regurgitation correlated with the dimensions of the mitral valve annulus, not with the site of left ventricular infarction (site of asynergy). The incidence of annular dilation with central mitral valve regurgitation in patients with ischemic heart disease is

thought to be very low; if annular dilation is present in such a patient, the condition can usually be attributed to concurrent myxomatous disease.

In a study of the pathogenesis of mitral regurgitation in humans, Van Dantzig and colleagues evaluated 188 patients admitted to the hospital with acute myocardial infarction with quantitative echocardiography. Significant mitral regurgitation (3+–4+) occurred in 13%. Left ventricular function, volume, shape, and mitral valvular features were measured and analyzed by stepwise logistic regression. In a regression analysis, only recurrent infarction, left ventricular sphericity index, and inferoposterolateral asynergy were independently associated with significant mitral regurgitation.

One of the important predictors of poor survival in patients with dilated cardiomyopathy is the left ventricular volume at end-diastole. Severe mitral regurgitation in the setting of dilated cardiomyopathy can substantially contribute to persistent left ventricular volume overload and increased left ventricular dimensions. Junker et al. reported on 57 patients with dilated cardiomyopathy (ischemic and nonischemic etiology) with and without mitral regurgitation. The overall incidence of mitral regurgitation was 60% in this population. Patients with functionally significant mitral regurgitation were in a higher New York Heart Association (NYHA) functional class, had a lower ejection fraction, larger left ventricular volume, higher left ventricular end-diastolic pressure, higher pulmonary capillary wedge pressure, and higher mean right atrial pressure. There were no significant differences observed in cardiac index or stroke index between patients with or without mitral regurgitation. Blondheim et al. reported that the incidence of mitral regurgitation (in 57% of patients in their study), even to a mild degree, was associated with a markedly decreased survival rate compared with patients with dilated cardiomyopathy without mitral regurgitation (22% vs. 60% at 32 ± 6 months). Finally, Hickey et al. also reported that moderate to severe mitral regurgitation in the presence of ischemic heart disease had a significantly adverse influence on long-term survival.

Surgical Treatment of Mitral Regurgitation

The surgical treatment of mitral regurgitation has evolved significantly since the early 1980s. Early methods to treat mitral regurgitation surgically simply involved valve replacement, with little understanding of the adverse consequences that valve replacement and interruption of annular–papillary continuity could have on short- and long-term left ventricular function. Two of the major advances in surgical treatment of mitral regurgitation have been the recognition of the importance of preserving mitral annular–papillary muscle continuity during valve replacement, and the development of techniques for mitral valve repair.

Numerous clinical and experimental studies have demonstrated the importance of preserving annular–papillary continuity of the mitral valve. As early as 1964, Lillehi and colleagues reported on the technique of preserving the papillary muscles and chordae tendineae and its benefits on left ventricular function after mitral valve replacement in humans. Coupled with early observations made by Rushmer et al. of the high incidence of postoperative "low cardiac output syndrome" after mitral valve replacement, Lillehi and colleagues introduced techniques of mitral valve replacement with preservation of the posterior (and anterior) mitral leaflet and chordae tendineae. In a series of 14 patients undergoing mitral valve replacement with chordal preservation, the observed operative mortality rate was 14%, which compared favorably with a historical mortality rate of 37%. The most important clinical evidence favoring chordal preservation has been reported by David et al. In a prospective study of the comparison of mitral valve replacement with or without chordal preservation, David and colleagues assessed left ventricular function in a small number of patients who had undergone conventional mitral valve replacement or chordal-preserving mitral valve replacement, before surgery and 3 to 6 months after surgery using radionuclide ventriculography. Patients entering the study were initially evaluated for mitral valve repair at the time of surgery. If mitral valve repair was judged to be not feasible, patients were alternately assigned at surgery to either conventional mitral valve replacement or chordal-preserving (both anterior and posterior leaflets) mitral valve cohorts. The two groups were similar in terms of age, valvular disease, preoperative functional class, and left ventricular function, as assessed by various load-dependent parameters. In both groups, left ventricular end-systolic volume, end-diastolic volume, and stroke volume decreased; however, ejection fraction decreased in the conventional mitral valve replacement group but was unchanged in the chordal-sparing mitral valve cohort. Furthermore, during maximal bicycle exercise, ejection fraction and stroke volume increased only in patients with an intact mitral subvalvular apparatus. Patients who had undergone conventional mitral valve replacement showed increased cardiac output during exercise with isolated increases in heart rate, without an increase in stroke volume. Natsuaki et al. investigated the importance of preserving the mitral subvalvular apparatus, comparing patients undergoing mitral valve replacement with preservation of the posterior chordae alone, preservation of both the anterior and posterior chordae, or mitral valve repair. These investigators observed significantly improved postoperative regional wall motion at the apical and diaphragmatic regions in patients who had undergone mitral valve replacement with preservation of both anterior and posterior chordae and mitral valve repair. Further evidence was provided by Spence et al., who measured peak isovolumic

left ventricular pressure and volume using an open-chest swine heart preparation on cardiopulmonary bypass and found that left ventricular systolic function was significantly impaired after severing the chordae tendineae. Studies by Hansen et al. and Sarris et al. using load-independent measurements of left ventricular contractility demonstrated that division of all chordae tendineae was accompanied by a 47% reduction in left ventricular E_{max} (maximum elastance) without a significant shift in V_o (ventricular volume at zero pressure).

The relative contributions of the anterior and posterior chordal groups to left ventricular function were investigated in another experiment by sequentially severing the anterior and posterior chordae tendineae in randomly assigned order. The contributions to maximum potential global left ventricular E_{max} were quantitatively similar. Thus, the contribution of each set of chordae was found to be additive in this study. Further, in an open-chest, *in situ*, isovolumic swine heart preparation, the effects of chordal detachment and subsequent reattachment on left ventricular function were assessed by load-independent measurements of E_{max}. All chordae were detached by severing the tips of both papillary muscles, resulting in a significant decline of left ventricular contractility. Left ventricular contractility was subsequently restored to baseline levels after reattachment of the native chordae by repair of the papillary muscles.

The techniques of mitral valve repair have been well described. As the advantages of mitral valve repair have become well recognized, mitral valvuloplasty for all forms of mitral valve disease has increasingly been used, significantly improving operative survival.

Except for anecdotal reports, surgical correction of mitral valve regurgitation in patients with dilated cardiomyopathy and severely impaired left ventricular function has not been seriously considered as an option to improve functional status in such patients. This is largely attributed to the presumed prohibitive operative mortality and poor survival in patients with severe left ventricular dysfunction.

Outcome after Surgery for Mitral Regurgitation

Mitral valve surgery for mitral regurgitation relieves symptoms, increases long-term survival, and prevents irreversible left ventricular dysfunction in 70% to 80% of patients with chronic mitral valve regurgitation. Surgical mortality depends on the patient's left ventricular function and also on associated co-morbid conditions such as older age and concomitant coronary artery disease. The 5-year survival rate for patients with significant mitral regurgitation secondary to coronary artery disease is approximately 30%. Postoperative improvement may even be expected in patients with heart failure refractory to medical therapy, as long as the cardiac index is greater than 1.5 L/minute/m^2 and left ventricular ejection fraction greater than 35%. In a large study evaluating mitral valve surgery for mitral regurgitation, Enriquez-Sarano and colleagues reported on the long-term outcome of 576 survivors of surgery for pure mitral regurgitation. For all patients, survival rates were 77% ± 2% and 56% ± 3% at 5 and 10 years, respectively. For those patients with ischemic mitral regurgitation, the survival rate was only 36% ± 6% at 10 years. The cumulative incidence of postoperative CHF was 23% ± 2% and 33% ± 3% at 5 and 10 years, respectively. In patients with ischemic mitral regurgitation, the incidence of postoperative heart failure was approximately 45% at 5 years, and only 10% to 15% for those with mitral regurgitation due to organic valvular disease. In those patients with a preoperative ejection fraction less than 50%, the incidence of postoperative heart failure was nearly 50% at 5 years. After the onset of CHF, survival was only 44% ± 4% at 5 years. Preoperative ejection fraction, presence of coronary artery disease, and NYHA functional class were independent predictors of postoperative heart failure. Thus, heart failure after surgical correction of mitral regurgitation occurs frequently, is predictable on the basis of preoperative left ventricular function, and occurs more frequently in patients with ischemic heart disease. The absence of symptoms early after suppression of the valvular regurgitation may be observed even in the presence of left ventricular dysfunction as a result of previously documented normalization of left atrial pressure, and is similar to what is observed in nonvalvular ventricular dysfunction.

Hospital mortality after mitral valve replacement and coronary artery bypass for ischemic mitral regurgitation has been reported to be as high as 40% in patients with a left ventricular ejection fraction of less than 35%. More recently, operative mortality for mitral valve surgery for ischemic mitral regurgitation with or without coronary artery bypass still approximates 10%. In cases where left ventricular function is severely impaired, the risk of death after mitral valve surgery is thought to be prohibitive, and heart transplantation has been recommended.

Because of the poor natural history of patients with end-stage cardiomyopathy, severe mitral regurgitation, and heart failure resistant to medical therapy, we have initiated a program to investigate the outcome of mitral valve repair in this population as an alternative to or bridge to heart transplantation. Between June 1993 and June 1996, 37 consecutive, nonrandomized patients with end-stage dilated cardiomyopathy and refractory severe mitral regurgitation underwent prospective evaluation after mitral valve repair for severe mitral regurgitation. Before surgery, all patients had NYHA Class III or IV limitations despite receiving maximal medical therapy, and had severe left ventricular dysfunction defined as an ejection fraction of less than 25% on left ventricular angiography or radionuclide angiography. Patients were excluded from this study if they showed evidence of primary mitral valvular disease, if significant mitral regur-

gitation preceded cardiomyopathy, if surgical intervention included revascularization of viable myocardium, or if they had significant aortic insufficiency. Mitral valve reconstruction was performed through a median sternotomy with standard cardiopulmonary bypass and arrest with hypothermic, blood cardioplegia in 33 patients. Mitral valve reconstruction was performed through a right thoracotomy with cardiopulmonary bypass and cold fibrillatory arrest in four patients who had a previous cardiac operation. All operations were performed with institutional approval and informed consent.

The age of the patients ranged from 33 to 78 years (mean, 62 ± 6 years). Eighteen patients had nonischemic dilated cardiomyopathy and 19 patients had end-stage ischemic cardiomyopathy without ongoing ischemia, as defined by negative dobutamine echocardiographic functional testing or negative positron emission tomography scanning. Before surgery, 24 patients were classified as NYHA Class IV and 13 as Class III. Mean duration of documented cardiomyopathy or symptomatic congestive heart failure was 6.6 ± 6.1 years. Preoperative ejection fraction ranged from 9% to 25% (mean, 16% ± 5%). At operation, all patients underwent mitral reconstruction by annuloplasty with implantation of a flexible remodeling ring (Duran Ring, Medtronic, Inc., Minneapolis, MN; or Physio Ring, Baxter, Inc., Irvine, CA). No patient required a complex repair (e.g., leaflet resection, leaflet/chordal turnover) at the time of the operation. All patients survived the mitral reconstruction procedure, despite their poor preoperative ventricular function. All patients were weaned from cardiopulmonary bypass with a phosphodiesterase inhibitor, amrinone, and norepinephrine. No patient required intraaortic balloon pumping or mechanical support. Intraoperative transesophageal echocardiography after annuloplasty and the discontinuation of cardiopulmonary bypass showed no mitral regurgitation in 33 patients and trivial to mild regurgitation in 4. One perioperative death occurred from right ventricular failure. The mean duration of hospitalization after the operation was 10 ± 4 days (range, 5–17 days). One-year actuarial survival was 82% (95% confidence interval, 73%–91%). There were eight late deaths (six sudden death, one heart failure, one secondary to complications from cholecystectomy). At a mean follow-up of 19 months (range, 1–24 months), all patients were in NYHA Class I or II.

Surgical correction of mitral regurgitation and accompanying volume overload has been effective in patients with mitral regurgitation and could also benefit patients with cardiomyopathy and secondary mitral regurgitation. In a study of 249 patients with mitral regurgitation who underwent preoperative angiographic assessment of left ventricular function, survival of surgically treated patients was significantly better than that of medically treated patients, despite greater functional and hemodynamic impairment in surgically treated patients before the operation. Unfortunately, many surgical studies have also shown that greater functional and hemodynamic impairment and reduced ejection fraction correspond to poor operative and in-hospital survival in patients undergoing mitral valve replacement for mitral regurgitation. The high operative mortality rate and poor outcome have prevented surgical correction for mitral regurgitation from becoming a routine treatment for patients with severely compromised left ventricular function.

Many studies have also shown, however, that mitral reconstruction, as opposed to replacement, results in improved rest and exercise ejection indexes. This improvement is mostly the result of a marked reduction in end-systolic stress and maintenance of a more ellipsoid chamber geometry. Many clinical studies have compared the results of mitral valve reconstruction with those of mitral valve replacement and have concluded that the preservation of the annular–chordal–papillary muscle continuity results in good maintenance of left ventricular function and geometry, which leads to better patient outcome.

Technically, mitral reconstruction with annuloplasty effectively corrected mitral regurgitation in these patients, a finding confirmed both on intraoperative transesophageal echocardiography and on follow-up transthoracic studies. Furthermore, despite high operative risks, there was only one operative or in-hospital death, and the actuarial survival rate was 82% at 1 year. Not only was survival improved, but functional status has changed remarkably in these patients. Importantly, clinical status has not worsened in any patient during follow-up. In addition, echocardiographic analyses revealed a strong trend toward decreased left ventricular volume after the operation, with a significant increase in ejection fraction and forward cardiac output. Improvement in echocardiographic parameters of ventricular function were not necessarily anticipated because left ventricular function has been shown to decrease after mitral valve replacement, presumably as a result of loss of chordal attachments and normal systolic ventricular shortening. Second, loss of the low-impedance left atrial chamber associated with correction of mitral regurgitation might be expected to cause further systolic impairment in patients with preexisting ventricular dysfunction. Left ventricular function improved, however, after surgery in these patients. This improvement implies that a component of ventricular decompensation observed before the operation was due to volume overload associated with severe mitral regurgitation superimposed on dilated cardiomyopathy. Possible mechanisms for the improvement in ventricular function include stabilization of the mitral annulus and left ventricular unloading that has induced a more favorable ventricular geometry. One study reports that remodeling of left ventricular geometry may be rapid and complete in patients with resultant regurgitant fractions of less than 30% after correction of mitral regurgitation. Our patients had a mean residual regurgitation

fraction of only 16% after the operation, which could favor rapid left ventricular remodeling. Furthermore, there is evidence from trials with left ventricular assist devices that unloading the dilated cardiomyopathic left ventricle encourages ventricular recovery.

MITRAL STENOSIS

Most patients presenting with hemodynamically significant mitral stenosis have preserved left ventricular wall thickness, left ventricular volume, and systolic and diastolic function in the absence of associated coronary artery disease. Symptoms of CHF in patients with mitral stenosis occur as a consequence of elevated pulmonary venous pressures secondary to obstruction of blood flow at the level of the mitral valve. Although unusual in this country today, fixed and elevated pulmonary vascular resistance may develop in patients with long-standing, hemodynamically significant mitral stenosis. As pulmonary vascular resistance rises, the pulmonary arteriolar bed becomes protected from transient increases in pressure associated with exertion; thus, pulmonary edema does not occur and patients subsequently experience fewer symptoms of dyspnea. These patients, however, eventually acquire symptoms of right heart failure, including peripheral coldness, cyanosis, hepatic enlargement, elevated jugular venous pressure, ascites, and peripheral edema. The risk that valve surgery poses to these patients is a consequence of pulmonary hypertension and right heart dysfunction—not failure of the left ventricle.

In some patients with long-standing mitral stenosis, important posterobasal regional wall motion abnormalities may develop because of a rigid mitral valve annulus and subvalvular apparatus. Significant left ventricular dysfunction in association with hemodynamically significant mitral stenosis is unusual, but does exist in a small proportion of patients. These patients tend to be elderly and have had long-standing mitral stenosis. They usually have severe posterobasal segmental wall contraction abnormalities, anterolateral segmental contraction abnormalities, or diffuse hypokinesis. The basis for the regional wall motion abnormalities may be related to diffuse scarring and retraction of the papillary muscles, or to markedly decreased compliance of the left ventricle. Chronic low cardiac output with significantly decreased coronary flow reserves may contribute to diffuse hypokinesis and decreased left ventricular compliance.

AORTIC REGURGITATION

Pathophysiologic Changes in Chronic Aortic Regurgitation

Regurgitation from the aorta into the left ventricle during diastole generates *both* a volume and pressure overload to the left ventricle. This leads to eccentric hypertrophy of the left ventricle (left ventricular wall thickness increases in proportion to the increase in ventricular diameter), such that the ratio between wall thickness and chamber radius remains normal. These observed changes during chronic aortic regurgitation allow the heart to maintain adequate ejection fraction despite increases in left ventricular end-diastolic volume. Patients with chronic aortic regurgitation may remain well compensated and asymptomatic until late in their clinical course, despite a substantial volume load on the left ventricle.

Natural History of Chronic Aortic Regurgitation

Bonow et al. reported on the natural history of 77 asymptomatic patients with normal left ventricular ejection fraction at rest and severe aortic regurgitation (3+ to 4+ aortic regurgitation by ventriculography, or pulse pressure > 70 mm Hg). During a mean follow-up of 49 months, no patient died and only 12 patients underwent aortic valve replacement, 11 of whom experienced an onset of symptoms and 1 of whom experienced ventricular dysfunction without symptoms. The proportion of patients who did not require operation was 90% ± 3%, 81% ± 6%, and 75% ± 7%, at 3, 5, and 7 years, respectively. Thus, in asymptomatic patients with normal left ventricular function, death is unusual, and less than 4% per year require aortic valve replacement because of the onset of symptoms or left ventricular dysfunction. In a more recent study, Bonow et al. reported on 104 asymptomatic patients with chronic severe aortic regurgitation and normal left ventricular ejection fraction at rest. Of these, 58% ± 9% remained asymptomatic with a normal ejection fraction after 11 years of follow-up (mean follow-up of 8 years), for an average attrition rate of less than 5% per year.

Thus, symptoms or onset of left ventricular dysfunction are not likely to develop in most patients with asymptomatic severe chronic aortic regurgitation. Chronic volume overload in aortic regurgitation, however, *eventually* leads to a deterioration in left ventricular systolic function. Ejection fraction and cardiac output decline, and end-systolic volume increases. The mechanism for onset of left ventricular dysfunction remains controversial, but may be associated with inadequate hypertrophy with afterload mismatch or primary myocardial dysfunction. Once symptoms of dyspnea, angina, presyncope, or syncope develop, the average survival is only 3 to 5 years.

Timing and Outcome of Surgery for Chronic Aortic Regurgitation

The decision to proceed with aortic valve surgery for chronic aortic regurgitation remains controversial and difficult because (a) a large number of patients do well long-term without surgery; (b) patients undergoing aortic valve surgery after the onset of severe left ventricular decompensation are less likely to improve symptomatically and are at increased risk for development of advanced heart failure within 5 years after surgery; and (c) asymptomatic patients with aortic regurgitation may progress to having irreversible left ventricular dysfunction without perceptible symptomatic deterioration. Asymptomatic or minimally symptomatic patients with aortic regurgitation should be identified early and offered aortic valve surgery before irreversible left ventricular dysfunction develops. Numerous studies have demonstrated that most symptomatic patients at risk of death from heart failure after operation have impaired systolic function before operation. A considerable number of studies since the early 1980s have attempted to define the optimal timing of aortic valve surgery for chronic aortic regurgitation. From these studies, a number of prognostic indices have been identified, including ejection fraction at rest or in response to exercise, duration of left ventricular dysfunction, fractional shortening, left ventricular dimensions at end-systole and end-diastole, end-systolic and end-diastolic volume index, and the ratio of end-diastolic radius to wall thickness. Henry et al. observed that preoperative echocardiographic measurements of the left ventricular end-systolic dimension (>55 mm) and percent fractional shortening (<25%) were strongly associated with late deaths due to CHF in 50 patients undergoing aortic valve replacement for isolated aortic regurgitation. Those patients with both a preoperative left ventricular end-systolic dimension greater than 55 mm and fractional shortening less than 25% were identified as a high-risk group, with 9 of 13 patients (69%) dying at operation or late from CHF. In contrast, of 32 patients with left ventricular end-systolic dimensions less than 55 mm, only 1 died at operation and 1 died late from congestive heart failure. After aortic valve replacement, significant reductions were noted in left ventricular end-diastolic dimensions. In most patients, this reduction occurred early (8–22 days) after aortic valve replacement. Cunha et al. reported that the 4-year survival rate after aortic valve surgery for chronic aortic regurgitation was 77% in patients with a preoperative fractional shortening of no more than 30%, and 96% for those patients with a fractional shortening greater than 30%. Thus, in symptomatic patients undergoing aortic valve surgery for aortic regurgitation, the postoperative survival rate, incidence of postoperative congestive heart failure, and likelihood of postoperative reversal of left ventricular dilation can be predicted on the basis of preoperative left ventricular systolic function, systolic size, and systolic wall stress. The prognostic information provided by echocardiographic assessment of left ventricular systolic dimension has been corroborated by several studies using measures of left ventricular systolic dimensions determined by angiography.

These same variables also identify asymptomatic patients with severe chronic aortic regurgitation and normal left ventricular systolic function who are likely to require aortic valve replacement over the course of the next 4 years because of the development of symptoms, or the onset of left ventricular dysfunction. Henry et al. prospectively followed 37 asymptomatic patients with significant isolated aortic regurgitation. They found that both left ventricular end-systolic dimension greater than 55 mm and fractional shortening less than 25% could be used to identify patients most likely to become symptomatic on follow-up and be referred for aortic valve surgery. In patients with an end-systolic dimension less than 40 mm at initial evaluation, the average rate of attrition is less than 5% per year. Bonow et al. demonstrated that no patient with an end-systolic dimension less than 40 mm died, experienced symptoms, or had left ventricular dysfunction. However, patients with an end-systolic dimension of 50 mm or more had a 19% likelihood per year of experiencing one of these cardiac events. Thus, when aortic valve replacement is delayed until the onset of symptoms, left ventricular dysfunction, or both, death before surgery is rare (limited to patients with marked ventricular dilatation), and postoperative survival should be excellent with substantial improvement in left ventricular dilatation and function.

Gaasch et al. demonstrated that the preoperative ratio of end-diastolic radius to wall thickness, an index of the ratio of left ventricular volume to mass, and a measure of the degree to which left ventricular muscle mass is appropriate for a given chamber volume, were strong echocardiographic predictors of whether regression of dilation and hypertrophy occurred after aortic valve replacement for chronic aortic regurgitation. Patients with a normal preoperative ratio of end-diastolic radius to wall thickness had a significant regression of left ventricular volume and mass after operation. Those with an increased ratio (≥ 4.0), however, had persistent left ventricular dilation and heart failure after surgery.

Left ventricular end-diastolic dimension also has considerable postoperative prognostic value after aortic valve surgery for aortic regurgitation. Henry et al. demonstrated that persistent left ventricular dilation (postoperative diastolic dimension ≥ 70 mm) identified patients at risk of subsequent death from heart failure. Patients with an end-diastolic dimension of 80 mm or more had a postoperative mortality rate of nearly 50%. Several echocardiographic studies have also shown that if a patient experiences a postoperative reduction in left ventricular end-diastolic dimension, this reduction usually occurs within the first 2 weeks to 2 months after operation, with little further change thereafter (up to 63 months post-surgery).

Although measuring left ventricular systolic dysfunction at rest is a sensitive means of detecting patients at risk, it is not specific. Improvement and even normaliza-tion of left ventricular systolic function can occur in patients after operation despite severe depression of systolic function before operation. Measuring left ventricular function during exercise and exercise capacity has also been used to determine timing of operation for aortic insufficiency and to provide prognostic information after surgery. Preserved exercise capacity before operation predicts improved survival after surgery and postoperative reversibility of left ventricular dysfunction. Furthermore, abnormal ejection fraction during exercise may precede the onset of symptoms or resting left ventricular dysfunction in many patients. Left ventricular dysfunction present only during exercise, however, should not be an indication for aortic valve surgery, although it may identify a group of patients who need to be observed closely for other evidence of left ventricular dysfunction. Bolen et al. identified a subgroup of patients with normal resting ejection fraction that decreased during angiotensin infusion; these patients had a larger regurgitant fraction and end-diastolic volume than did patients whose ejection fraction was maintained. Thus, the patients who experienced left ventricular dysfunction during this intervention appeared to have reached their limit of preload reserve and were unable to compensate for any further increase in afterload. The prognostic significance of this abnormal response is unknown. Studies during supine exercise have indicated that two thirds of symptomatic patients with a normal resting ejection fraction have abnormal ejection fraction responses during exercise.

In summary, patients with hemodynamically significant aortic regurgitation and symptoms of CHF (NYHA Class III or IV), angina, or syncope should undergo aortic valve surgery. Asymptomatic or minimally symptomatic patients, on the other hand, require serial assessments of left ventricular size and function to determine the optimal timing of surgery. An exercise tolerance test ensures that patients are not masking symptoms by limiting activity. Asymptomatic patients with left ventricular enlargement are observed serially as long as left ventricular function remains normal. Aortic valve surgery is recommended if left ventricular function deteriorates by radionuclide or echocardiographic measures. Noninvasive studies like serial M-mode echocardiograms are used to follow left ventricular size and function and help predict which patients will likely have persistent postoperative left ventricular dysfunction and a poor long-term prognosis. Asymptomatic patients with normal ventricular size should be tested yearly for deterioration of the resting left ventricular function (ejection fraction < 40%), increases in the end-systolic dimension to greater than 55 mm, or decreases in left ventricular fractional shortening to less than 25%, with the understanding that waiting for symptomatic decompensation will compromise postoperative outcome. The rate of progression of left ventricular dysfunction should also be considered when scheduling aortic valve replacement, with rapid progression suggesting the need for earlier surgery. Shorter preoperative duration of left ventricular dysfunction predicts the postoperative return of normal function. Coronary angiography is performed in patients older than 45 years of age to assess the need for concomitant coronary artery revascularization.

AORTIC STENOSIS

The natural history of aortic stenosis is not completely understood given the advent of aortic valve replacement, but compared with aortic insufficiency, valvular aortic stenosis is characterized by a more malignant course in terms of survival after development of symptoms. Ross and Braunwald concluded that the average survival in patients with significant aortic stenosis was 1 to 2 years after the onset of heart failure, 2 to 3 years after the onset of syncope, and 4 to 5 years after the onset of angina. Frank et al. reported on 15 patients with a catheterization-proven valve area of 0.7 cm²/m² who refused surgery. The 3-, 5-, and 10-year mortality rates were 36%, 52%, and 90%, respectively. Chizner et al. reported on 23 patients with significant aortic stenosis and a mean peak-to-peak catheter gradient of 69 ± 33 mm Hg. Their mortality rates at 1, 2, 5, and 11 years were 26%, 48%, 64%, and 94%, respectively. Okeefe et al. followed 50 symptomatic, unoperated patients with severe aortic stenosis in whom surgery was declined or deferred. Average age of the population was 77 years, and 65% had associated coronary artery disease. Actuarial survival rates were 55%, 37%, and 25% at 1, 2, and 3 years, respectively, compared with an age-matched general population with survival rates of 93%, 85%, and 77%. All the deaths were due to cardiac problems except for one patient with aortic stenosis. Horstkotte and Loogen reported an average survival after the onset of symptoms of 23 months in 35 patients who had refused surgery and had an aortic valve area less than 0.8 cm² documented by cardiac catheterization. The mean survival after the onset of angina was 45 months, 27 months after the onset of syncope, and only 11 months after the onset of heart failure. The 5-year mortality rate was 82%, and all patients were dead at 12 years of follow-up.

The transition from the asymptomatic to symptomatic stage of aortic stenosis has a profound effect on the natural history of this disease. The subsequent clinical course of hemodynamically significant aortic stenosis becomes malignant. Of patients with severe, hemodynamically significant aortic stenosis (valve area ≤ 0.7 cm²), symptoms develop in 40% within 1.5 to 2.0 years of diagnosis. The actuarial probability of remaining free of angina, syncope, or dyspnea was 86% at 1 year and 62% at 2 years. Three patients died of sudden death. In each case, however, death was preceded by the onset of symptoms by 3 to 5 months. Doppler flow velocity and ejection fraction were independent predictors of cardiac events. Thus, patients with asymptomatic, hemodynami-

cally significant aortic stenosis are at significant risk for the development of cardiac events within 2 years of the onset of symptoms. While they are asymptomatic, however, the risk of sudden death is low. Kelley et al. observed 51 asymptomatic patients with severe aortic stenosis (Doppler-derived peak systolic gradient of ≥ 50 mm Hg). During an average follow-up of 17 ± 9 months, 41% of patients became symptomatic and 16% died. Only two of the initially asymptomatic patients died of cardiac causes, and in each case, death was preceded by the onset of symptoms.

Kennedy et al. studied 66 patients with symptomatic or minimally symptomatic moderate aortic stenosis (aortic valve area 0.7–1.2 cm²). At 4 years of follow-up, 59% of patients remained free of death or aortic valve replacement. Fourteen patients had died, and 21 underwent aortic valve replacement for progression of disease or symptoms. Multivariate and univariate predictors of complications of aortic stenosis included ejection fraction, aortic valve area index, left ventricular end-diastolic pressure, and left ventricular end-systolic and end-diastolic volume indices.

The natural history of mild aortic stenosis (aortic valve area > 1.5 cm²) is benign. Horstkotte and Loogen followed 142 patients with mild aortic stenosis. At 10 years of follow-up, aortic stenosis remained mild in 88% of patients and progressed to moderate aortic stenosis in 4%, whereas 8% of patients required aortic valve replacement. At 20 years of follow-up, the aortic stenosis remained mild in 63% and progressed to moderate stenosis in 15%, whereas 22% of patients underwent aortic valve replacement or had severe aortic stenosis. Davies et al. studied the rate of progression of mild aortic stenosis in 65 patients. In 60 patients, the aortic valve gradient increased from a median of 10 mm Hg (range, 0–60 mm Hg) to a median of 52 mm Hg (range, 15–120 mm Hg) over an interval of 1 to 17 years (mean, 7 years). The mean rate of increase in gradient (assuming a linear rate of increase) was 6.5 mm Hg per year. This increase was significantly faster in patients with aortic valve calcification or aortic regurgitation present at the time of the initial study. The rate of progression was not related to age, sex, or initial gradient. Thus, the progression of mild or moderate aortic stenosis is variable and in some cases may be rapid. The probability of progression cannot be assessed in a given patient, and regular follow-up is therefore indicated. Peter et al. studied the rate of progression of aortic stenosis in 49 patients. During a follow-up period of 32 months (range, 11–66 months), maximal pressure gradient rose from 38 ± 15 mm Hg to 60 ± 20 mm Hg in the entire group, with a median increase of 7.2 mm Hg per year. In 43% of patients, an increase of greater than 10 mm Hg per year was observed. This subgroup of patients were significantly older (64 vs. 53 years) and had a significantly increased prevalence of coronary artery disease (38% vs. 7%).

Patients with severe aortic stenosis and severe left ventricular dysfunction probably derive clinically important benefits from aortic valve replacement. It is particularly important for these patients because left ventricular function often begins deteriorating early in the course of the disease, and may reach a point where valve replacement can no longer produce clinical improvement. This consideration does not apply in general to aortic stenosis because most such patients have symptoms and undergo surgery when left ventricular function is still normal or only mildly to moderately impaired. Second, when impaired left ventricular function develops in aortic stenosis, the relief of pressure overload almost always restores normal function or at least produces considerable improvement. Significant concomitant coronary artery disease, however, can obscure whether left ventricular dysfunction is derived from ischemic heart disease, valvular heart disease, or both. Carabello et al. observed 14 patients with critical aortic stenosis (valve area ≤ 0.4 cm^2/m^2) and a history of advanced CHF, left ventricular ejection fraction less than 45% (mean ejection fraction 28% $\pm$ 3%), and no other valvular lesions or concomitant coronary artery disease. The operative mortality rate was 21% (3 of 14 patients), and 1 of 11 surviving patients showed no long-term symptomatic improvement. Compared with survivors with major clinical improvement, nonsurvivors and patients with no symptomatic improvement had significantly lower ejection fractions for any given wall stress, suggesting that depressed intrinsic contractility may have produced the low ejection fraction rather than the afterload mismatch observed in the group of patients with clinical improvement. Further, a mean systolic aortic valve gradient of 30 mm Hg or less was predictive of a poor outcome regardless of aortic valve area.

Despite early symptomatic improvement after aortic valve replacement for aortic stenosis, there is a real and significant incidence of late recurrence of CHF symptoms. In patients who had no functional disability 1 year after aortic valve replacement, the recurrence of CHF noted 10 years after follow-up depended on whether they had had advanced symptomatic disease before the operation. Almost two thirds of deaths occurring more than 12 years after aortic valve replacement are caused by CHF. Thus, the degree of preoperative myocardial fibrosis resulting from aortic stenosis, which correlates with the degree of hypertrophy, may ultimately determine the long-term prognosis. Preoperative data are significantly predictive of left ventricular performance more than 10 years after operation, and impaired function in turn depends closely on residual hypertrophy. Preoperative factors predictive of late death after aortic valve replacement include peak-to-peak systolic gradient, cardiothoracic index, left ventricular failure, prosthetic orifice diameter of 15 mm or less, age, ventricular ectopic beats, male gender, and antianginal or antiarrhythmic treatment.

In summary, the natural history of symptomatic, severe aortic stenosis is malignant and aortic valve replacement is clearly indicated in the appropriate-risk patient. The risk of sudden death in a truly asymptomatic patient with severe aortic stenosis is not well defined, but appears to be approximately 1% to 2%. Thus, aortic valve replacement is not strictly indicated in the asymptomatic patient with severe aortic stenosis to prevent sudden death. In most of these patients, however, symptoms do develop rapidly; when this occurs, aortic valve replacement is indicated. Asymptomatic patients with severe aortic stenosis and impaired left ventricular function should be advised to undergo aortic valve replacement. The course of disease in patients with symptomatic, moderate aortic stenosis is progressive, and a significant mortality rate exists at 4 years after diagnosis. Thus, these patients require close follow-up, and aortic valve replacement is indicated in the appropriate-risk patients. The natural history of patients with mild aortic stenosis or asymptomatic, moderate aortic stenosis is relatively benign; thus, aortic valve replacement may not be indicated. These patients, however, require close follow-up to observe the progression of their disease.

SELECTED REFERENCES

Boltwood CM, Tei C, Wong M, Shah PM. Quantitative echocardiography of the mitral complex in dilated cardiomyopathy: the mechanism of functional mitral regurgitation. *Circulation* 1983;68:498–508.

Bonow RO, Dodd JT, Maron BJ, et al. Long-term changes in left ventricular function and reversal of ventricular dilatation after valve replacement for chronic aortic regurgitation. *Circulation* 1988;78:1108–1120.

Bonow RO, Lakatos E, Maron BJ, Epstein SE. Serial long-term assessment of the natural history of asymptomatic patients with chronic aortic regurgitation and normal left ventricular systolic function. *Circulation* 1991;84:1625–1635.

Bonow RO, Picone AL, McIntosh CL, et al. Survival and functional results after valve replacement for aortic regurgitation from 1976 to 1983: impact of preoperative left ventricular function. *Circulation* 1985;72:1244–1256.

Bonow RO, Rosing DR, Kent KM, Epstein SE. Timing of operation for chronic aortic regurgitation. *Am J Cardiol* 1982;50:325–336.

Bonow RO, Rosing DR, McIntosh CL, et al. The natural history of asymptomatic patients with aortic regurgitation and normal left ventricular function. *Circulation* 1983;68:509–517.

Carabello BA, Green LH, Grossman W, et al. Hemodynamic determinants of prognosis of aortic valve replacement in critical aortic stenosis and advanced congestive heart failure. *Circulation* 1980;62:42–48.

David TE, Burns RJ, Bacchus CM, et al. Mitral valve replacement for mitral regurgitation with and without preservation of chordae tendineae. *J Thorac Cardiovasc Surg* 1984;88:718–725.

David TE, Uden DE, Strauss HD. The importance of the mitral apparatus in left ventricular function after correction of mitral regurgitation. *Circulation* 1983;68[Suppl]:II-76–II-82.

Hendren WG, Nemec JJ, Lytle BW, et al. Mitral valve repair for ischemic mitral insufficiency. *Ann Thorac Surg* 1991;52:1246–1252.

Henry WL, Bonow RO, Borer JS, et al. Observations on the optimum time for operative intervention for aortic regurgitation: I. evaluation of the results of aortic valve replacement in symptomatic patients. *Circulation* 1980;61:471–483.

Henry WL, Bonow RO, Rosing DR, Epstein SE. Observations on the optimum time for operative intervention for aortic regurgitation: II. serial echocardiographic evaluation of asymptomatic patients. *Circulation* 1980;61:484–492.

Horstkotte D, Loogen F. The natural history of aortic valve stenosis. *Eur Heart J* 1988;9[Suppl E]:57–64.

Kay GL, Kay JH, Zubiate P, Yokoyama T, Mendez M. Mitral valve repair for mitral regurgitation secondary to coronary artery disease. *Circulation* 1986;74[Suppl 1]:88–98.

Lund O. Preoperative risk evaluation and stratification of long-term survival after valve replacement for aortic stenosis. *Circulation* 1990;82: 124–139.

Rankin JS, Livesey SA, Smith LR, et al. Trends in surgical treatment of ischemic mitral regurgitation: effects of mitral valve repair on hospital mortality. *Semin Thorac Cardiovasc Surg* 1989;1:149–163.

Tsakiris AG, Rastelli GC, Amorim D, Titus JL, Wood EH. Effect of experimental papillary muscle damage on mitral valve closure in intact anesthetized dogs. *Mayo Clin Proc* 1970;45:275–285.

Van Dantzig JM, Delemarre BJ, Koster RW, Bot H, Visser CA. Pathogenesis of mitral regurgitation in acute myocardial infarction: importance of changes in left ventricular shape and regional function. *Am Heart J* 1996; 131:865–871.

Myocardial Replacement Therapies

Management of End-Stage Heart Disease, edited by Eric A. Rose and Lynne Warner Stevenson. Lippincott–Raven Publishers, Philadelphia ©1998.

CHAPTER 14

Cardiac Allotransplantation

Daniel J. Goldstein and Eric A. Rose

EPIDEMIOLOGY OF END-STAGE CONGESTIVE HEART FAILURE

With a nationwide prevalence of three million cases, an incidence of more than 400,000 per year, and a fatality rate of 250,000 per year, heart failure represents a public health problem of enormous proportions. Heart failure is the only form of heart disease that is increasing in frequency; in fact, annual mortality rates for heart failure far exceed those due to human immunodeficiency virus (HIV) infection and breast cancer. It is widely recognized as the most expensive diagnosis-related group financed by the Health Care Finance Administration, and it is singly responsible for one million hospitalizations per year, with in-patient costs estimated at $8 billion and total costs exceeding $35 billion. Although emerging medical therapies have improved survival and quality of life for patients with mild to moderate heart failure, approximately 60,000 patients eventually contract end-stage heart failure unresponsive to maximal medical therapy. Despite the exciting recent laboratory and clinical developments in the fields of mechanical support, xenotransplantation, and ventricular reduction, cardiac allotransplantation remains the only hope for long-term survival for many of these ill patients.

HISTORICAL PERSPECTIVE

In 1960, Lower and Shumway described the surgical technique for cardiac transplantation; 7 years later, Barnard successfully performed the first human cardiac transplantation. A flurry of activity followed, and within a short time, several transplantation centers were established worldwide. The initial enthusiasm for cardiac transplantation soon waned because of prohibitive perioperative mortality and poor survival rates. Except for

Department of Surgery, Columbia-Presbyterian Medical Center, New York, New York 10032

occasional clinical efforts at Stanford University, the field of cardiac transplantation remained dormant until the early 1980s, when cyclosporine A was introduced. The advent of cyclosporine A signaled the arrival of specific immunotherapy, and with it came improved survival rates, broadened interest, and increases in patient recruitment. Unfortunately, because of these successes, the demand for donor organs has now outstripped supply, and a paradoxic rise in mortality has occurred as more patients are dying while awaiting transplantation.

EVALUATION OF POTENTIAL CANDIDATES FOR TRANSPLANTATION

Inclusion Criteria

Over 2,000 patients underwent cardiac transplantation in 1995, representing only a fraction of the potential recipient pool. At the moment, donor hearts are given first to those patients in whom medical therapy has failed and those most disabled by the ravages of congestive heart failure (CHF).

At present, patients eligible for cardiac transplantation must have end-stage cardiac disease with a life expectancy of less than 1 year; inoperable coronary artery disease (CAD) with intractable anginal symptoms; or malignant ventricular arrhythmias unresponsive to conventional medical or surgical therapies. Currently, whenever myocardial viability is detected in patients with severe left ventricular dysfunction, serious consideration is given to surgical revascularization; similar deliberations are made for patients with severe valvular heart disease and coexisting cardiomyopathy in whom valvular replacement may outweigh the risks of heart transplantation.

Patients with New York Heart Association (NYHA) Class III or IV heart failure refractory to maximal medical therapy are considered eligible for transplantation if left ventricular ejection fraction is less than 20% and functional capacity is severely impaired, as assessed by determination of $\dot{V}O_{2max}$. Studies performed at our institution showed $\dot{V}O_{2max}$ to be a reliable indicator of outcome, predicting a survival benefit in patients with a pre-transplantation $\dot{V}O_{2max}$ of 14 mL/kg/minute or less.

At many institutions, a growing number of patients undergoing transplantation have received a left ventricular assist device as a bridge to transplantation. All potential candidates for mechanical support must first meet transplantation inclusionary criteria.

Exclusion Criteria

The allotransplantation criteria used at our center were formulated to avoid performing transplantation on patients in whom the risk of death from transplant failure or from co-morbid conditions is too great to justify the use of a scarce and valuable organ. In general, any coexistent systemic illness that limits survival independent of heart disease is considered a possible contraindication to transplantation.

Significant end-organ dysfunction, evidenced by reduction in creatinine clearance, elevation in serum creatinine and total bilirubin, or significant coagulopathy, is also considered a contraindication to transplantation, as are active infection, recent pulmonary infarction, excessive obesity, active mental illness or psychosocial instability, and drug, tobacco, or alcohol abuse. Because severe pulmonary hypertension is associated with right heart failure and death after transplantation, pulmonary vasoreactivity (with sodium nitroprusside or inhaled nitric oxide) must be demonstrated before a patient is put on the waiting list. Finally, because of the rigorous immunosuppressive regimens and the possibility that these regimens will be intensified during episodes of acute rejection, transplantation is not offered to patients with active or recent malignancy or the presence of antibodies to HIV. Patients with distant history of treated malignancy are considered adequate candidates for transplantation, as are some patients with unrespectable primary cardiac tumors localized to the heart.

Donor Criteria

Acceptance criteria for heart donors include age under 65 years and no evidence of malignancy, septicemia, or antibodies to HIV or hepatitis B or C. Cardiac function is evaluated by electrocardiography and echocardiography, and potential donors with prolonged cardiac dysfunction or a low cardiac output are excluded. In male donors older than 45 and female donors older than 50 years of age, cardiac catheterization is recommended. Finally, the harvest team should examine the donor organ before proceeding with organ harvest.

As our experience with transplantation has grown, we and others have extended the criteria for acceptable donor hearts. This expansion of criteria is the result of (a) increased understanding and improved management of perioperative complications; (b) the ongoing critical shortage of donor organs; and (c) the increasing demand for donor organs. We and others have begun to accept donors who are older and who have less-than-ideal hemodynamic profiles for transplantation in patients in desperate conditions.

IMMUNOSUPPRESSION AND ANTIBIOTIC PROPHYLAXIS

Since the late 1970s, three major immunosuppressive protocols have evolved at our institution. From 1977 to early 1983, double immunotherapy was used with corticosteroids and azathioprine. Between 1983 and 1985, the protocol was modified to include cyclosporine instead of azathioprine in the double-drug regimen. Since then, triple therapy has been instituted with cyclosporine, azathioprine, and steroids.

Our current protocol includes oral azathioprine and intravenous steroids given before surgery, and oral cyclosporine titrated to creatinine clearance. Cyclosporine dosage is adjusted to maintain serum cyclosporine levels near 200 ng/mL and to maintain a serum creatinine of 175 μmol/L or less. After the first 6 postoperative months, cyclosporine levels are targeted to 150 ng/mL. One year after surgery, levels are maintained near 100 ng/mL. Prednisone (1 mg/kg/day) is begun immediately after surgery and tapered to 0.1 to 0.15 mg/kg/day by 3 months after surgery. Azathioprine (2 mg/kg/day) is adjusted to maintain the white blood cell count ($>4,000/mm^3$) and platelet count ($>100,000/mm^3$).

Antibiotic prophylaxis is administered to all cardiac transplant recipients. In the perioperative period, bacterial prophylaxis with vancomycin and aztreonam is given. Patients who are positive for the purified protein derivative test receive isoniazid and pyridoxine. Viral prophylaxis consists of annual influenza A and B vaccines and cytomegalovirus (CMV) prophylaxis. Prevalence of CMV infection is monitored monthly in both urine and buffy coat cultures. All patients receive 5 mg/kg of acyclovir beginning during surgery. After operation, the patient should receive 400 to 800 mg of acyclovir orally three times per day for up to 1 year. Recipients of CMV-positive donor organs receive 500 mg/kg of Gammagard (Baxter Healthcare Co., Glendale, CA), once a week for 4 weeks, and then once every 2 weeks for 4 weeks. All blood products given to transplant recipients are irradiated and either screened as CMV negative or transferred through a Pall filter. Antiprotozoal prophylaxis consists of trimethoprim–sulfamethoxazole once daily for a year, while antifungal prophylaxis includes nystatin daily for 3 months.

SURVIVAL

Actuarial survival rates for the 20-year experience with 887 patients undergoing cardiac allotransplantation at our institution are represented in Figure 1. The effect of the three different immunosuppressive protocols on graft survival is depicted in Figure 2. The current actuarial survival rate at 1 year is 76%, 61% at 5 years, and 42% at 10 years, comparable with the worldwide data of the Registry of the International Society for Heart and Lung Transplantation (ISHLT), which indicate 1- and 5-year survival rates of 78% and 67%, respectively. As in other series, the most frequent causes of death within the first year of cardiac transplantation were acute rejection and infection, whereas graft CAD or allograft vasculopathy were the leading causes of death after the first year.

Complications

Rejection

Episodes of acute rejection, diagnosed by routine endomyocardial biopsy or the new onset of clinical symptoms or alterations in cardiac function, are a common occurrence in the first year after transplantation. Although the prevalence of rejection has declined in the

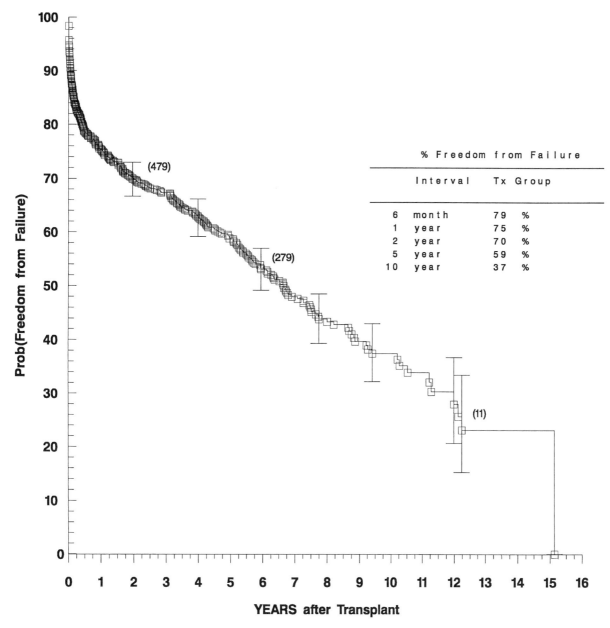

FIG. 1. Kaplan-Meier survival curve depicting the 20-year experience with cardiac allotransplantation at Columbia-Presbyterian Medical Center.

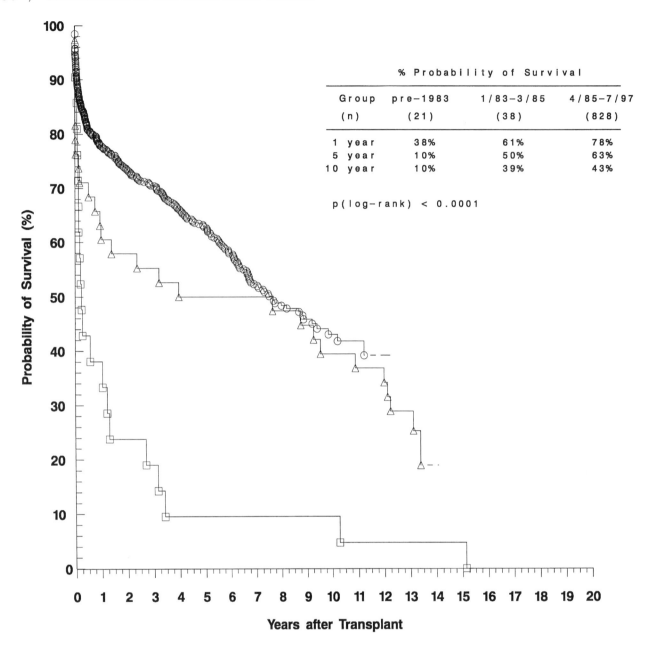

FIG. 2. Effect of immunosuppression regimen on survival after cardiac allotransplantation. The squares represent the 21 patients who underwent transplantation before 1983 under cyclosporine–azathioprine immunosuppression (precyclosporine era). The triangles correspond to the early cyclosporine (plus corticosteroid) experience. The circles represent the experience with triple-drug (cyclosporine–azathioprine–cortocosteroids) immunosuppressive therapy.

era of immunosuppressive triple therapy, an analysis of our experience revealed an actuarial freedom from rejection of 45% at 1 year, with nearly 80% of first-year rejections occurring within the first 3 months after transplantation. Interestingly, there were no significant differences in rejection frequency and actuarial freedom from rejection between primary transplant and retransplanted patients. Our algorithm for treatment of rejection has been published previously. Briefly, low-grade (I or II) and clinically asymptomatic Grade III rejection is treated with oral steroid boost therapy, which is followed by weekly endomyocardial biopsy until histologic resolution is confirmed. In cases of persistent rejection, a second steroid boost is given intravenously. Patients not responding to a second steroid dose and all patients manifesting hemodynamic instability receive intravenous OKT3 or antithymocyte globulin (if hypersensitive to OKT3). In our reported experience, 52% and 36% of rejection episodes have responded to oral and intravenous steroid therapy, respectively. The remainder of the patients are being treated with specific anti–T-cell or anti–B-cell modalities.

Graft Atherosclerosis

Accelerated graft CAD represents a major limitation to long-term survival in cardiac transplant recipients. The advent of intravascular ultrasound and coronary flow measurements has helped decipher some of the mechanisms underlying the development of transplant arteriopathy.

Angiographic evidence of graft CAD has been reported in as many as 45% of cardiac transplant patients surviving more than 3 years, and is associated with a fivefold increased risk for other cardiac events, such as myocardial infarction, heart failure, or sudden death. Although the exact pathogenic origin of graft CAD is not known, both immunologic and nonimmunologic mechanisms have been proposed for the development of the diffuse, concentric myointimal proliferation characteristic of this process. The observation that patients with graft CAD possess elevated plasma levels of the interleukin-2 receptor, a marker of acute allograft rejection, suggests that acute allograft rejection and graft CAD may be related immune processes. Because improvements in the immunologic control of acute rejection have not yielded a decreased incidence of graft CAD, however, and because clinical studies investigating the link between rejection and CAD have produced conflicting results, this association has remained a matter of controversy.

In other studies, several nonimmunologic risk factors for the development of graft CAD have been identified, including donor age, gender, cold ischemic time, and recipient obesity and hyperlipidemia. These observations, together with the known effects of cyclosporine and steroids on weight gain and lipid metabolism, suggest

that patients with frequent episodes of acute rejection might be at higher risk for graft CAD.

Finally, CMV infection has been identified as a risk factor for graft CAD in two clinical studies. Although precise mechanisms are unclear, it has been suggested that CMV infection promotes graft CAD through endothelial cell activation, modulation of lipid metabolism, or immunologic stimulation.

Current approaches in the prevention of graft CAD include aggressive treatment of acute rejection as well as eliminating possible risk factors through weight loss and lipid-lowering strategies, even though no objective data exist demonstrating the beneficial impact of these interventions on graft vasculopathy. Pharmacologic therapies proposed for the prevention and treatment of graft CAD have included platelet-modifying agents and calcium channel blockers. Although early enthusiasm for the use of aspirin and dipyridamole has been tempered by equivocal long-term results, short-term studies using quantitative angiography and intravascular ultrasound have confirmed the ability of diltiazem to prevent and even induce regression of graft CAD.

The outlook for patients with accelerated CAD is poor. Retransplantation remains the most definitive treatment for these patients, but the shortage of donor organs, ethical issues, long waiting times, and suboptimal results have all limited the use of retransplantation. In fact, the 1995 ISHLT Registry reports that only 2.6% of total cardiac transplantation procedures were retransplantations.

In a published study, we have reported 14 cases of cardiac retransplantation (including 1 in a patient who received a third transplant), among 431 patients transplanted over 14 years. Indications for retransplantation included graft CAD in eight cases, acute rejection in five cases, and intraoperative graft failure in one case. One- and 2-year survival rates were 71% and 60%, respectively, which are similar to those reported by Karwande et al. Despite reports of inferior survival rates in retransplanted patients, we found no differences in linearized acute rejection rates or actuarial survival in retransplanted patients compared with those in patients receiving a primary transplant, and have encountered similar results in our experience with cardiac retransplantation in pediatric patients.

Transplant surgeons continue to perform retransplantation because few alternatives exist. Transplant vasculopathy is usually diffuse and involves both proximal and distal coronary vessels and is therefore not often amenable to surgical intervention. Despite this difficulty, percutaneous coronary atherectomy, angioplasty, and, most recently, laser transmyocardial revascularization have all been used in selected patients with some success. Surgical revascularization has been attempted in a small group of patients with mixed results. The combined experience with these modalities suggests a 25% perioperative mortality; long-term results are not yet available. It is unclear whether these techniques will have a significant impact on the treatment of graft CAD. Use of intravascular ultrasound, quantitative angiography, and coronary flow measurements of distal coronary beds may evolve to the extent that we are able to identify early, asymptomatic transplant vasculopathy amenable to revascularization. If this occurs, coronary bypass surgery may become an important, and certainly more practical, alternative to retransplantation.

Lymphoproliferative Disorders

Posttransplantation lymphoproliferative disorders (PTLDs) represent a spectrum of abnormal B-lymphocyte growths that develop after organ transplantation and immunosuppression and are often associated with Epstein-Barr virus infection. Ranging in severity from atypical lymphoid hyperplasia associated with a mononucleosis-like syndrome to malignant lymphoma with metastatic potential, PTLDs have been shown to respond to reductions in immunosuppression as well as to systemic chemotherapy.

A high index of suspicion is necessary to diagnose PTLDs. The diagnosis requires tissue biopsy, which must be submitted to immunohistochemical and flow cytometry analysis. The management of these disorders is tailored to the clinical presentation. For patients with mononucleosis-like illness and minor lesions, immunosuppression is reduced and antiviral agents and supportive care are instituted. Even patients with monoclonal lesions may respond to this therapy. Reduction of immunosuppression alone has led to remission in 42% to 50% of solid organ transplant recipients, although Penn estimates a more pessimistic figure of 31%. Patients with true lymphomas are less likely to respond to these conservative measures. In such patients, use of chemotherapy has been suggested; however, reported experience with this treatment is limited to a few small series from individual institutions.

As reported in a retrospective analysis, 19 of 516 (4%) patients receiving cardiac allografts over a 9-year period at our institution contracted PTLDs involving the lungs, gastrointestinal tract, lymph nodes, or multiple extranodal sites. Although no correlation was found between immunosuppression dosing and PTLD incidence or site of involvement, patients with PTLDs involving the lungs and gastrointestinal tract showed superior responses and improved survival after reduction of immunosuppression compared with patients with involvement of other extranodal sites. In this series, overall 1- and 5-year survival rates were 89.5% and 52.6%, respectively, compared with 84.2% and 68.4% in age- and sex-matched non-PTLD control subjects.

Much remains to be learned about these disorders. Promising advances in the management of PTLDs with the use of new immunotherapies like anti–B-cell antisera may improve long-term survival in transplant recipients. It is clear that the treatment of PTLDs should remain in the hands of experienced transplant physicians who have the difficult task of maintaining a careful balance between allograft function, tumor control, and patient survival.

COSTS

As the demand for cardiac replacement has outpaced the available donor supply, the number of patients on waiting lists has grown significantly. The resulting increases in waiting times have resulted in a greater proportion of severely ill patients awaiting and receiving transplants. In fact, the percentage of United Network for Organ Sharing Status I patients who are undergoing transplantation is consistently increasing, whereas the number of Status II (out-patient for the most part) patients undergoing transplantation is decreasing. Although success rates and long-term survival have not been affected by this trend, the costs of transplantation have risen substantially.

One factor that has contributed to these rising costs is the prolonged preoperative hospitalization required by Status I patients (inotropic or mechanical support dependent). In a study from the St. Louis Health Center, mean pretransplantation charges for Status I and Status II patients were $109,116 versus $250 respectively; this dramatic difference in cost was largely due to the difference in hospital stay: a mean of 25 days of pretransplantation intensive care unit stay for Status I patients versus 0 days for Status II patients.

We performed a cost analysis of the cardiac transplantation program at Columbia-Presbyterian and found that the average total hospital and postdischarge charges per patient had nearly tripled over 4 years, from $45,000 in 1988 to $121,000 in 1992. These increases were accompanied by nearly twofold increases in average pretransplantation and posttransplantation hospital lengths of stay, and a dramatic increase in the proportion of transplant recipients who were bound to intensive care units before surgery.

In this era of cost containment, high technologies destined for the care of a few are increasingly being questioned. Transplantation centers—motivated in part by the managed care industry—are looking for different ways to reduce costs. To this end, institution of home dobutamine programs, restructuring of organ procurement billing, and revision of current waiting list practices are being studied.

As pointed out by Sapirstein, society will eventually have to take a hard look at cardiac transplantation and other expensive interventions and assign definite yet emotionally acceptable limits to extending the lives of patients with end-stage heart failure. Undoubtedly, the future of cardiac transplantation will be determined in part by issues unrelated to the success of the procedure or the excellent quality of life it provides.

FUTURE DIRECTIONS

Although the current success of heart transplantation can be largely attributed to the use of cyclosporine, continued improvements in immunosuppression regimens, diagnosis and treatment of rejection, and management of critically ill patients have allowed survival rates to remain favorable even though patients who undergo transplantation today are in general sicker than they were a few years ago.

Whereas in the past, reducing perioperative mortality and conquering the rejection barrier were the most pressing obstacles standing in the way of successful transplantation, attention to the long-term complications of transplantation has moved into the forefront.

This paradigm shift is most evident in the ongoing efforts in three distinct areas. First and foremost, transplant physicians are struggling to understand the development of allograft vasculopathy, the leading cause of death among transplant recipients surviving more than 1 year. It is hoped that understanding the pathogenesis of transplant arteriopathy will elucidate the relative contribution of immune and nonimmune mechanisms to the development of the disease, and accordingly lead to tailored therapies.

Because retransplantation is a very limited option, conventional interventions like angioplasty, coronary bypass, and valvular replacement, as well as newer therapies like laser transmyocardial revascularization, are likely to play an increasing role in the management of patients with advanced transplant vasculopathy.

Second, efforts will be increasingly directed at the management of PTLDs. Advances in immunotherapy and manipulation of immunosuppressive regimens will likely improve treatment options for patients with PTLDs—particularly those with monoclonal lesions. Therapeutic algorithms to balance allograft survival and tumor control are likely to evolve so that the long-term outlook for transplant recipients with PTLDs is improved.

Last, in an effort to thwart cyclosporine-induced renal dysfunction, new regimens based on lower cyclosporine dosing or replacement with new agents like FK506 and mycophenolate mofetil are likely to be investigated.

We believe progress in the field will improve long-term survival and quality of life for the lucky few who receive precious donor hearts. Therefore, the donor organ shortage will continue to limit the widespread application of this therapy. Thus far, efforts at changing the public's attitudes toward organ donation have failed. As a result, the search for alternatives to cardiac replacement will continue unabated.

SELECTED REFERENCES

CONSENSUS Trial Study Group. Effects of enalapril on mortality in severe congestive heart failure. *N Engl J Med* 1987;316:1429–1435.

Costanzo-Nordin MR. Cardiac allograft vasculopathy: relationship with acute cellular rejection and histocompatibility. *J Heart Lung Transplant* 1992;11:S90–S104.

Gao SZ, Schroeder JS, Alderman EL, et al. Prevalence of accelerated coronary artery disease in heart transplant survivors: comparison of cyclosporine and azathioprine regimens. *Circulation* 1989;80[Suppl]:III-100–III-105.

Halle A, DiSciascio G, Massin E, et al. Coronary angioplasty, atherectomy, and bypass surgery in cardiac transplant patients. *J Am Coll Cardiol* 1995;26:120–128.

Hosenpud J, Novick R, Breen T, et al. The registry of the International Society of Heart and Lung Transplantation: twelfth official report—1995. *J Heart Lung Transplant* 1995;14:805–815.

Mancini DM, Eisen H, Kussmaul W, et al. Value of peak exercise oxygen consumption for optimal timing of cardiac transplantation in ambulatory patients with heart failure. *Circulation* 1991;83:778–786.

Michler RE, McLaughlin MJ, Chen JM, et al. Clinical experience with cardiac retransplantation. *J Thorac Cardiovasc Surg* 1993;106:622–631.

Miller LW, Donohue TJ, Wolford TA. The surgical management of allograft coronary disease: a paradigm shift. *Semin Thorac Cardiovasc Surg* 1996;8:133–138.

Nalesnik MA. Posttransplantation lymphoproliferative disorders: current perspectives. *Semin Thorac Cardiovasc Surg* 1996;8:139–148.

Sarris GE, Moore KA, Schroeder JS, et al. Cardiac transplantation: the Stanford experience in the cyclosporine era. *J Thorac Cardiovasc Surg* 1994;108:240–252.

Schocken DD, Arrieta MI, Leaverton PE, Ross EA. Prevalence and mortality rate of congestive heart failure in the United States. *J Am Coll Cardiol* 1992;20:301–306.

Schroeder JS, Gao SZ, Alderman EL, et al. A preliminary study of diltiazem in the prevention of coronary artery disease in heart transplant recipients. *N Engl J Med* 1993;328:164–170.

Shapiro RS, Chauvenet A, McGuire W, et al. Treatment of B-cell lymphoproliferative disorders with interferon-alpha and intravenous gammaglobulin. *N Engl J Med* 1988;318:1334.

Ventura HO, Mehra MR, Smart FW, Stapleton DD. Cardiac allograft vasculopathy: current concepts. *Am Heart J* 1995;129:791–798.

Votapka TV, Swartz MT, Reedy JE, et al. Heart transplantation charges: status 1 versus status 2 patients. *J Heart Lung Transplant* 1995;14:366–372.

Management of End-Stage Heart Disease, edited by Eric A. Rose and Lynne Warner Stevenson. Lippincott–Raven Publishers, Philadelphia ©1998.

CHAPTER 15

Xenotransplantation

John H. Artrip, Oktavijan P. Minanov, Silviu Itescu, and Robert E. Michler

With the development of increasingly effective immunosuppressive agents, organ transplantation has become the best therapeutic option available for patients with end-stage organ disease. Despite this success, the supply of human donor organs remains inadequate to meet the demand (Table 1). According to the United Network of Organ Sharing (UNOS) Scientific Registry, over 67,000 patients were listed for transplantation during 1995. Yet, throughout the year, only 20,000 organs were transplanted from 8,540 donors, whereas 3,500 patients listed died waiting for an organ. The 5-year period between 1990 and 1995 witnessed over a 70% increase in the number of patients awaiting organ transplantation. Efforts to increase donation rates, such as educational programs and "required request" legislation have not dramatically improved donation rates, as measured by a disappointing 28% increase in donors over the same period. If supply and demand continue to grow at the same rate, by the year 2000, nearly 100,000 Americans will be in need of organ transplantation, with a mere 11,000 donors available for transplantation that year.

The situation appears even more bleak for patients with end-stage heart disease. At the end of 1995, nearly 6,600 patients were listed for heart transplantation, almost a 50% increase from 1990. Yet, during the same 5-year period there was only a 15% increase in heart donation rates. Of all Americans listed for heart transplantation each year, approximately 35% receive transplants, whereas nearly 20% to 30% die before a donor is found. For members of certain populations, such as children, or patients who are UNOS Status II or have the O blood type, the likelihood of being transplanted is even worse.

With 1-year survival rates exceeding 90% at the best centers, it is more likely for a patient to die on the waiting list than to die within the first year after transplantation.

The severe shortage of hearts has prompted several investigators to develop alternative strategies to human heart transplantation. These strategies include mechanical and biologic devices (xenografts) implanted either temporarily ("bridge" therapy to allotransplantation) or permanently ("destination" therapy replacing allotransplantation). Of the mechanical devices under development, the most progress has been made with the left ventricular assist device. Left ventricular assist devices have been successfully applied as bridge therapy and have been approved for destination therapy in human clinical trials. Major limitations of left ventricular assist devices and other mechanical devices include their large size, requirement of an external power supply, and risk of thromboembolism, anemia, bleeding, and infection. Xenografts obviate these problems, but replace them with

TABLE 1. *Statistics for U.S. transplantation from the United Network for Organ Sharing (UNOS) database for kidney, liver, pancreas, heart, and lung, 1990–1995*

Year	Organ transplantions[a]	Donors[b]	Waiting list[c]	Deaths[d]
1990	15,459	6,637	21,914	1,982
1991	16,187	6,947	24,719	2,382
1992	16,605	7,092	29,415	2,602
1993	18,258	7,759	33,352	2,918
1994	19,018	8,140	37,609	3,072
1995	20,064	8,540	43,854	3,448

[a]All U.S. transplantations including kidney, liver, pancreas, heart and lung.
[b]All U.S. donors including cadaveric and living related.
[c]The UNOS OPTN waiting lists on the last day of each year.
[d]All U.S. deaths in patients awaiting organ transplantation.

J. H. Artrip, S. Itescu, and R. E. Michler: Department of Surgery, Columbia-Presbyterian Medical Center, New York, New York 10032

O. P. Minanov: Department of Surgery, University of North Carolina, Chapel Hill, North Carolina 27514 the morbidity of rejection and the need for more intensive immunosuppression.

HISTORY OF CLINICAL XENOTRANSPLANTATION

The development of vascular techniques by Alexis Carrel in the early 1900s endowed surgeons with the basic skills necessary to transplant organs. Between 1902 and 1912, there were several attempts at human xenotransplantation. Kidney xenografts taken from nonprimate donors, such as rabbit, pig, goat, and lamb, were placed in uremic patients: all transplantations ended acutely in rejection. The first attempt to use a nonhuman primate donor was by Unger, who, in 1910, performed a chimpanzee-to-human kidney transplant. The graft clotted immediately and the patient died within 36 hours.

Transplant surgeons would have to wait over 50 years before the understanding of immunology was sufficient to make transplantation possible. In 1959, the first immunosuppressive agent, 6-mercaptopurine, was introduced into clinical transplantation. Shortly thereafter, the introduction of two potent agents, azathioprine in 1961 and corticosteroids in 1963, provided surgeons with immunosuppression effective enough to undertake human transplantation again. During the early 1960s, organ transplantation became a clinical reality; however, ethical repercussions of human organ donation combined with an inadequate definition of brain death immediately imposed a shortage of donor organs. Surgeons were pressed to use either ethically questionable volunteer donors or poorly preserved postmortem cadaveric organs.

Confronted by this dilemma, Reemtsma performed six chimpanzee-to-human renal transplantations in 1963. Despite an immunosuppressive regimen consisting of actinomycin, azathioprine, and steroids, graft survival was prolonged up to 9 months. A year later, Starzl performed six baboon-to-human renal transplantations using azathioprine and steroid immunosuppression, and achieved graft survival up to 2 months. In the same year, Hardy performed the first heart transplantation using a chimpanzee donor and achieved graft survival for 2 hours. Four years later, Cooley performed a sheep-to-human and Ross performed a pig-to-human heart xenotransplantation in dying recipients: both grafts failed immediately on reperfusion. Over the next two decades, various attempts at clinical xenotransplantation were unable to achieve extended survival, and the appeal of xenotransplantation declined. Not until the introduction of cyclosporine during the 1980s would surgeons again seriously confront the cross-species barrier. In 1984, Bailey performed a baboon-to-human heart transplantation in a female infant (Baby Fae) using cyclosporine-based immunosuppression. Despite ABO incompatibility, the cardiac xenograft survived for 20 days. In 1992 and 1993, Starzl performed two baboon-to-human liver xenotransplantations using potent FK506-based immunosuppression and achieved graft survival of 70 and 26 days.

Despite powerful new immunosuppressive techniques and a better understanding of graft rejection, the fact remains that the longest surviving xenograft was transplanted over 30 years ago, and survival was only 9 months. With such slow progress, why do transplant physicians continue to pursue successful cross-species transplantation? The answer is straightforward: the severe shortage of human donors results in the death of nearly 30% of waiting recipients, and the need for donors continues to grow as more patients are identified and retransplantation lists continue to grow.

IMMUNOLOGIC BARRIERS TO XENOTRANSPLANTATION

Biologic organ replacement, whether by allograft or xenograft, poses the immunologic problem of rejection. In human allotransplantation, the predominant antigenic differences between donor and recipient are confined to the major histocompatibility and blood group antigens. In contrast, a xenograft is likely to express a multitude of antigens that are not expressed by human cells and are likely to elicit antixenograft immunity in human recipients.

Preformed Xenoreactive Antibody and Hyperacute Xenograft Rejection

A considerable obstacle to cross-species transplantation has been hyperacute rejection, in which graft rejection occurs within minutes to hours after reperfusion of the donor organ (Figure 1). Hyperacute rejection occurring in allotransplantation is mediated by preformed antibodies directed against donor major histocompatibility or blood group antigens. Although no effective therapy exists once the rejection process has been initiated, careful preoperative cross-matching can usually avoid hyperacute rejection. Hyperacute rejection occurring in xenotransplantation is mediated by preformed antibodies directed against xenogeneic antigens on donor endothelium. Cross-species combinations innately susceptible to hyperacute rejection are labeled "discordant," whereas combinations less susceptible to hyperacute rejection are labeled "concordant."

In the pig-to-primate model of discordant xenotransplantation, the xenoreactive antibodies are directed against the oligosaccharide, galactose α1,3-galactose (Gal α1,3-Gal). Gal α1,3-Gal synthesis requires the enzyme α1,3-galactosyltransferase. This glycosylation enzyme is responsible for the generation of Gal α1,3-Gal residues on both glycoproteins and glycolipids found on the surface of porcine endothelium. The α1,3-galactosyl-

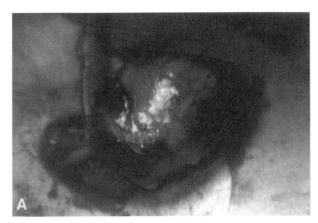
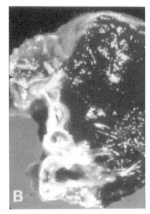
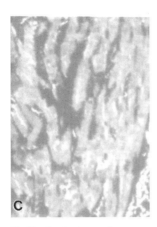

FIG. 1. Pig-to-baboon heterotopic heart transplantation. **A:** Hyperacute rejection. **B:** Explanted specimen showing massive tissue swelling. **C:** Interstitial edema and hemorrhage (10× magnification).

transferase enzyme is present in active form in lower mammals and New World monkeys. Human beings, apes, and Old World monkeys (collectively referred to as platyrrhines) have an inactivated form of the α1,3-galactosyltransferase gene, and do not express this enzyme. Without the enzyme, platyrrhines are unable to synthesize Gal α1,3-Gal and possess naturally occurring antibodies specific for this oligosaccharide.

The importance of this antibody–antigen system in initiating hyperacute rejection has been corroborated by several lines of experimentation. Administration of the Gal α1,3-Gal carbohydrate, which competes with the membrane-bound sugar for xenoreactive antibody, markedly reduces primate serum cytotoxicity to pig kidney cells and transplanted hearts. Enzymatic removal of Gal α1,3-Gal epitopes from porcine endothelium prevents binding of the xenoreactive antibodies and the activation of complement. Furthermore, transfection of a COS cell with cDNA for α1,3-galactosyltransferase confers to the transfected cell the susceptibility to complement lysis by natural human xenoreactive antibody.

Although both immunoglobulin (Ig) class G and M anti-αgal antibodies are present in primate serum, IgM is the primary mediator of hyperacute rejection. Because of its pentameric structure, IgM anti-αgal antibodies are more effective activating complement on porcine endothelial cells. Selective depletion of IgM but not IgG prolonged organ survival is an *ex vivo* model of pig-to-human heart xenotransplantation; moreover, infusion of purified human IgG into cynomolgus monkeys prevented hyperacute rejection of porcine xenografts by competing with IgM for complement binding.

Anti-αgal antibodies develop within a few months of human life. The antibody response is believed to result from antigenic exposure to gut microorganisms expressing Gal α1,3-Gal epitopes on their bacterial surface. In the perinatal period, newborn humans whose gastrointestinal tracts have not yet been colonized by bacteria do not have anti-αgal IgM antibodies. However, placental transfer of maternal IgG leads to detectable levels of anti-αgal IgG in the fetal circulation. Because of its larger size and the inability of IgM to pass the blood–placenta barrier, maternal anti-αgal IgM is not present in the fetal circulation.

In studies using newborn baboons in the absence of immunosuppression, pig cardiac xenografts survived for approximately 3.4 days without hyperacute rejection. Histologic examination of the explanted xenografts demonstrated only a mild degree of microscopic hemorrhage and thrombosis, whereas immunofluorescent examination demonstrated no evidence of immunoglobulin (IgM or IgG) and complement (C3, C4, C5b, or membrane attack complex [MAC]; Figures 2, 3). The absence of natural IgM xenoreactive antibody in newborn primates permits prolonged graft survival; however, the transplanted xenograft is susceptible to a "delayed" rejection process.

Inducible Xenoreactive Antibody and Acute Vascular Rejection

Although allogeneic and concordant xenogeneic combinations usually lack preformed donor-specific antibodies, a heavy exposure to donor antigens may induce a humoral response. An inducible humoral response to alloantigens has been implicated in severe types of acute allograft rejection, which are marked by histopathologic findings of severe vascular destruction. Analogous to acute vascular rejection in allogeneic combinations, concordant xenogeneic combinations are susceptible to a form of rejection that is unresponsive to T-cell immunosuppression and occurs too late to be hyperacute rejection. In a series of heterotopic heart transplantations from the cynomolgus monkey to the baboon, graft rejection correlated with the development of cytotoxic antibodies specific to donor lymphocytes. Immunosuppression tar-

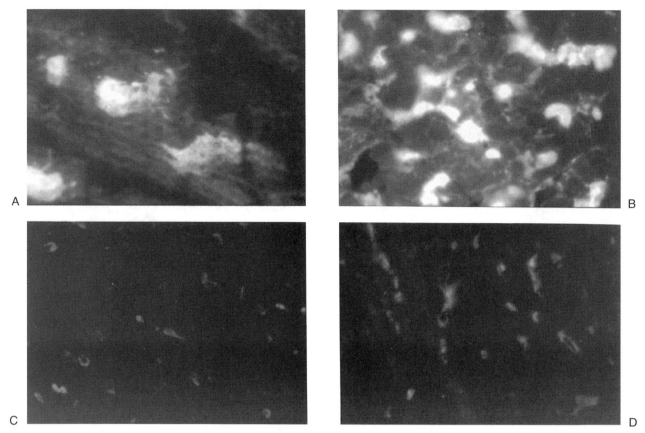

FIG. 2. Immunofluorescent staining of hyperacutely rejected pig-to-adult baboon heterotopic heart transplants (10× magnification). Specimens stain strongly for immunoglobulin M (IgM) **(A)**, C3 **(B)**, C4 **(C)**, and membrane attack complex (MAC) **(D)**.

geting the inducible humoral component, such as total lymphoid irradiation, significantly extended graft survival. The induction of lymphocytotoxic antibodies and the added benefit of humoral-directed therapies imply an important role for humoral immunity. The antigenic targets and the exact mechanism by which this rejection occurs are unknown; however, the humoral response may be directed against donor histocompatibility antigens that are upregulated by cytokines produced by a local inflammatory response.

The presence of preformed xenoreactive antibodies in discordant combinations has limited xenograft survival to the hyperacute period. Efforts to reduce preformed xenoreactive antibody with plasmapheresis or immunoadsorption have reduced xenoreactive antibody levels to less than 5% of pretreatment levels; however, the recipients rapidly reform xenoreactive antibody and are subject to delayed humoral rejection. Newborn primates lack preformed xenoreactive antibody; therefore, newborn baboons heterotopically transplanted with porcine xenografts survived beyond the hyperacute period. Measurement of serum xenoreactive antibodies showed a marked decrease in IgG levels at the time of graft rejection, which was consistent with their binding to xenoantigens on the

pig graft. Some authors have suggested that the binding of xenoreactive antibody to endothelial cells induces conformational changes, resulting in the release of heparan sulfate and creation of a local precoagulant environment.

Cellular Xenograft Rejection and Delayed Xenograft Rejection

A unique form of cellular rejection appears to occur in highly disparate xenogeneic combinations. This type of rejection (termed "delayed xenograft rejection") occurs approximately 3 to 5 days after transplantation and precedes classic T-cell rejection. In a series of heterotopic heart transplantations using the discordant guinea pig-to-rat combination, treatment of the rat recipients with cobra venom factor was used to mitigate complement directed hyperacute rejection. Immunophenotypic analysis of the acutely rejected xenograft showed tissue infiltration with macrophages and natural killer (NK) cells. In other studies using the porcine-to-newborn baboon model to avert hyperacute rejection, histologic examination of the rejected hearts demonstrated a dense mononuclear infiltrate extending from the subepicardial region into the

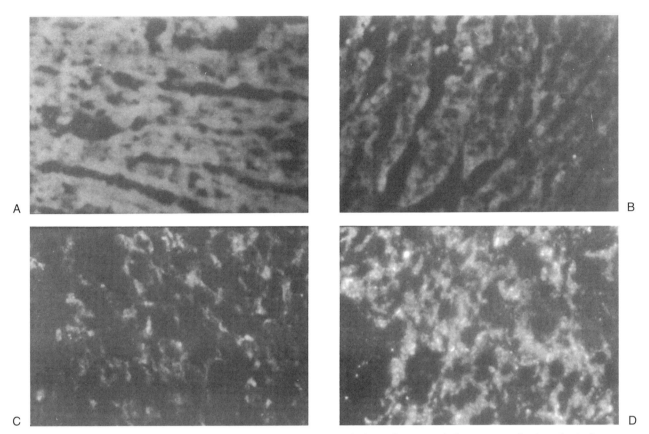

FIG. 3. Immunofluorescent staining of a pig-to-newborn baboon heterotopic heart transplant explanted at 96 hours (10× magnification). Specimens stain weakly for immunoglobulin M (IgM) **(A)**, C3 **(B)**, C4 **(C)**, and membrane attack complex (MAC) **(D)**.

myocardium (Figure 4). Immunophenotypic analysis of the infiltrate showed that it consisted primarily of macrophages and NK cells (Figure 5).

In vitro studies examining the cellular response to porcine endothelium demonstrated that primate peripheral blood mononuclear cells exhibit NK cell activity against pig aortic endothelial cells, and after activation with interleukin-2 (IL-2), the NK activity is greatly enhanced. Pretreatment of human mononuclear cells with anti-CD2 monoclonal antibody significantly inhibited the NK-specific lysis, whereas antibodies directed against other NK cell surface structures, such as CD11a, CD18, CD16, CD8, or CD57, did not inhibit NK-specific lysis. CD2 molecules on the surface of human NK and T cells

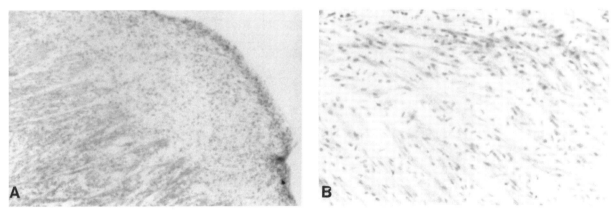

FIG. 4. Hematoxylin and eosin staining of a pig-to-newborn baboon heterotopic heart transplant explanted at 96 hours. **A:** Cellular infiltrate extending from epicardium into myocardium (10× magnification). **B:** Mononuclear cells predominate (20× magnification).

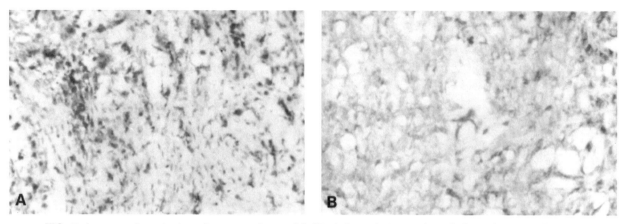

FIG. 5. Immunophenotyping of mononuclear cell infiltrate in a pig-to-newborn baboon heterotopic heart transplant explanted at 96 hours, showing strongly positivity for CD68 (macrophages) **(A)**, and moderate positivity for CD16 (natural killer cells) **(B)**.

bind two structurally related ligands, CD58 and CD48, expressed by endothelial cells. Although the porcine ligand for CD2 has not been defined, it is likely to be homologous to the human CD48 or CD58 molecules. Because interactions between CD2 and its ligands on pig aortic endothelial cells are likely to be of direct clinical significance in the human NK cell response against pig xenografts, determining a way to decrease these interactions may be useful in prolonging xenograft survival.

T-Cell Immunity with Xenografts

Cellular rejection in less disparate xenografts shows striking similarity to acute allograft rejection. Acute allograft rejection progresses over the course of days and commonly occurs 1 to 2 weeks posttransplantation. Biopsies taken during an acute rejection episode show a heavy lymphocytic infiltrate. Analogous to the findings in acute allograft rejection, immunopathologic examination of explanted cardiac xenografts from the concordant combination cynomolgus monkey-to-baboon revealed an extensive lymphocytic infiltrate consisting of CD8 and CD4 T cells. Lymphocytes propagated from the xenograft biopsy specimens demonstrated specific cytotoxicity against donor target cells. Furthermore, naïve T cells cultured with xenogeneic splenocytes developed an accelerated (memory) proliferative response after reexposure to xenogeneic tissue.

In vitro studies such as the mixed lymphocyte reaction and cell-mediated lympholysis assays suggest that the classic T-cell response to xenogeneic cells may be weaker than the response to allogeneic cells. In allorejection, recipient T-cell activation occurs through the direct interaction between T cells and donor target cells. The process requires that T-cell receptors ($\alpha\beta$ or $\gamma\delta$), coreceptors (CD4 or CD8), and adhesion molecules (lymphocyte function-associated antigen-1, LFA-1, and CD2) recognize their respective ligands on allogeneic

donor target cells. Widely disparate species combinations, such as mouse to human, have a weak direct response. The diminished xenogeneic response likely reflects the structural incompatibilities between the recipient molecules and their respective ligands on the murine target cells. In contrast, other species combinations, such as pig to human, have a pronounced direct T-cell response. After exposure to porcine endothelium, CD4 T cells demonstrate enhanced proliferation and IL-2 production. Furthermore, T-cell proliferation is inhibited by monoclonal antibodies directed against porcine human leukocyte antigen-like molecules or adhesion molecules (LFA-1 and CD2), implying direct T-cell activation by pig endothelial cells.

The indirect pathway of T-cell activation could account for the vigorous *in vivo* and *in vitro* cellular response to pig tissue. Xenoantigens processed by recipient antigen-presenting cells and subsequently presented to recipient T cells would lead to T-cell activation by avoiding molecular incompatibilities between foreign and native tissue. In support of a prominent indirect pathway, human macrophages produce over 10 times as much IL-1β after culture with porcine endothelial cells than with allogeneic cells. Finally, interruption of antigen presentation using anti-CD4 or anti-DR antibodies diminished the T-cell proliferative response to xenoantigens.

Strategies for Overcoming the Immunologic Barrier

Despite the advances in immunosuppressive therapies, conventional cyclosporine-based immunosuppression is unable to overcome the immunologic barrier of xenotransplantation. As outlined earlier, hyperacute rejection has three essential components: (a) preformed xenoreactive antibody, (b) a functional complement system, and (c) xenoreactive antigen on donor endothelium. Strategies directed at countering any one of these components could mitigate hyperacute rejection. Plasmapheresis and various immunoadsorption techniques, such as immunoaffinity columns or perfusing the recipient's blood through a second donor organ, have been used to reduce preformed xenoreactive antibody. Infusion of intravenous Gal α1,3-Gal sugar derivatives or treatment with anti-idiotypic antibodies directed against anti-αgal have been used to deactivate the xenoreactive antibody. Strategies targeting the complement system have used cobra venom factor to deplete the C3b component of complement, soluble complement receptor (soluble CR1) to bind the C3b and C4b components of complement, and intravenous immunoglobulin specific for complement components C5 and C6. Each of these strategies only delays rejection, however, until the antibody or complement can function again.

Efforts in molecular biology have focused on genetically engineering animal donors to express human proteins in their tissue. Transgenic pigs that express human complement regulatory proteins (CRPs) on their endothelium have been developed. CRPs such as membrane cofactor protein (MCP [CD46]), decay accelerating factor (DAF [CD55]) and homologous restriction factor (CD59) protect endothelial cells from inadvertent injury by activated complement. MCP and DAF inhibit the formation of C3-convertase and CD59 inhibits the C8 and C9 components of MAC. Although still under debate, it appears that endogenous CRPs are species specific and inhibit homologous complement more effectively than heterologous complement. For this reason, xenografts are especially vulnerable to complement-mediated injury.

Human DAF and CD59 have been variably expressed in transgenic pigs using microinjection of minigene constructs. Minigene constructs contain the gene of interest, transcription and translation initiation and termination sequences, and a promoter or regulatory region. After microinjection, the minigene randomly integrates into the genomic DNA. The expression of the genetic construct critically depends on the site of integration and promoter sequence used. Transgenic cardiac grafts expressing DAF transplanted into cynomolgus monkey recipients have survived a median of 5.1 days in the absence of immunosuppression and over 60 days with potent immunosuppression. Transgenic cardiac grafts expressing both DAF and CD59 survived 30 hours in splenectomized and immunosuppressed baboon recipients. The genetic construct used the α- and β-globulin promoters, resulting in the expression of the human CRPs on hematopoietic cell lines. The resistance to hyperacute rejection depended on translocation of the CRPs to endothelial cells, and lasted only a short time after xenotransplantation. Current efforts use tissue-specific promoters such as von Willebrand factor or β-actin for high-level endothelial cell expression.

Microinjection of yeast artificial chromosomes (YACs) may overcome the major difficulties of minigene constructs. YAC constructs contain the entire gene of interest and the native 5' and 3' flanking regions encoding the promoter and regulatory regions. YAC constructs are much larger than the minigene constructs, permitting a greater repertoire of splice variants, and may be independent of integration site. The larger size, however, results in a lower net yield of founder animals. YAC technology has been used to develop transgenic pigs expressing human MCP.

An alternative approach involves genetically modifying donor endothelium to eliminate or reduce xenoreactive antigen expression. The Gal α1,3-Gal epitopes have successfully been eliminated in mice by genetically "knocking out" the galactosyltransferase necessary for its synthesis. Embryonic stem cells needed to manipulate higher mammals in a similar way are not yet available. Reducing the expression of Gal α1,3-Gal epitopes may be possible by redirecting precursor molecules through an alternative synthetic pathway. H-transferase (α1,2-fucosyltransferase) competes with α1,3-galactosyltransferase for the substrate N-acetyl lactosamine and diverts the synthesis of Gal α1,3-Gal epitopes to the H-antigen of the universal donor blood group O. Transgenic mice and pigs expressing the H-transferase gene have been developed and show a decrease in the level of Gal α1,3-Gal epitopes.

If hyperacute rejection can be avoided, the xenograft would then become susceptible to induced antibody response and subsequent endothelial cell activation. The inducible antibody response requires that anti–B-cell agents be an essential component of the immunosuppression. In addition to trials using the more common anti–B-cell agents, such as azathioprine and cyclophosphamide, experimental trials have been performed using 15-deoxyspergualin, brequinar, leflunomide, and mycophenolate mofetil (MMF). These agents, in combination with steroids and the anti–T-cell agents cyclosporine or FK506, have extended graft function in various rodent xenotransplantation models from days to weeks. MMF may be especially promising in concordant xenotransplantation. A comparison between azathioprine and MMF in cynomolgus monkey-to-baboon heterotopic cardiac transplantation demonstrated animals treated with MMF have longer graft survival.

Special strategies will need to be developed to suppress NK cell-mediated xenograft rejection. Monoclonal anti-CD2 antibody, which disrupts an important accessory molecule for NK cell adhesion, may be of benefit together with therapy aimed at blocking other NK cell ligands. Immunosuppression directed at the cellular elements of T-cell activation and effector cell cytotoxicity would be expected to follow similar strategies used with allotransplantation. If the indirect pathway of T-cell activation proves important, however, novel immunosuppressants that inhibit antigen-presenting cells may prove effective.

INFECTIOUS DISEASE POTENTIAL

Because nonhuman primates may harbor potentially dangerous microorganisms like human immunodeficiency virus (HIV), the possibility of disease transmission through xenotransplantation has become a concern. The possibility of seeding the recipient with potentially pathogenic organisms, especially in the setting of immunosuppression, creates a unique environment for infectious organisms. Agents that are nonpathogenic in their natural hosts may be lethal when placed in another species. For example, herpes B virus has low pathogenicity in its native host, the macaques, but when this virus is transmitted to nonmacaque primates, it causes a neurologic syndrome with an approximate mortality of 70%. Nonhuman primates, such as baboons, carry the greatest known potential for infectious disease transmission. Animals harboring potentially pathogenic microorganisms must be excluded as donors.

The risks with recognized zoonotic pathogens can be reduced, if not eliminated, by controlling the donor vendor source, using screening tests, and by adhering to strict sterilization procedures during organ procurement and grafting. If the appropriate guidelines are maintained, risk of an infectious disease being transmitted after xenotransplantation will be similar to that of allotransplantation.

Potential donor animals should undergo routine physical examinations and should have viral/bacterial cultures obtained of blood, throat, stool, and urine. We believe that the following organisms represent an absolute contraindication to using an animal as a donor for a human heart transplant, and that all potential donor animals should be screened for them initially, as well as undergoing periodic surveillance testing:

Retroviruses
  Simian T-lymphotropic virus (STLV) 1—as high as 40% seropositivity in baboons
  Simian immunodeficiency virus (SIV)—unexpected in baboons
  Simian retrovirus 1, 2, and 5—less common but a definite possibility in baboons
  Human T-lymphotropic virus (HTLV) 1 and 2—HTLV 1 cross-reacts with STLV
  HIV 1 and 2—would not anticipate HIV 1 infection, but certainly if found would be of concern; HIV 2 presence would likely represent cross-reaction with SIV
Herpesviruses
  Macaque herpes B virus (*Herpesvirus simiae*)—unexpected in baboons
Hepatitis A, B, C, and D—antigen positive or hepatitis C antibody positive
Encephalomyocarditis virus—can be found in U.S. primates and it may have affected the myocardium in a detrimental fashion even in animals who have recovered from the infection
Monkey pox—unexpected in the United States
Simian hemorrhagic fever—unexpected in the United States
Filovirus (Marburg and Ebola)—unexpected in the United States and in baboons
Lymphocytic choriomeningitis—can be present
Orthoreovirus—has been associated with encephalitis in baboons
T. gondii—parasite that can be latent in heart muscle, found in 16% to 35% of the baboon population; risk for transmission is at least the same as with human heart transplants, and perhaps higher because the immunosuppression may be higher with xenotransplantation
M. tuberculosis—baboons need to be tuberculin tested, and positive animals excluded

Under the supervision of the Centers for Disease Control and Prevention, institutional review boards and animal care committees need to establish guidelines to screen and monitor donor animals and organ recipients. If the appropriate guidelines are met, the risk of infectious disease transmission after xenotransplantation will be reduced.

DONOR SELECTION

Nonhuman Primates

Nonhuman primates have been favored as organ donors by those wishing to minimize genetic disparity between donor and human recipients. Because of its genetic similarity with humans, the chimpanzee would seem the most logical alternative to human organ donors. Although blood group distribution and size of the chimpanzee are compatible with human recipients, chimpanzees are unavailable as donors. The chimpanzee is an endangered species and international regulations forbid its capture and importation. At present, there are only about 2,000 chimpanzees in colonies in the United States, and their use in biomedical research is confined to research involving HIV and hepatitis.

The next most logical choice is the baboon. Unlike the chimpanzee, the baboon is not endangered and is available in large numbers in sub-Saharan Africa. Because risk of transmitting an infectious disease may be greater with wild animals, however, the undomesticated baboon is not suitable for use as a donor. Baboons bred in domestic colonies would be more suitable donors, but only a few hundred such baboons live in the United States. In addition, the universal donor group O is exceedingly rare in the baboon, which could exclude type O recipients. Finally, the baboon grows to a weight of approximately 35 kg, limiting use of its organs to pediatric patients.

Porcine Donors

Although nonhuman primates represent the best alternative to human allografts, their limited numbers, the size discrepancy, and ethical concerns have renewed enthusiasm for using domesticated farm animals as organ donors. The pig is available in large numbers (approximately 90 million are slaughtered each year in the United States) and has a cardiac anatomy, size, and physiology similar to those of humans. Ethical concerns about using pig heart donors would likely be less vociferous than those regarding the use of nonhuman primates. Considering these factors, the pig appears to be the most suitable donor for xenotransplantation; yet surmounting the immunologic barriers of rejection remains a great limitation.

XENOTRANSPLANTATION AS A BRIDGE TO ALLOTRANSPLANTATION

In our opinion, heart xenotransplantation must first undergo human clinical trials as a "bridge" to allotransplantation. Although bridge therapy does not alleviate the organ shortage, it allows for early investigation into human xenotransplantation and may potentially improve the recipients' clinical condition before allotransplantation. Bridge therapy with mechanical assist devices has been beneficial not only as temporary support, but by actually improving hepatic, renal, and other end-organ function before allotransplantation. Bridge therapy with xenografts offers the greatest potential benefit for patients who are not candidates for mechanical devices.

The question has been raised whether bridge therapy with xenografts could potentially sensitize the recipient's immune system and jeopardize further allotransplantation. "Bridging" studies using the primate cynomolgus monkey-to-baboon heterotopic heart transplant model found no evidence of accelerated rejection in subsequent allografts. Histologic examination of the explanted allografts showed no differences between baboon recipients that underwent prior xenotransplantation and those that did not.

ETHICAL ISSUES AND PUBLIC POLICY

Discussion of the advances in cardiac xenotransplantation must be accompanied by a discussion of the ethical debates about this procedure. Many have raised the question of whether our using animals in this capacity is ethical. Rene Descartes, the 17th century mathematician and philosopher, held that animals are mere automations of life and void of feelings, emotions, and the capacity to suffer. Taking this line of reasoning, humans can treat animals as they wish. At the other extreme are objections based on religious or metaphysical beliefs that hold the rights of all living creatures to be equal. From this line of reasoning, humans are morally responsible for actions taken against another living being, and the use of any animal, living tissue, or even cell culture in scientific endeavors is not justified. Clearly, neither position is held by the majority of people in the United States, and neither should be adopted by policy makers.

During the mid-1980s, the case of Baby Fae brought attention to questions surrounding xenotransplantation and the use of animals in scientific research. Kushner and Belliotti noted in their examination of the case of Baby Fae that for unequal treatment of the two groups to be moral, it must be justified. Justification for the unequal treatment of the baboon donor and the infant Baby Fae requires a morally relevant difference between humans and animals. If the moral difference between humans and animals is the capacity for human emotional relationships, then the donation of organs by nonhuman primates or pigs for transplantation may be acceptable.

Even with the acceptance of a moral distinction between humans and animals, the next logical question becomes whether it is justified to use primates in this manner. Ethical justification requires that the benefits of the procedure be sufficient to warrant the harm against the animal. What level of success justifies scientists to continue their pursuit? And, what level of success is needed to warrant clinical application? Clearly, these questions will need to be addressed on an individual basis and will need to be readdressed with each scientific advancement in this field.

In light of scientific advancements, as well as the ethical issues surrounding xenotransplantation, several governmental agencies have begun examining this topic. The American Institute of Medicine and the British Nuffield Council on Bioethics have formed a committee to discuss the science, ethics, and public policy on xenotransplantation. The following important recommendations were made:

- Guidelines for addressing the infectious disease risks for human trials of xenotransplantation must encompass four major areas: (a) screening source animals for the presence of infectious organisms, (b) surveillance throughout the lifetime of recipients and periodic surveillance of their contacts, (c) establishment of tissue banks containing samples from source animals and recipients, and (d) establishment of national and local registries of patients receiving xenotransplants.
- Institutional review boards and animal care committees are required to conform to the national guidelines for minimizing and continued surveillance of infectious risks.
- IA mechanism must be established to ensure coordination between the federal agencies and other entities involved in the development, oversight, and evaluation of national guidelines.
- When the science base for specific types of xenotransplants is judged sufficient and the appropriate safeguards are in place, well chosen human xenotransplan-

tation trials using animal cells, tissues, and organs would be justified.

THE FUTURE OF XENOTRANSPLANTATION

The desperate shortage of human donor hearts, the limited use of mechanical assist devices, and the recent successes in xenotransplantation justify the future clinical application of cardiac xenografts. In the near future, clinical xenotransplantation will achieve its goal of extended graft survival. Although reservations have been voiced because the initial recipients will likely be patients for whom no therapeutic alternative exists, one must also recall:

> To do nothing, or to prevent others from doing anything, is itself a type of experiment, for the prevention of experimentation is tantamount to the assumption of responsibility for an experiment different from the one proposed (Shimkin).

SELECTED REFERENCES

Alter BJ, Bach FH. Cellular basis of the proliferative response of human T cells to mouse xenoantigens. *J Exp Med* 1990;171:333–338.

Bailey LL, Nehlsen-Cannerella SL, Concepion W, et al. Baboon-to-human cardiac xenotransplantation in a neonate. *JAMA* 1985;254:3321–3329.

Blakely ML, Van der Werf, Berndt MC, et al. Activation of intragraft endothelial and mononuclear cells during discordant xenograft rejection. *Transplantation* 1994;58:1059–1066.

Brauer RB, Baldwin WM, Wang D, et al. Functional activity of anti-C6 antibodies in C6-deficient rats reconstituted by liver allografts: ability to inhibit hyperacute rejection of discordant cardiac xenografts. *Transplantation* 1996;61:588–594.

Bravery CA, Batten P, Yacoub M, et al. Direct recognition SLA- and HLA-like class II antigens on porcine endothelium by human T cells results in T cell activation and release of IL-2. *Transplantation* 1995;60:1024–1033.

Calne RY. Organ transplantation between widely disparate species. *Transplant Proc* 1970;2:550–556.

Caplan AL. Is xenografting morally wrong? *Transplant Proc* 1992;24:722–727.

Chen JM, Michler RE. Heart xenotransplantation: lessons learned and future prospects. *J Heart Lung Transplant* 1993;12:869–875.

Consenza CA, Cramer DV, Tuso PJ, et al. Combination therapy with brequinar sodium and cyclosporine synergistically prolongs hamster-to-rat cardiac xenograft survival. *J Heart Lung Transplant* 1994;13:489–497.

Cooley DA, Hallman GL, Bloodwell RD, et al. Human heart transplantation: experience with 12 cases. *Am J Cardiol* 1968;22:804–810.

Diamond LE, McCurry KR, Martin MJ, et al. Characterization of transgenic pigs expressing functionally active human CD59 on cardiac endothelium. *Transplantation* 1996;61:1241–1249.

Evans RW, Orians CE, Ascher NL. The potential supply of organ donors: an assessment of the efficiency of organ procurement efforts in the United States. *JAMA* 1992;267:239–246.

Fodor WL, Williams BL, Matis LA, et al. Expression of a functional human complement inhibitor in a transgenic pig as a model for the prevention of xenogeneic hyperacute organ rejection. *Proc Natl Acad Sci USA* 1994;91:11153–11157.

Frazier OH, Rose EA, Macmanus Q, et al. Multicenter clinical evaluation of the HeartMate 1000 IP left ventricular assist device. *Ann Thorac Surg* 1992;53:1080–1090.

Galili U, Macher BA, Buehler J, et al. Human natural anti-α-galactosyl IgG: the specific recognition of α(1,3) linked galactose residues. *J Exp Med* 1985;162:573–582.

Galili U, Shohet SB, Kobrin E, et al. Man, apes, and old world monkeys differ from other mammals in the expression of α-galactosyl epitopes on nucleated cells. *J Biol Chem* 1988;263:17755–17762.

Hardy JD, Kurrus FE, Chavez CM, et al. Heart transplantation in man: developmental studies and report of a case. *JAMA* 1964;188:1132.

Itescu S, Kwiatkowski P, Wang SF, et al. Circulating human mononuclear cells exhibit augmented lysis of pig endothelium following activation with IL-2. *Transplantation* 1996;62:1927–1933.

Kaplon RJ, Michler RE, Xu H, et al. Absence of hyperacute rejection in newborn pig-to-baboon cardiac xenografts. *Transplantation* 1995;59:1–6.

Koren E, Milotic F, Neethling FA, et al. Monoclonal antiidiotypic antibodies neutralize cytotoxic effects of anti-αGal antibodies. *Transplantation* 1996;62:837–843.

Kroshus TJ, Bolman RM, Dalmasso AP. Selective IgM depletion prolongs organ survival in an ex vivo model of pig-to-human xenotransplantation. *Transplantation* 1996;62:5–12.

Kroshus TJ, Rollins SA, Dalmasso AP, et al. Complement inhibition with anti-C5 monoclonal antibody prevents acute cardiac tissue injury in an ex vivo model of pig-to-human xenotransplantation. *Transplantation* 1995;60:1194–1202.

Kushner T, Bellotti R. Baby Fae: a beastly business. *J Med Ethics* 1985;11:178–183

Langford GA, Cozzi E, Yannoutsos N, et al. Production of pigs transgenic for human regulators of complement activation using YAC technology. *Transplant Proc* 1996;28:862–863.

Leventhal JR, Dalmasso AP, Cromwell JW, et al. Prolongation of cardiac xenograft survival by depletion of complement. *Transplantation* 1993;55:857–866.

Leventhal JR, Flores HC, Gruber SA, et al. Evidence that 15-deoxyspergualin inhibits natural antibody production but fails to prevent hyperacute rejection in a discordant xenograft model. *Transplantation* 1992;54:26–31.

Leventhal JR, John R, Fryer JP, et al. Removal of baboon and human antiporcine IgG and IgM natural antibodies by immunoadsorption. *Transplantation* 1995;59:294–300.

Levin HR, Oz MC, Chen JM, et al. Reversal of chronic ventricular dilation in patients with end-stage cardiomyopathy by prolonged mechanical unloading. *Circulation* 1995;91:2717–2720.

Magee JC, Collins BH, Harland RC, et al. Immunoglobulin prevents complement mediated hyperacute rejection in swine-to-primate xenotransplantation. *J Clin Invest* 1995;96:2404–2412.

McCurry KR, Kooyman DL, Alvarado CG, et al. Human complement regulatory proteins protect swine-to-primate cardiac xenografts from humoral injury. *Nat Med* 1995;1:423–427.

Michler RE, Chen JM, Mancini DM, et al. Sixteen years of cardiac transplantation: the Columbia-Presbyterian Medical Center Experience 1977–1993. In: Terasaki PI, ed. *Clinical transplants 1993*. Los Angeles: UCLA Tissue Typing Laboratory, 1994.

Michler RE, McManus RP, Smith CR, et al. Prolongation of primate cardiac xenograft survival with cyclosporine. *Transplantation* 1987;44:632–636.

Michler RE, Shah AS, Itescu S, et al. The influence of concordant xenografts on the humoral and cell-mediated immune responses to subsequent allografts in primates. *J Thorac Cardiovasc Surg* 1996;112:1002–1009.

Michler RE, Xu H, O'Hair DP, et al. Newborn discordant cardiac xenotransplantation in primates: a model of natural antibody depletion. *Transplant Proc* 1996;28:651–652.

Minanov OP, Itescu S, Neethling FA, et al. Anti-gal IgG antibodies in sera of newborn humans and baboons and its significance in pig xenotransplantation. *Transplantation* 1997;63:182–186.

Murray AG, Khodadoust NM, Pober JS, et al. Porcine aortic endothelial cells activate human T cells: direct presentation of MHC antigens and costimulation by ligands for human CD2 and CD28. *Immunity* 1994;1:57–63.

Neething FA, Koren E, Ye Y, et al. Protection of pig kidney cells from the cytotoxic effect of anti-pig antibodies by α-galactosyl oligosaccharides. *Transplantation* 1994;57:959–963.

Norin AJ, Roslin MS, Panza A, et al. TLI induces specific B-cell unresponsiveness and long-term monkey heart xenograft survival in cyclosporine-treated baboons. *Transplant Proc* 1992;24:508–510.

O'Hair DP, McManus RP, Komorowski R. Inhibition of chronic vascular rejection in primate cardiac xenografts using mycophenolate mofetil. *Ann Thorac Surg* 1994;58:1311–1315.

Oriens CE, Evans RW, Ascher NL. Estimates of organ-specific donor availability for the United States. *Transplant Proc* 1993;25:1541–1542.

Parker WR, Bruno D, Holzknecht ZE, Platt JL. Xenoreactive natural antibodies: isolation and initial characterization. *J Immunol* 1994;153: 3791–3803.

Platt JL, Lindman BJ, Chen H, et al. Endothelial cell antigens recognized by xenoreactive human natural antibodies. *Transplantation* 1990;50:817–822.

Pruitt SK, Kirk AD, Bollinger RR, et al. The effect of soluble complement receptor type 1 on hyperacute xenograft rejection of porcine xenografts. *Transplantation* 1994;57:363–370.

Reemtsma K. Xenotransplantation: a brief history of clinical experiences: 1900–1965. In: Cooper DKC, Kemp E, Reemtsma K, White *DJG,* eds. *Xenotransplantation.* New York: Springer-Verlag, 1991:10–12.

Reemtsma K, McCracken BH, Schlegel JU, et al. Renal Heterotransplantation in man. *Ann Surg* 1964;160:384–410.

Rollins SA, Kennedy SP, Chodera AJ, et al. Evidence that activation of human T cells by porcine endothelium involves direct recognition for LFA-1 and CD2. *Transplantation* 1994;57:1709–1716.

Rosengard AM, Cary NR, Langford GA, et al. Tissue expression of human complement inhibitor, decay-accelerating factor, in transgenic pigs. *Transplantation* 1995;59:1325–1333.

Ross DN. Pathological findings in patients who have died. In: Shapiro H, ed. *Experience with human heart transplantation.* Durban: Butterworths, 1969:227–228.

Sandrin MS, Fodor WL, Mouhtouris E, et al. Enzymatic remodeling of the carbohydrate surface of a xenogenic cell substantially reduces human antibody binding and complement-mediated cytolysis. *Nat Med* 1995, 12: 1261–1267.

Sandrin MS, Vaughan HA, Dabkowski PL, et al. Anti-pig IgM antibodies in human serum react predominantly with Gal α1,3-Gal epitopes. *Proc Natl Acad Sci USA* 1993;90:11391–11395.

Sharma A, Okabe J, Birch P, et al. Reduction in the level of Gal (alpha 1,3)Gal in transgenic mice and pigs by the expression of an alpha(1,2)-fucosyltransferase. *Proc Natl Acad Sci USA* 1996;93:7190–7195.

Shaw AS, Itescu S, O'Hair DP, et al. Importance of cell-mediated immune responses in rejection of concordant heart xenografts in primates. *Transplant Proc* 1996;28:775–776.

Shimkin MR. The problem of experimentation on human beings: the research worker's point of view. *Daedalus* 1969;98:463–479.

Spital A. The shortage of organs for transplantation: where do we go from here? *N Engl J Med* 1991;325:1243–1246.

Starzl TE. Clinical xenotransplantation. *Xenotransplant* 1994;1:3–7.

Starzl TE, Fung JJ, Tzakis A, et al. Baboon-to-human liver transplantation. *Lancet* 1993;341:65–71.

Starzl TE, Marchioro TL, Peters GN, et al. Renal heterotransplantation from baboon to man: experience with 6 cases. *Transplantation* 1964;2: 752–776.

Tearle RG, Tange MJ, Zannettino ZL, et al. The α1,3-galactosyltransferase knockout mouse: implications for xenotransplantation: *Transplantation* 1996;61:13–19.

Thomas F, Araneda D, Quarantillo P. Long-term survival of disparate cardiac xenografts: induction of tolerance and humoral accommodation. *Transplant Proc* 1994;26:1220–1223.

United Network for Organ Sharing Scientific Registry. *UNOS Facts and Statistics, Annual Report, November 1996.*

Van den Berg CW, Morgan BP. Complement-inhibiting activities of human CD59 and analogues from rat, sheep, and pig are not homologously restricted. *J Immunol* 1994;152:4095–4105.

Watier H, Guillaumin J-M, Piller F, et al. Removal of terminal *a*-galactosyl residues from xenogeneic porcine endothelial cells. *Transplantation* 1996;62:105–113.

White DJG, Braidley P, Dunning J, et al. *Hearts from pigs transgenic for human DAF are not hyperacutely rejected when xenografted to primates.* Presented at the Third International Congress on Xenotransplantation, Boston, 1995.

Xiao F. Chong A, Foster P, et al. Leflunomide controls rejection in hamster-to-rat cardiac xenografts. *Transplantation* 1994;58:828–834.

Xu H, Edwards NM, Chen JM, et al. Newborn baboon serum lacks natural anti-pig xenoantibody. Transplantation *1995;59:1189–1194.*

Xu H, Edwards NM, Chen JM, et al. Age-related development of human anti-pig xenoantibody. J Thorac Cardiovasc Surg 1995;110: 1023–1029.

Ye Y, Neethling FA, Niekrasz M, et al. Evidence that intravenously administered *a*-galactosyl carbohydrates reduce baboon serum cytotoxicity to pig kidney cells and transplanted pig hearts. *Transplantation* 1994;58: 330–337.

Management of End-Stage Heart Disease, edited by Eric A. Rose and Lynne Warner Stevenson. Lippincott–Raven Publishers, Philadelphia ©1998.

CHAPTER 16

Left Ventricular Assist Devices

Michael Argenziano and Mehmet C. Oz

The first attempts at mechanical cardiac assistance were made almost 70 years ago. Subsequent work culminated in the development of the heart–lung machine, which was introduced by Gibbons in 1953. The next successful circulatory assist device, the intraaortic balloon pump (IABP), was developed by Moulopoulos in 1961 and first applied clinically in 1967. Still the most common form of mechanical cardiac assistance, the IABP is used in patients with reversible (usually ischemic) cardiogenic shock and as a bridge to transplantation.

Several efforts to develop long-term ventricular assist devices (VAD) and total artificial hearts were initiated in the United States as early as 1950. These initiatives were formally organized in 1964 under the National Institutes of Health Artificial Heart Program. The first successful clinical use of a left ventricular assist device (LVAD) occurred in 1966, when DeBakey supported a patient with postcardiotomy failure for 4 days using an extrathoracic left heart bypass system. After this accomplishment, however, progress was relatively slow. It was not until 1978 that the first patient was bridged to cardiac transplantation by a VAD at the Texas Heart Institute. This patient survived for 5 days on a pneumatically powered LVAD until a donor organ became available.

New prosthetic materials, engineering advances, and increasing clinical experience have resulted in a new generation of ventricular assist systems. These devices have been used successfully for both short- and long-term support. Although now used widely as bridges to transplantation, such devices will almost certainly be used as a long-term form of cardiac replacement in the near future.

INDICATIONS FOR SUPPORT

Hemodynamic eligibility criteria for mechanical cardiac assistance, especially in acute failure, are based on

the characteristics of cardiogenic shock first outlined by Norman et al. These include cardiac output less than 2.0 L/minute/m², systolic blood pressure less than 90 mm Hg, left or right atrial pressures greater than 20 mm Hg, systemic vascular resistance greater than 2,100 dynes-second/cm, and urine output less than 20 mL/hour (in adults). In patients meeting these criteria despite maximal pharmacologic inotropic therapy, death will likely occur if mechanical cardiac assistance is not instituted. Intraaortic balloon counterpulsation is usually tried first, and can often successfully support patients if implemented early. Many others, however, require more direct hemodynamic support with a VAD. Depending on the mechanism and extent of myocardial dysfunction, patients may require left, right, or biventricular support. In addition, the duration of support depends on a variety of factors, including the etiology and acuteness of heart failure, the patient's transplantation eligibility, and available device options. For the purposes of this chapter, indications for mechanical ventricular assistance are classified according to the acuteness of heart failure.

Acute Ventricular Failure

The two major acute indications for VADs are postcardiotomy cardiogenic shock and myocardial infarction. Patients undergoing cardiac surgical procedures are at risk for myocardial injury secondary to ischemia during cross-clamping, reperfusion injury, cardiac arrhythmias, and metabolic abnormalities. When patients are unable to be weaned off cardiopulmonary bypass, VAD support may often be initiated. Postcardiotomy shock patients can be divided into two groups: (a) those who had persistent or exacerbating dysfunction before surgery (unlikely to be weaned off device support); and (b) those who had adequate ventricular function before surgery (may recover sufficiently to tolerate device removal). In the latter group, a few days of temporary support (usually with an external pulsatile or centrifugal pump system) should be enough to

Division of Cardiothoracic Surgery, Columbia University College of Physicians and Surgeons, New York, New York 10032 assess whether the myocardial damage is reversible, especially if cardiac enzymes, electrocardiography, and echocardiography show the injury to be limited. In patients younger than 65 years of age without permanent end-organ dysfunction, device support can be justified even if myocardial recovery is not expected, because they can be bridged to transplantation with a long-term LVAD.

Patients in cardiogenic shock due to acute myocardial infarction are difficult to manage, and their survival may depend on the rapid institution of circulatory support. Cardiogenic shock usually occurs when greater than 40% of the ventricular mass is lost to infarction. Without mechanical assistance, this condition is associated with a mortality rate of more than 80%. Because early revascularization of ischemic myocardium has been shown to improve survival, some patients have been supported with emergent percutaneous extracorporeal membrane oxygenation (ECMO) or standard cardiopulmonary bypass until angioplasty or coronary bypass surgery could be performed. In those without hemodynamic stabilization, this form of support can be converted to bridge to transplantation support by implantation of a long-term device.

Chronic Heart Failure

Because waiting times on the transplantation list are increasing, many patients with chronic heart failure require IABP and high-dose pharmacologic support in order to survive. In the absence of an immediately available donor organ, LVAD support allows establishment of hemodynamic stability, reversal of end-organ dysfunction, and the opportunity for nourishment and physical rehabilitation. Even in the absence of acute hemodynamic deterioration, LVAD support may be useful in patients with slowly progressive cardiac deterioration because it can prevent and even reverse end-organ dysfunction due to chronic hypoperfusion. Although patients on LVAD support are classified as United Network for Organ Sharing (UNOS) Status I, most of these patients are in better condition than other Status I transplantation candidates without mechanical devices, enjoying a significantly higher rate of survival to transplantation, as well as an improved survival rate after transplantation. Overall, approximately 70% of LVAD patients are successfully bridged to transplantation, and of those transplanted, the actuarial survival rate at 1 year is 80%, a rate comparable with that of conventional transplant recipients and superior to that of the sicker subset of UNOS Status I recipients.

VENTRICULAR ASSIST DEVICES

Intraaortic Balloon Pump

Introduced in 1968 for the hemodynamic stabilization of patients with complicated myocardial infarction and cardiogenic shock, the IABP is the simplest and most widely used form of short-term mechanical ventricular assistance. The IABP supports the failing heart by augmenting diastolic coronary perfusion while decreasing ventricular afterload during systole. Although the magnitude of improvement in coronary perfusion has been debated, the pump does decrease left ventricular stroke work, reducing myocardial oxygen consumption by 10% to 20%.

Although the IABP is widely considered to be the first line of mechanical circulatory support, the effectiveness of this device is limited in two important ways. First, the device itself provides only modest augmentation of cardiac output; thus, its effectiveness depends on the presence of some degree of native cardiac function. Second, the need for systolic–diastolic synchronization makes the device much less effective in the presence of arrhythmias. The mortality rate of patients supported by the IABP remains high, ranging from 7% to 86%. This rate underscores the limited applicability of IABP in patients with severe cardiac dysfunction. We have discontinued using the IABP to support patients chronically as a bridge to transplantation, especially if the etiology of heart failure is nonischemic.

Extracorporeal Centrifugal Pumps

Centrifugal pumps have been available since 1977, when they were introduced as an alternative to roller pumps for cardiopulmonary bypass. Although these devices have been approved by the U.S. Food and Drug Administration (FDA) only for short-term cardiopulmonary bypass, they are frequently used as VADs because of their widespread availability, low cost, and simplicity. These devices can be used as left, right, or biventricular assist devices by modifying the cannulation scheme. The most commonly used external centrifugal pump is the Biomedicus Biopump (Medtronic Biomedicus, Inc., Eden Prairie, MN), which consists of an acrylic pump head with inlet and outlet ports oriented at right angles to each other. The impeller, composed of a stack of parallel cones, is driven through magnetic coupling by an external motor and console. Rotation of the impeller creates a constrained vortex, which drives blood flow in proportion to rotational speed. An electromagnetic flowmeter positioned along the outflow cannula measures instantaneous blood flow. Because of the centrifugal nature of blood flow, this pumping system is less traumatic to blood elements than is the roller pump. In an *in vitro* trial comparing available centrifugal pump systems with a roller pump, the Biomedicus pump caused significantly less hemolysis than the Sarns/3M centrifugal system (3M Healthcare, Ann Arbor, MI) or the roller pump.

A major advantage of the Biomedicus pump is its versatility. Left ventricular assistance is accomplished by placing the uptake cannula in the left atrium or ventricle through the left interatrial groove, left atrial appendage, left atrial free wall, or left ventricular apex, and the return cannula is placed in the ascending aorta using standard cannulation techniques. Right ventricular assistance is achieved by placing the uptake cannula in the right atrium through the free wall or atrial appendage, and the return cannula into the pulmonary artery. This device is also frequently used in ECMO circuits, which consist of femoral venous and arterial cannulation sites and the addition of a membrane oxygenator and heat exchanger.

The Biomedicus pump has been used both in postcardiotomy cardiogenic shock and as a bridge to transplantation in patients who cannot be weaned from the device. In one report, of the 41 patients (representing 1% of the total cardiac surgery population) who required ventricular assistance for postcardiotomy cardiogenic shock, 44% of LVAD patients, 14% of right ventricular assist device (RVAD) patients, and 55% of biventricular ventricular assist device (BiVAD) patients were successfully weaned from support, with an overall survival rate of 20%. In another series, of 37 patients receiving ventricular assistance with the Biomedicus pump (either for inability to separate from cardiopulmonary bypass or for postcardiotomy cardiogenic shock), 38% were weaned from support and 11% underwent cardiac transplantation, with an overall survival rate to discharge of 39%.

Several centers have reported their experience with Biomedicus VAD support as a bridge to transplantation. In one series, seven of nine patients supported for up to 3 days received successful transplantation. Golding et al. reported that three of six patients supported as long as 31 days survived transplantation. In the latter report, the frequency of left atrial and left ventricular thrombus formation after left atrial cannulation led the investigators to recommend direct left ventricular cannulation for patients bridged to transplantation.

There are several disadvantages to the use of the Biomedicus centrifugal pump. They include the need for systemic heparinization, the limited duration of support, the frequent development of profound interstitial edema, and the need for continuous supervision by specially trained personnel. This latter requirement can cost over $1,000 per day, a particularly limiting factor in most hospitals in which perfusion services are a scarce resource. Although some centers have used these devices without systemic heparinization for periods of hours, longer periods of support seem to require maintenance of the activated clotting time at a minimum of 200 seconds. Similarly, although extended periods of support have been reported, results have been better in patients supported for less than a week. Undoubtedly this result is due to the gradual development of interstitial edema because of the progressive accumulation of extracellular fluid. Because the centrifugal pump is preload dependent, significant volume infusion is required to replace fluid lost to the interstitial space due to increases in capillary permeability. It has been suggested that this inflammatory response may be related, in part, to the nonpulsatile nature of centrifugal flow, because it is less prevalent when pulsatile devices are used.

In summary, centrifugal pumps have been used most frequently in patients unable to be weaned from cardiopulmonary bypass and in patients with postcardiotomy cardiogenic shock. In these patients, clinical results available from the International Society for Heart and Lung Transplantation/American Society for Artificial Internal Organs (ISHLT/ASAIO) Combined Registry indicate a 25.4% hospital discharge rate for centrifugal pump support (n = 863).

Extracorporeal Pulsatile Devices

Pneumatically driven external pulsatile assist devices may be used for univentricular or biventricular support for patients with postcardiotomy cardiogenic shock or as a bridge to transplantation. Like centrifugal devices, an external power supply and console limit patient mobility, and insertion of the device can be performed without cardiopulmonary bypass in selected cases. Unlike centrifugal pump systems, however, pulsatile devices are designed to allow sternal closure, and their use results in a low incidence of thromboembolism. These devices are more costly than centrifugal devices; however, specially trained personnel are not needed to maintain the device, offsetting some of the cost. In addition, these devices are better suited technically for long-term support because they use more secure cannulation techniques and are more portable. The two external pulsatile devices currently available are the Abiomed BVS 5000 (Abiomed Cardiovascular, Inc., Danvers, MA) and the Pierce-Donachy/Thoratec device (Thoratec Laboratories Corporation, Berkeley, CA).

Abiomed BVS 5000

The Abiomed BVS 5000 (Figure 1) is an extracorporeal, pneumatically driven, pulsatile assist device introduced clinically in 1988 for left, right, and biventricular support. The vertically oriented pump houses two individual polyurethane chambers, a gravity-filled "atrial" chamber, and an air-driven "ventricular" chamber. Unidirectional flow is maintained by three-leaflet polyurethane valves, necessitating continuous systemic heparinization (to an activated clotting time of 180 seconds after surgical bleeding is controlled). Stroke volume is maintained at 80 mL, and maximum device output is 5.5 L/minute. In the auto mode, ventricular rate is based on venous return, which can be augmented by lowering the pump column toward the floor. In the weaning mode, the desired extent of assistance can be titrated in 0.1-L/minute increments. Venous return cannulae are placed in the right or left

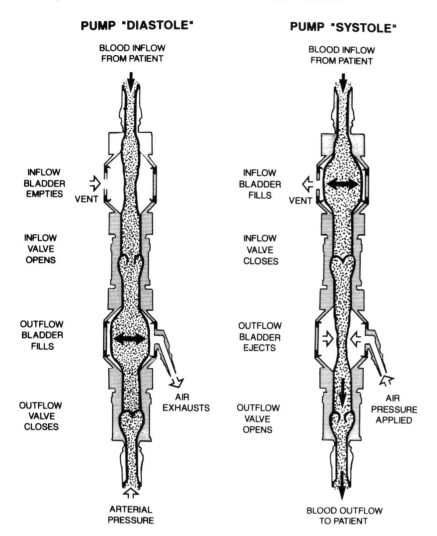

PUMP "DIASTOLE"

BLOOD INFLOW
FROM PATIENT

INFLOW
BLADDER
EMPTIES   VENT

INFLOW
VALVE
OPENS

OUTFLOW
BLADDER
FILLS

OUTFLOW   AIR
VALVE   EXHAUSTS
CLOSES

ARTERIAL
PRESSURE

PUMP "SYSTOLE"

BLOOD INFLOW
FROM PATIENT

INFLOW
BLADDER
FILLS   VENT

INFLOW
VALVE
CLOSES

OUTFLOW
BLADDER
EJECTS

OUTFLOW   AIR
VALVE   PRESSURE
OPENS   APPLIED

BLOOD OUTFLOW
TO PATIENT

FIG. 1. Abiomed BVS 5000 extracorporeal pulsatile pump. (Courtesy of Abiomed Cardiovascular, Inc., Danvers, MA.)

atrium and outflow cannulae (with attached Dacron grafts) are anastomosed to the main pulmonary artery or aorta. All cannulae are wrapped in Dacron and externalized below the costal margin, allowing sternal closure. Further advantages of the Abiomed system include elimination of the need for continuous supervision by a perfusionist because the simplified operation can be overseen by a nurse.

Initial experience with the Abiomed device was encouraging, with four of five postcardiotomy patients weaned from device support and three of these patients discharged from the hospital. A larger series followed that compared Abiomed support (n = 26) with Biomedicus support (n = 37) in patients with postcardiotomy cardiac failure. Although 38% of patients were weaned from support, 11% underwent transplantation, and 39% were discharged in the Biomedicus group, Abiomed patients were weaned successfully in 62% of cases, underwent transplantation in 12%, and discharged in 62%. These results led the authors to recommend pulsatile Abiomed support over centrifugal Biomedicus support for postcardiotomy cardiogenic shock.

Although the Abiomed BVS 5000 has received only premarket approval for use in postcardiotomy cardiac failure, it has also been applied as a bridge to transplantation. In one series, six patients had this device implanted for up to 11 days while awaiting transplantation. All received allografts and four were discharged. At another center, of eight patients in cardiogenic shock who were bridged to transplantation, six underwent successful transplantation, with a mean support duration of 3.5 days.

Pierce-Donachy/Thoratec Device

The Thoratec VAD system (Figure 2) is an extracorporeal pneumatic device constructed of a polycarbonate housing that surrounds an inner seam-free polyurethane sac. This blood-pumping sac, as well as the inflow and outflow cannulae, is made from a special polyurethane elastomer with extensive flex-life and thromboresistance. The external pneumatic drive console provides alternating positive and negative air pressure, which empties and fills the prosthetic ventricle through Bjork-Shiley Monostrut outlet and inlet valves, with a stroke volume of 65

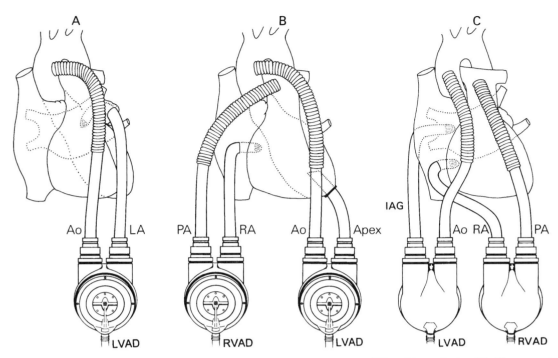

FIG. 2. Thoratec ventricular assist system used for left ventricular **(A)** or biventricular **(B, C)** support. (Courtesy of Thoratec Laboratories Corporation, Berkeley, CA.)

mL and a maximum flow rate of 7 L/minute. The device may be set in one of three modes: asynchronous (fixed rate), volume (fill-to-empty), and synchronous (timed to the electrocardiogram). In the commonly applied volume mode, the device adjusts the pumping rate according to the patient's venous return. The prosthetic ventricle is placed paracorporeally on the anterior abdominal wall and communicates with the cardiac chambers and great vessels through polyurethane cannulae, which traverse the subcostal chest wall. Inflow cannulae are placed in the left atrium or left ventricular apex, and the outflow cannula is attached to a 14-mm Dacron outflow graft that is sewn to the ascending aorta. Similar cannulae are used for right atrial and pulmonary artery cannulation when the Thoratec VAD is used for right ventricular assistance. Because of a significant risk of thromboembolism, all patients are maintained on anticoagulants, including heparin, warfarin, or dipyridamole.

Pennington and colleagues reported a series of 48 patients supported by the Thoratec VAD. Thirty of these patients had postcardiotomy cardiac failure and received left (n = 14), right (n = 7), or biventricular (n = 9) assistance for up to 22 days. Fifteen patients were weaned from the device and 11 (37%) were discharged. As of April, 1993, 145 total patients had received Thoratec VAD support because they could not be weaned from cardiopulmonary bypass or had postcardiotomy heart failure. Thirty-seven percent of these patients were successfully weaned from device support, and 21% left the hospital alive.

In Pennington and colleagues' original report, 11 patients were supported as a bridge to transplantation for up to 75 days, and 5 were transplanted successfully. Subsequently, Farrar and Hill reported a multiinstitutional study in which the Thoratec VAD was used as a bridge to transplantation in 193 critically ill heart transplant candidates at 41 medical centers in 8 countries. Of these patients, 129 (67%) received heart transplants and 105 (54%) were discharged from the hospital. Mean duration of support was 27 days and ranged from 1 to 248 days, with no significant association between length of assistance and mortality during support or after transplantation. Seventy-four percent of the patients received biventricular support. Bleeding occurred in 42% of patients and led to death in 7%, and infection occurred in 36% of recipients and led to death in 8%. End-organ dysfunction also occurred with significant frequency (renal failure in 36%, hepatic failure in 24%, transient hemolysis in 19%), and 10% of patients died of multiorgan failure. In a separate analysis, these investigators identified elevations in blood urea nitrogen and previous cardiac operations as predictors of poor outcome in bridge-to-transplantation patients.

Long-term Implantable Devices

Although a variety of VADs can be used as bridges to myocardial recovery or transplantation, most patients with end-stage heart failure cannot benefit from these devices because the donor organ pool is relatively constant. The ultimate goal of assist device research, therefore, is to develop a portable, implantable system that can provide long-term support in patients with end-stage heart disease on an out-patient basis. There are currently two such long-term implantable LVAD systems in use: the Novacor LVAS (Baxter Healthcare Corporation, Novacor Division, Oakland, CA), and the HeartMate LVAD (Thermo Cardiosystems, Woburn, MA). Although these devices are now used as bridges to transplantation, clinical experience with these devices should enable permanently implantable support devices to be developed.

Novacor LVAS

The Novacor LVAS was first developed by Portner in 1979, and consists of an implanted blood pump, an electromagnetic energy converter, and an extracorporeal control unit (Figure 3). The blood pumping surface is composed of seamless, smooth polyurethane (Biomer; Ethicon, Inc., Somerville, NJ) bonded to two symmetrically opposed pusher plates housed within a fiberglass-reinforced shell. Bovine pericardial tissue valves (Baxter-Edwards, Irvine, CA) are used to ensure unidirectional flow, and the pump has a maximum stroke volume of 70 mL and can pump in excess of 10 L/minute. The external control console provides power and automatic control through a percutaneous lead and air vent. The device can be operated in three modes: synchronous counterpulsation (based on internal position sensors), electrocardio-

gram-triggered synchronous operation, and fixed-rate operation. In most patients, the device is operated in the synchronous counterpulsation mode. In this mode, the device triggers pump systole when it senses a decreased pump filling rate near the end of native ventricular systole. The unit is responsive over a wide range of heart rates and preload conditions. The device is implanted through median sternotomy on cardiopulmonary bypass, and the pump/drive unit is positioned between the posterior rectus sheath and the rectus abdominis muscle below the left costal margin. The inflow cannula in placed into the left ventricular apex, the outflow cannula is anastomosed to the ascending aorta, and the percutaneous vent line is tunneled subcutaneously toward the right lower quadrant of the abdomen. Because of an overall thromboembolic rate of 8% to 10%, Novacor patients are anticoagulated with perioperative dipyridamole and heparin/warfarin once perioperative bleeding subsides.

Although experience with the Novacor LVAS is not as extensive as with the Thoratec device, as of April 1996, it had been implanted clinically in 434 patients. Two hundred fifty-two of the patients had wearable systems (personal communication, Linda Strauss, Novacor Division, Baxter Healthcare Corporation), with results similar to those with the Thoratec (despite longer-term support), including a 61% successful transplantation rate and a 56% hospital discharge rate. In a report from the University of Pittsburgh, 12 of 29 patients receiving the Novacor device underwent long-term circulatory support, and of these, 10 (83%) were successfully transplanted and discharged from the hospital. The disadvantages of this implantable system include its limitation to left ventricular support, the large size of the pump/drive unit (which limits its use in patients weighing less than 60 kg), and the requirement for anticoagulation.

HeartMate LVAD

The HeartMate LVAD is an implantable, pulsatile blood pump that is available in pneumatically driven (implantable pneumatic [IP]) or electrically powered (vented electric [VE]) models. The pneumatic pump, introduced in 1986, is fabricated from titanium and houses a flexible, textured polyurethane diaphragm bonded to a rigid pusher plate, which is actuated pneumatically from a portable, external console (Figure 4). The VE model has been available since 1991, and uses the same pusher plate mechanism and has similar flow characteristics, but features a low-speed torque motor that drives the pusher plate through a pair of nested helical cams. Two small tubes exit the device and reside outside the patient, one carrying the power cable to the external portable battery pack or bedside console, and the other acting as an air vent. Both models use 25-mm porcine xenograft valves (Medtronic-Hancock, Minneapolis, MN) within inlet and outlet Dacron graft conduits, and

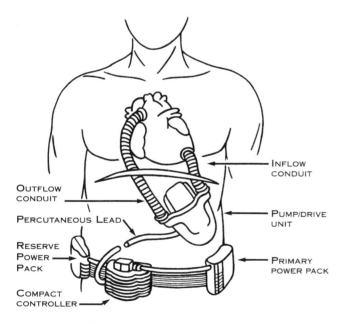

OUTFLOW CONDUIT

PERCUTANEOUS LEAD

RESERVE POWER PACK

COMPACT CONTROLLER

INFLOW CONDUIT

PUMP/DRIVE UNIT

PRIMARY POWER PACK

WEARABLE N100 LVAS

FIG. 3. Novacor implantable left ventricular assist system (wearable N100 model). (Courtesy of Baxter Healthcare Corporation, Novacor Division, Oakland, CA.)

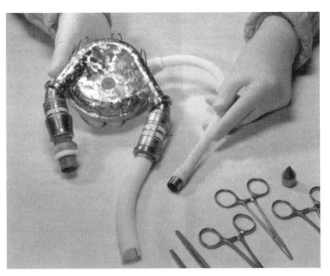

FIG. 4. The Thermo Cardiosystems HeartMate left ventricular assist device. (Courtesy of Thermo Cardiosystems, Woburn, MA.)

are capable of a maximum stroke volume of 85 mL and a maximum pump output of approximately 11 L/minute. Both pumps can be operated in a fixed-rate or automatic mode, and the pneumatic device can also be synchronized with the electrocardiogram.

The blood-contacting portion of the titanium housing incorporates sintered titanium microspheres, and the flexible diaphragm is covered with integrally textured polyurethane to promote the adherence of cellular blood elements and the formation of a pseudointimal layer (Figure 5). This biologic lining may be responsible for a reduction of thromboembolic risk, and consequently, HeartMate patients do not receive anticoagulation, and most do not receive antiplatelet agents. Although patients at our institution formerly received aspirin, our current protocol includes no anticoagulant or antiplatelet therapy

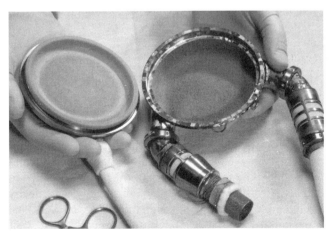

FIG. 5. The HeartMate interior blood-contacting surfaces. (Courtesy of Thermo Cardiosystems, Woburn, MA.)

of any kind. The device is implanted using median sternotomy and cardiopulmonary bypass. A core of myocardium is removed from the left ventricular apex, and an inlet cannula is inserted and secured after passage through a cruciate incision in the diaphragm. The outlet graft is passed over the diaphragm and anastomosed to the ascending aorta, and the device is positioned intraabdominally or preperitoneally in the left upper quadrant. Finally, the driveline is tunneled subcutaneously to the left lower quadrant.

The major indication for institution of HeartMate support has been as a bridge to transplantation, and clinical results have been encouraging. Worldwide, hundreds of devices have been implanted. In the United States, 157 devices had been implanted as of November, 1993, with successful transplantation in 70% and hospital discharge in 47% to 65%. An FDA-approved multiinstitutional study of transplantation candidates meeting standard criteria of cardiac decompensation compared 75 patients receiving the HeartMate IP-LVAD with 33 patients receiving only medical therapy. The 1-year survival rate in patients successfully implanted with the LVAD was 91%, versus 67% in non-LVAD patients, and 71% versus 36%, respectively, were transplanted successfully. Based on these results, the FDA approved the IP-LVAD for commercial use in October, 1994 as a bridge to heart transplantation. Clinical trials of the VE-LVAD are in progress.

In a report from the Cleveland Clinic, of 27 patients receiving the HeartMate LVAD, 18 (67%) had undergone transplantation and were discharged, with 7 deaths (26%) occurring before transplantation. In the most recent report from the Texas Heart Institute, of 19 patients who had been supported with the pneumatic HeartMate for longer than 30 days, 16 (84%) underwent transplantation, and 2 died of multiorgan failure. In the 16 patients, 1- and 2-year survival rates after transplantation were 100%, compared with the 0% 1-year survival rate in matched control patients not receiving LVAD support.

Experience with the HeartMate LVAD at our institution has produced similar results. At the Columbia-Presbyterian Medical Center, 104 patients underwent insertion of the TCI HeartMate LVAD between August 1990 and October 1997. Eighty-three patients (80%) were male and the mean age at time of implant was 50 ± 13 years. Indications for LVAD insertion were end-stage heart failure resulting from ischemic cardiomyopathy, idiopathic cardiomyopathy, myocarditis, and idiopathic hypertrophic subaortic stenosis. Fifty percent of the devices used were IP, and 50% were VE. Mean duration of support was 99 ± 99 days. Hemodynamic parameters, as well as indices of renal and hepatic function, improved significantly after LVAD insertion. Sixty-seven patients (64%) have undergone successful cardiac transplantation, 6 were weaned off LVAD support, and 7 await transplantation.

PATIENT SELECTION

Regardless of the etiology of heart failure, evaluation of potential LVAD candidates includes estimation of hemodynamic performance, end-organ function, and other comorbidities that could limit survival. Many, but not all candidates for mechanical circulatory assistance meet criteria for ventricular failure similar to those outlined by Norman et al., including cardiac output less than 2.0 L/minute/m^2, systolic blood pressure less than 90 mm Hg, atrial pressures greater than 20 mm Hg, systemic vascular resistance greater than 2,100 dynes-second/cm, and urine output less than 20 mL/hour. In such patients, severe cardiac dysfunction persists despite maximal pharmacologic inotropic and vasodilatory support, IABP counterpulsation, and aggressive treatment of arrhythmias, acidosis, hypovolemia, and hypothermia. Exclusionary criteria for LVAD support have traditionally included chronic renal failure, severe peripheral vascular or symptomatic cerebrovascular disease, severe hepatic or pulmonary disease, metastatic malignancy, significant blood dyscrasias, and uncontrollable infection. In addition, although many critically ill patients exhibit reversible neurocognitive deficits, evidence of permanent central nervous system injury eliminates patients from consideration. Because LVAD support can sometimes reverse end-organ dysfunction if instituted before the onset of permanent damage, the application of these exclusionary criteria should be followed at the surgeon's discretion.

Because VADs are currently approved only as bridges to ventricular recovery or transplantation, any patient with acute myocardial injury associated with a poor chance of ventricular recovery should be considered for device insertion only if selection criteria for transplantation are met. In these cases, advanced age, history of recent malignancy, and psychosocial instability are additional contraindications. For these reasons, it is useful to classify potential device support candidates into one of two major categories: bridge to recovery (postcardiotomy shock or acute myocardial infarction) and bridge to transplantation (progressive heart failure and cardiogenic shock in a patient eligible for transplantation). Although patients in these two groups may overlap, data from the ISHLT/ASAIO Combined Registry indicate that of patients receiving mechanical assistance for postcardiotomy shock, only 8% are transplantation candidates.

Bridge to Recovery

Despite advances in myocardial preservation and surgical techniques, the incidence of postcardiotomy cardiogenic shock has remained relatively stable, occurring in 1% to 7% of patients. In addition, a substantial proportion of myocardial infarctions are complicated by cardiogenic shock or life-threatening arrhythmias. Because of the high mortality of these complications, proper selection of patients for device support can increase survival in VAD patients. In patients receiving LVADs for postcardiotomy shock, a number of risk factors have been shown to affect survival, including unsuccessful operation, perioperative myocardial infarction, biventricular failure, and advanced age.

Although the outcome of mechanical cardiac assistance for postcardiotomy shock is unrelated to the original surgical procedure, a technically unsuccessful operation makes myocardial recovery unlikely. Nonetheless, patients who have undergone a technically unsuccessful operation should be considered for LVAD insertion if they are eligible for transplantation.

Although the rate of successful weaning from mechanical support is not affected by age, patients older than 70 years of age have a decreased overall survival rate. Although myocardial recovery is possible in older patients, their lower physiologic reserve increases their risk for multiorgan dysfunction and mortality after weaning. Consequently, 34% of patients younger than 39 years of age survive to hospital discharge, whereas only 13% of patients older than 70 years of age do so.

Other factors have been suggested as contraindications to VAD support, including perioperative coagulopathy, ventricular arrhythmias, preoperative infection, and reoperation. Perioperative coagulopathy usually occurs secondary to prolonged cardiopulmonary bypass time, and analysis of the Combined Registry database reveals that although prolonged bypass time (>6 hours) does negatively affect VAD survival, the severity of perioperative coagulopathy does not because it is usually correctable after surgery. This analysis also suggests that perioperative bleeding is more common in patients supported with centrifugal than pulsatile pumps, and that the former group has a lower rate of successful weaning. Although arrhythmias are detrimental to patients on IABP support, this has not been the case for VADs. Finally, although preoperative infection and reoperation pose theoretic risks, preoperative bacteremia and previous thoracic surgery have not been found to affect survival to a statistically significant extent.

Bridge to Transplantation

Because patients receiving mechanical ventricular assistance as a bridge to transplantation usually have chronic rather than acute heart failure and must satisfy relatively stringent transplantation requirements, they are often less critically ill than patients requiring support for postcardiotomy shock. However, bridge-to-transplantation patients often have end-organ dysfunction related to long-term cardiac insufficiency, are usually chronically debilitated, and must withstand the rigors of a second operation (transplantation) with the attendant risks of postoperative immunosuppressive regimens. For these reasons, effective selection of patients can be challenging, and requires a screening method specifically suited to this special patient population.

Although several authors have studied the risk factors for patients undergoing long-term LVAD support, these results have yielded only lists of "high-risk" characteristics rather than specific guidelines on how to stratify patients according to probability of survival. Based on our initial experience with 54 LVAD recipients, we have developed a screening system that can be used on patients at the time of initial evaluation. This system consists of a small number of readily evaluable factors and is easy to apply. Factors associated with increased mortality, including oliguria, ventilator dependence, and hepatic dysfunction resulting in coagulopathy, are assigned relative weights (see Figure 6 on p. 209), along with factors that present technical limitations during device insertion, such as reoperation and right heart failure (manifested by elevated central venous pressure). Patients are subsequently given risk factor points based on the presence or absence of these risk factors. The total score is used to estimate the patient's risk of mortality during or after device implantation. In our experience, this practical screening scale accurately predicts which patients are unlikely to survive device insertion (risk score > 7). We use this scale to guide discussions about the suitability of individual patients and to identify which hurdles the patient must clear before receiving a device (e.g., reversal of oliguria). Although it is not an absolute criterion for selection of LVAD recipients, most of the later patients in our series (and particularly the survivors) scored less than 5 points on this screening scale.

Device Selection

Although patient selection is the most critical determinant of survival during mechanical ventricular assistance, selection of a device appropriate for each patient is also important. Device selection is usually based on availability, indication for support, and the potential for reversibility of cardiogenic shock. Available support options differ with respect to ease of insertion and operation, pulsatility of flow, maximum duration of support, the need for anticoagulation, the potential for patient mobility, and the ability to provide biventricular support. Therefore, a clear set of expectations should exist for each patient in whom ventricular assistance in begun, based on the potential for myocardial recovery, the presence of coexisting morbidity, and the eligibility for transplantation. To this end, patients can be classified into one of two groups: (a) postcardiotomy failure or acute cardiogenic shock, and (b) chronic progressive heart failure, although occasional cross-over between groups may occur.

Postcardiotomy Failure/Acute Cardiogenic Shock

Patients who cannot be weaned from cardiopulmonary bypass after cardiac surgery require a device that can provide continuous circulatory support for a minimum of 48 hours in the anticipation of myocardial recovery. Ideally, the device should be easily replaceable by another system if recovery does not occur. Initial attempts at weaning from cardiopulmonary bypass, especially after myocardial revascularization procedures, usually involve insertion of an IABP. When the IABP is not sufficient to separate the patient from the bypass circuit, extracorporeal VADs may be used. Use of centrifugal pumps, the cheapest available option, is limited by technical constraints including mechanical deterioration, fibrin deposition, hemolysis, and endorgan dysfunction. In addition, cannulae cannot be well secured to the vessels, and their positioning precludes sternal closure, a critical requirement for patient mobilization and prevention of hemorrhagic and infectious complications.

For short-term (<1 week) assistance, we have used the Abiomed external pulsatile device, reserving the centrifugal systems for smaller patients (body surface area < 1.3 m²). In our experience, patients without evidence of myocardial recovery after several days of support are not likely to be successfully weaned from mechanical support. At this stage, decisions regarding long-term support options must be made. If long-term univentricular support is required, an implantable pulsatile LVAD can be used. In patients requiring biventricular assistance or (rarely) isolated right ventricular assistance, the right ventricle can be supported for extended periods with the Abiomed heterotopic pulsatile system or the Thoratec paracorporeal system.

Patients with acute cardiogenic shock outside the operating room, as after myocardial infarction, secondary to viral or postpartum myocarditis, or during interventional cardiology procedures, have a potential for myocardial recovery similar to that of the postcardiotomy group. Because these patients are not on cardiopulmonary bypass, however, circulatory support must be instituted rapidly if death or irreversible organ damage is to be averted. Although emergent insertion of the IABP is often useful in these situations, especially in patients with ongoing ischemia, other devices, such as the Hemopump (Medtronic, Minneapolis, MN) and the CPS portable ECMO system (Bard, Inc., Murray Hill, NJ), can provide rapid and complete circulatory support until cardiopulmonary bypass or centrifugal support can be instituted. Unfortunately, the survival rate in these patients is in general poor. Of all studied risk factors, patients who experience cardiac arrest before implantation have the highest risk for death after LVAD placement. Finally, in cases where the etiology of failure (CHF) is not clear or is suspected to require medium-term support (as for viral or postpartum cardiomyopathy), immediate insertion of a heterotopic pulsatile system (Abiomed BVS 5000) may be a reasonable choice, particularly in nontransplantation centers. Implantable pulsatile systems may also useful in these situations; such devices ultimately allow greater patient mobility.

Chronic Progressive Heart Failure

Because of a limited donor organ supply, most patients with progressive congestive heart failure (CHF) are excluded from the transplantation waiting list because of age, end-organ dysfunction, or other criteria. Of the estimated 60,000 Americans who might benefit from mechanical circulatory support, less than 4,000 are currently on transplantation waiting lists and therefore eligible for LVAD insertion. Although many patients awaiting transplantation are on pharmacologic regimens and therefore hemodynamically stable, the frequency of acute or subacute decompensation occurring before a suitable donor can be found results in a waiting list mortality rate of approximately 30%. When these patients require mechanical ventricular assistance, an implantable device should be used because myocardial recovery is not likely and long-term bridging to transplantation may be required. Trials of long-term device use have now begun and, if successful, will expand the patient population eligible for long-term VAD support.

SURGICAL CONSIDERATIONS

Short-term Devices

Technical aspects of extracorporeal mechanical support are similar among the various available centrifugal pump systems. For left heart support, the left atrium is cannulated through the atrial appendage or dome, or the right superior pulmonary vein, with return through cannulation of the ascending or transverse thoracic aorta. For centrifugal pump systems, the inflow cannula is typically a 32- or 34-Fr venous cannula, and the aortic cannula is typically left in place from the primary open heart procedure. With the Abiomed system, inflow is from a 46- or 36-Fr inflow cannula with outflow through a 14-mm Dacron-coated graft sewn to the ascending aorta. For right ventricular assistance, an arterial cannula is placed in the pulmonary artery, and venous inflow established using the preexisting cardiopulmonary bypass cannulation site.

To initiate left heart support and separate the patient from the cardiopulmonary bypass circuit, cardiopulmonary bypass flow is gradually decreased. When left atrial pressure rises to 15 to 20 mm Hg, assist flow is begun. Cardiopulmonary bypass is discontinued, and the venous line is clamped but left in place in case right ventricular support is required after the initiation of left heart assistance. After exclusion of air from the circuit, assist flow is increased incrementally, and volume administration is guided by pump flow rates and left heart filling pressures.

Most patients have some degree of right ventricular failure when left heart assistance is initiated. If the left ventricular bypass circuit cannot maintain flows above 2.0 L/minute/m^2 despite maximal inotropic support and inhaled nitric oxide (NO), right ventricular assistance is initiated. Early hemodynamic stability is critical; thus, in cases of acute heart failure, BiVAD use is strongly encouraged. For biventricular assistance, the flow rates of the two pumps must be adjusted incrementally to ensure adequate delivery of preload to the left-sided pump without overloading the left ventricle. This is best accomplished by slowly increasing right-sided flow, and, as left atrial pressures rises, increasing left-sided flow until rates greater than 2.2 L/minute/m^2 are achieved. Subsequently, transesophageal echocardiography is used to monitor left heart filling. Although the benefits of pulsatile over nonpulsatile flow are debated, many investigators routinely use IABP support to provide pulsatility in patients on centrifugal pumps. The external pulsatile devices eliminate the need for this potentially risky procedure.

After establishment of adequate hemodynamic support, the device cannulae are brought out through the midline incision, and the skin, but not the sternum, closed around them. If longer cannulae are used, it is possible to exit them from the subcostal region, which allows sternal closure, although we usually leave the sternum open to facilitate reexploration, the diagnosis of tamponade, and the preservation of the sternum for eventual closure at the time of device removal. Finally, after discontinuation of cardiopulmonary bypass, heparinization is reversed with protamine. After returning to the intensive care unit, the patient is not anticoagulated until bleeding has subsided. Then heparin is administered to maintain the activate clotting time above 160 to 200 seconds. The advent of heparin-coated surfaces may allow extended periods of perfusion without systemic heparinization; however, these circuits will probably remain prone to clotting, particularly at low flow rates.

Implantable Pulsatile Devices

Similar implantation techniques are used for the two currently available implantable ventricular assist systems, the Novacor and the HeartMate. The Novacor device has typically been placed in a preperitoneal pocket posterior to the rectus muscle, whereas the HeartMate was initially positioned intraperitoneally. Because of occasional complications and theoretic concerns, including bowel perforation or obstruction, subsequent diaphragmatic hernia, and wound dehiscence, the HeartMate can also be implanted in the preperitoneal position. In this section, we describe our technique for implantation of the HeartMate device, which is roughly representative of techniques used in general for both this device and the Novacor system.

Before heparinization, a plane is developed in the preperitoneal plane by dividing the linea alba and sharply separating the preperitoneal fat and peritoneum from the posterior rectus sheath and the transversalis muscle at its diaphragmatic insertion. Drivelines are tunneled to an exit point in the left lower quadrant. After heparinization, the aorta and right atrium are cannulated and cardiopulmonary bypass is instituted. Aprotinin is usually administered early in the procedure, except in patients who have recently received aprotinin therapy; in such patients, administration is delayed until arterial access has been established to cope with the potential for anaphylaxis. A vent is placed through the apex of the left ventricle and, without placing a cross-clamp or administering cardioplegia, a silicone inflow cuff is sutured to the left ventricular apex (Figure 6). The apex is cored and any visualized thrombus is removed. The device is placed in the pocket and the inflow cannula brought through the diaphragm and secured to the apical inflow cuff. The outflow graft is anastomosed to the right lateral aspect of the ascending aorta using a running 4-0 polypropylene suture. The patient is placed in a steep Trendelenburg position and the device vented through a needle hole in the outflow graft and ascending aorta. To reduce the risk of air embolism, the aortic root is visualized by transesophageal echocardiography while the device is manually operated, allowing complete evacuation of air.

After cardiopulmonary bypass flow is decreased, the LVAD is activated, initially at a low fixed rate to ensure adequate filling, then at higher fixed rates. Finally, the device is set at the auto mode. Right heart function is maximized with intravenous dobutamine, milrinone, and dopamine, and inhaled NO is used in cases refractory to these agents. Patients with the HeartMate device are not anticoagulated after surgery, whereas patients receiving the Novacor system receive intravenous heparin or oral warfarin after perioperative bleeding has subsided.

The removal of long-term implantable devices can be challenging, and poses different problems depending on whether the device is being removed because of transplantation, device replacement, or device weaning. Many of the problems associated with device removal can be avoided by taking precautionary steps at the time of implantation. These steps include avoiding entry into pleural spaces, which prevents adherence of lung tissue around the outflow graft, and placing a polytetrafluoroethylene pericardial sheet (Gore-tex; W. L. Gore & Assoc., Flagstaff, AZ) over the right ventricle and outflow graft (if it lies directly in the midline), which facilitates the reoperative sternotomy.

At explantation, the upper abdomen is opened and the heart dissected free from the posterior sternal plate. The outflow graft is retracted posteriorly and laterally, and the sternum is divided with an oscillating saw. After a dissection plane has been established laterally, the vena cavae, right atrium, and aorta are exposed by incising the fibrous cast surrounding the outflow graft. If technical difficulties are anticipated, vascular exposure for cardiopulmonary bypass is obtained in the groin, but cannulae are not inserted until the chest is opened and the central vessels ruled out as cannulation sites. Groin cannulation should be avoided if possible because there is a high incidence of problematic seromas in the transplant population. After central cannulation, LVAD flow is reduced to 1 L/minute to prevent entrainment of air from the empty ventricle. Once full cardiopulmonary bypass flow is attained, the device is inactivated and the outflow graft clamped and divided. The left ventricle is decompressed by placing a bypass sucker into the LVAD through the divided outflow graft, and the inflow cannula is removed from the ventricular apex. The LVAD driveline is divided with a rib cutter and removed. The diaphragmatic and fascial defects are repaired with running 0 polypropylene sutures. The skin and subcutaneous tissues at the driveline exit site are allowed to heal by secondary intention. Heart transplantation proceeds as per routine.

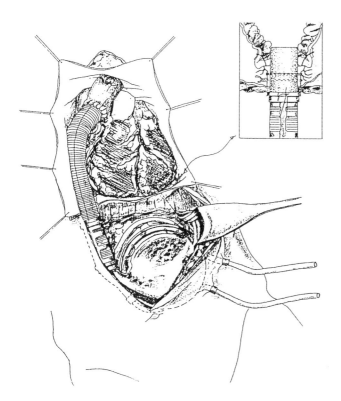

FIG. 6. HeartMate implantation, with left ventricular assist device in preperitoneal pocket. Inset shows positioning of the inflow cannula in the left ventricular apex.

PERIOPERATIVE MANAGEMENT

Bleeding

Regardless of the device used for ventricular assistance, bleeding complications may occur, limiting the success of implantation. Although often multifactorial in nature, hemorrhage may result from the excess fibrinolysis and platelet activation associated with mechanical circulatory support. Prolonged and extensive blood loss and subsequent blood product administration may lead to increases in pulmonary vascular resistance through activation of cytokine pathways, increasing the risk for right ventricular failure and postoperative mortality. Aprotinin, a bovine serine protease inhibitor, has been used successfully to decrease the complications associated with perioperative blood product transfusions and reoperations for the control of bleeding. Its efficacy and safety in cardiac surgical patients have been demonstrated by a number of investigators.

In a multiinstitutional study of 142 TCI HeartMate LVAD recipients, aprotinin use was found to be safe and effective in decreasing postoperative blood loss and intraoperative transfusion requirements. Forty-two patients receiving aprotinin lost an average of 1.5 L of blood after surgery, whereas patients not receiving aprotinin (n = 100) lost an average of 4.0 L of blood after surgery. Consequently, an average of 4.8 units of packed cells were transfused in the aprotinin group, compared with 8.2 units in patients not receiving the antifibrinolytic agent. Interestingly, the rate of perioperative right ventricular failure requiring RVAD placement was lower in patients receiving aprotinin (9.5%, vs. 18% in non–aprotinin-treated patients). This result is not surprising because the association between perioperative blood loss and right ventricular failure was also observed in this study (mean blood loss of 10.5 L in patients receiving RVADs vs. 2.4 L in others). Although overall survival was not affected by the use of aprotinin in this study, the 7-day mortality rate was significantly lower in aprotinin-treated patients (12%) than in non–aprotinin-treated patients (28%). Despite various reports of the nephrotoxic effects of this agent, this study observed only a small, transient elevation in serum creatinine levels, with no evidence of permanent renal sequelae. Finally, although thrombotic complications related to the procoagulant activity of aprotinin are a theoretic concern, the rate of thromboembolic events was approximately the same in the aprotinin group (2.4%) and the nonaprotinin group (4.0%). Encouraged by these findings, we now administer perioperative aprotinin to all patients undergoing LVAD placement and removal.

Right Ventricular Failure

Right-sided circulatory failure occurs in at least 20% of patients requiring LVAD support. Although native left ventricular function does not significantly contribute to cardiac output after LVAD placement, factors influencing right ventricular function, including air embolism, poor intrinsic contractility, myocardial stunning, elevated pulmonary vascular resistance, cardiac arrhythmias, and volume status, are critical in the maintenance of adequate right ventricular output and LVAD filling. The ability of the impaired right ventricle to supply an adequate volume of blood to the left ventricle is directly related to pulmonary vascular resistance (PVR). PVR is often elevated in patients with chronic CHF, and may be further increased in the early postoperative period by the effects of cardiopulmonary bypass due to thromboxane A_2.

Evidence suggests that PVR may be increased by impairments in the release of NO by the pulmonary vascular endothelium. Endothelial dysfunction related to cardiopulmonary bypass may be responsible for further perioperative elevations in PVR. In patients receiving LVADs for advanced heart failure, pulmonary hypertension often limits the adequacy of device filling, and may be exacerbated by transfusion-induced cytokine release during extensive bleeding. In such cases, patients may require institution of biventricular mechanical support. Concomitant central venous pressure elevations also lead to increases in venous bleeding.

Right Ventricular Assist Device Placement

During periods of right ventricular dysfunction or elevated PVR, aggressive volume loading can improve LVAD flow, using the right ventricle as a passive conduit to the left heart. In addition, the intraoperative management of right ventricular failure often includes the use of pulmonary vasodilator and inotropic agents. When these treatments fail or are associated with prohibitive decreases in systemic vascular tone, mechanical right ventricular assistance may be required. Although success has been reported with pulmonary artery balloon counterpulsation, more powerful methods of right ventricular support are usually needed. Short-term support can be achieved with a nonpulsatile device such as the Biomedicus Biopump, although we prefer the pulsatile support provided by the Abiomed device. Cannulation sites are usually the right atrial appendage and the main pulmonary artery.

In a report of the worldwide Thoratec experience, 78% of all patients undergoing support received biventricular devices, with survival rates of 63% in LVAD patients and 52% in BiVAD patients. In striking contrast, of 142 patients supported with the TCI HeartMate LVAD in another report, only 22 (15%) received RVADs; all but 1 of the 22 died. The discrepancy between these results is probably due to the looser requirements for biventricular support with the Thoratec, because the device is easily configured for this purpose. On the other hand, patients receiving implantable LVAD systems are less likely to receive heterotopic or external pump support of the right ventricle at the time of LVAD placement because such support significantly complicates perioperative care. Therefore, only the most critically ill LVAD recipients receive RVADs. Despite these considerations, the success of the Thoratec in RVAD patients emphasizes the importance of early recognition and treatment of existing or potential right ventricular failure after LVAD placement, especially because RVAD placement at the time of LVAD insertion is associated with a far lower morbidity rate than implantation a few days later.

We have defined right ventricular failure as a decrease in right ventricular function or output requiring insertion of an RVAD, administration of inhaled NO for elevated PVR, or pharmacologic inotropic support for greater than 10 days. In our experience, one third of patients undergoing support with an LVAD met one of these criteria for right ventricular failure. Twenty-two percent of the patients with right ventricular failure required only medical inotropic support, whereas RVAD insertion was required in only four cases, and was life saving in two of these. Four patients (21%) died from RVF, and three died from other causes. Overall, 12 patients (63%) survived, 9 have undergone transplantation, and 3 await transplantation.

Nitric Oxide

Nitric oxide, initially described as an endothelium-derived relaxant factor, has been implicated in a wide variety of physiologic and pathophysiologic processes. Inhaled NO has been shown to cause pulmonary vasodilatation in primary pulmonary hypertension, in pulmonary hypertension secondary to congenital heart disease, and in adult respiratory distress syndrome. At our institution, inhaled NO is used in all LVAD patients manifesting right ventricular dysfunction or increased pulmonary vascular resistance during and after weaning from cardiopulmonary bypass. A stock NO gas mixture (800 ppm; Airco, Riverton, NJ) is mixed through the ventilator circuit to achieve a concentration of 20 ppm. The mixture is then titrated to a maximum of 80 ppm, reducing PVR, which allows sufficient LVAD filling. To date, we have used this agent in over ten patients, with successful reversal of right ventricular failure and improvements in LVAD filling and output. Although RVAD placement was required for right ventricular failure in 4 of 54 patients (7.4%) receiving LVADs before we began using inhaled NO, none of the subsequent 18 LVAD recipients has required biventricular mechanical support. In patients with right heart failure, regardless of the means of acute support, volume unloading is critically important because these patients may experience a volume overload of more than 15% of their body weight. When aggressive diuresis cannot rapidly remove large quantities of fluid, we have used arterial or venous ultrafiltration.

In summary, although transient right ventricular dysfunction with or without pulmonary hypertension is common after LVAD insertion, pharmacologic inotropic support can usually maintain adequate right ventricular output and LVAD flows until the right ventricle can recover and PVR can decrease. In cases of right ventricular failure refractory to inotropic agents, we have used RVAD support and, most recently, inhaled NO to achieve adequate LVAD filling and output. Postoperative aggressive volume unloading is critically important.

Postbypass Vasodilatory Shock

Vasodilatory shock is defined as systemic hypotension and organ hypoperfusion caused by loss of vascular tone, or "vasomotor collapse." It is characterized by low systemic vascular resistance and normal or elevated cardiac output. Clinical conditions classically associated with vasodilatory shock include sepsis and anaphylaxis, but cardiopulmonary bypass with pump oxygenation may also induce a systemic inflammatory response and, in many patients, a state of vasodilatory shock.

Vasodilatory shock induced by cardiopulmonary bypass is usually mild, requiring moderate amounts of pressor support during weaning and through the next 24 to 36 hours. In some patients, however, profound vasodilatory shock develops, requiring high-dose catecholamine and fluid therapy. Severe forms of this condition are more common after extensive cardiac surgical procedures, particularly those requiring prolonged cardiopulmonary bypass time. For example, patients who undergo LVAD insertion for end-stage cardiac failure usually receive perioperative catecholamine pressor therapy. Unfortunately, this therapy is associated with several adverse effects, including renal, coronary, and gastrointestinal hypoperfusion, peripheral vascular ischemia, and increased cardiac work and oxygen consumption. These effects promote lactic acidosis, leading to myocardial depression and catecholamine receptor insensitivity. The factors responsible for the loss of vascular tone in these cases are unknown, but we believe that a deficiency in the vasoconstrictor hormone vasopressin may play a role.

Arginine vasopressin (AVP) is an endogenous peptide with both renal (V_2 receptor) and vasomotor (V_1 receptor) effects. Exogenous AVP is an intriguing pressor that increases arterial pressure when sympathetic nerve function is impaired, but has no effects on normal subjects in doses up to 0.26 U/minute. A rat model of septic shock has shown that whereas the vasoconstrictor action of norepinephrine is decreased, that of vasopressin is markedly increased. Furthermore, we have shown that some patients in septic shock have abnormally low serum AVP levels and demonstrate a pressor response to very low doses of intravenous vasopressin. In addition, AVP has been used successfully in a few patients with severe postbypass vasodilatory shock. In these patients, minute physiologic doses of AVP were administered (0.007–0.05 U/minute), suggesting a vasopressin hypersensitivity.

In an ongoing, prospective trial at our institution, 9 of 13 patients undergoing LVAD implantation have exhibited signs of moderate to severe vasodilatory shock requiring catecholamine support on weaning from bypass. Intravenous arginine vasopressin (Pitressin; Parke-Davis, Morris Plains, NJ) was administered to these patients in the small dose of 0.1 U/minute. Within 15 to 30 minutes, seven of the nine patients were weaned completely off exogenous catecholamine pressors, with a 37% mean increase in arterial pressure. The eighth patient required 24 hours of AVP therapy to eliminate catecholamine support, and the ninth patient, who initially could not be separated from bypass because of severe vasodilatation, was successfully weaned off bypass after 15 minutes of AVP infusion.

Blood Product Administration

Evidence obtained from animal and human studies indicates that posttransfusion alloimmunization against the major histocompatibility complex is induced by the contaminating leukocytes in blood products. Furthermore, a number of studies in humans have demonstrated that the rate of human leukocyte antigen allosensitization can be reduced with the use of leukocyte-poor blood products. In one report, patients transfused with leukocyte-filtered products had an allosensitization rate of 11.7%, whereas those receiving conventional transfusions were alloimmunized in 31.4% of cases. On the basis of these data, we now pass all blood products, particularly platelet concentrates, through leukocyte filters.

POSTOPERATIVE MANAGEMENT

Arrhythmias

The incidence of malignant ventricular arrhythmias is high in patients with cardiomyopathy and remains so after LVAD implantation, perhaps secondary to ischemia, intrinsic arrhythmogenicity associated with ventricular dilatation, or effects of necessary inotropic agents. The sewing ring used to secure the LVAD inflow cannula to the ventricular apex may also serve as a local focus of abnormal electrical activity. It has been suggested that a major limitation of LVADs may be their inability to maintain adequate pump output during episodes of serious arrhythmias due to decreased right ventricular output. We have previously reviewed the courses of LVAD recipients at our institution to identify the incidence of malignant ventricular arrhythmias and determine whether univentricular support was adequate to maintain sufficient cardiac output during these events.

In our most recent report, 9 of 58 patients (16%) receiving LVADs had ventricular tachycardia or fibrillation before device implantation, and 11 (19%) had malignant arrhythmias after LVAD insertion. A study of the first nine of the latter group of patients revealed small hemodynamic changes during the course of the arrhyth-

mia (mean arterial blood pressure decrease of 3 ± 16 mm Hg), with decreases in LVAD flow of 1.6 ± 0.9 L/minute. Two patients with early arrhythmias and severe perioperative right ventricular dysfunction experienced dangerous decreases in LVAD flow (to 2.3 and 3.0 L/minute), which improved with correction of the arrhythmia by electrical cardioversion. Six patients (67%) were fully ambulatory, and although most reported lethargy, there were no syncopal episodes. All patients were placed on low-dose heparin during their arrhythmias, and seven patients underwent successful electrical cardioversion. The others responded to pharmacologic therapy or overdrive pacing. No deaths or thromboembolic events occurred in the 11 patients with arrhythmias.

Our experience demonstrates that malignant ventricular arrhythmias are remarkably well tolerated in patients supported with LVADs alone, especially after the decreases in pulmonary vascular resistance that occur within 48 to 72 hours after LVAD insertion. Arrhythmias should be suspected in patients who demonstrate sudden decreases in LVAD flow, with or without changes in arterial blood pressure. Although malignant ventricular arrhythmias are usually not life-threatening in LVAD patients, especially after the early postoperative period, this complication should be managed aggressively to improve LVAD output and the clinical status of the patient, and to avoid the potential adverse sequelae of thrombus formation or further right ventricular myocardial injury from prolonged fibrillation.

Anticoagulation

Even though bleeding is a more common problem than thromboembolism in patients supported with mechanical assist devices, most such patients receive continuous anticoagulation therapy after perioperative coagulation parameters have normalized. Patients supported by centrifugal or external pulsatile pump systems are heparinized to maintain the activated clotting time above 150 to 200 seconds, although limited experience with the Carmeda coating system suggests that centrifugal support without systemic anticoagulation is potentially feasible. Patients supported with the Thoratec and Novacor pulsatile systems are often given perioperative dextran and dipyridamole, and after bleeding has subsided, a partial thromboplastin time of greater than 50 seconds or a prothrombin time of greater than 18 seconds is maintained with heparin or warfarin, respectively.

Because of the HeartMate's integrally textured blood-contacting surface, a biologic pseudointima composed of blood-derived cellular components forms relatively rapidly. It is thought that the elimination of the blood–device interface by this biologic lining as well as the wandering vortex design are responsible for the low thromboembolic risk associated with this device. Thus, patients with this device do not receive postoperative anticoagulants. In many centers, HeartMate patients receive only aspirin or dipyridamole. At our center, these patients receive no anticoagulant or antiplatelet therapy at all.

Antimicrobial Prophylaxis

At our institution, all patients undergoing LVAD insertion receive antimicrobial prophylaxis. Intravenous vancomycin, aztreonam, and fluconazole are given before surgery and continued for 3 days. In addition, patients with fungal colonization receive a full 10-day course of fluconazole. Patients showing clinical signs of infection during support, including fever, chills, catheter-site erythema, drainage from the driveline or LVAD pocket, or leukocytosis, are pancultured and receive empiric broad-spectrum antibiotic therapy. Subsequent therapy is tailored to the infectious source and responsible organism.

Ventricular Recovery and Device Weaning

The potential for ventricular recovery in patients with cardiogenic shock secondary to postcardiotomy failure or acute myocardial infarction depends on a variety of factors, including the cause of heart failure, preexisting ventricular function, and adequacy of operative repair or revascularization during the primary procedure. Using this information, the degree of myocardial recovery is assessed with weaning trials, in which centrifugal device flow is reduced while hemodynamic and echocardiographic parameters are evaluated. It usually becomes clear over the course of a few days which patients will recover sufficiently to allow device removal and which will require longer-term support. In addition to hemodynamic stability during device weaning, other clinical clues that may be helpful in determining the patient's status include cardiac isoenzyme levels and the severity of electrocardiographic abnormalities.

In patients with acute decompensation of chronic heart failure or cardiogenic shock due to subacute processes, such as viral or idiopathic cardiomyopathy, assessment of ventricular recovery is more difficult. In viral, postpartum, and many cases of idiopathic cardiomyopathy, the degree and time course of ventricular functional deterioration are variable, and the condition may subside or even improve after weeks to months of support. Most patients with chronic dilated cardiomyopathy receive assist devices as bridges to transplantation; however, the success of pharmacologic agents such as angiotensin-converting enzyme inhibitors, nitrates, and beta blockers in halting and even reversing maladaptive ventricular dilation (through "reverse remodeling") has led to the suggestion that long-term mechanical unloading may improve ventricular function sufficiently to allow device explantation without transplantation. This hypothesis is supported by studies that document a normalization of myocardial fiber orientation and regression of myocyte hypertrophy in hearts supported with the LVAD.

This hypothesis was tested at our center in seven patients undergoing cardiac transplantation for New York Heart Association Class IV heart failure due to idiopathic dilated cardiomyopathy. All patients had comparable levels of ventricular dilation and dysfunction. Four of these patients were supported medically before transplantation, and three received LVADs as bridges to transplantation. All patients underwent echocardiography during support and *ex vivo* analysis of diastolic properties at the time of transplantation. As expected, patients supported by LVADs experienced significantly greater ventricular unloading than medically treated patients, as assessed by estimation of ventricular pressures and volumes. Furthermore, when the native hearts of these patients were analyzed at the time of transplantation, medically treated hearts had diastolic properties consistent with chronic dilatation, whereas hearts that had been mechanically unloaded exhibited a significant leftward shift in the end-diastolic pressure–volume relationship, indicating a reversal of dilatation.

Encouraged by these data as well as the occasional echocardiographic observation of native ventricular function (aortic valve opening during LVAD systole), we have explanted LVADs in three patients who demonstrated hemodynamic stability during LVAD weaning before transplantation. All three patients were hemodynamically stable after explantation, with ejection fractions greater than 55% despite minimal pharmacologic support. Although two patients remain well with no evidence of recurrent ventricular dysfunction at 4 and 18 months after explantation, the third patient died of acute cardiac decompensation 6 months after explantation. Because this experience indicates that short-term hemodynamic stability after explantation is not necessarily an indicator of long-term cardiac function, we are exploring other means of identifying ventricular recovery in these patients. Based on a report describing the successful use of serum anti-beta$_1$ receptor antibody levels to predict ventricular recovery in a small number of LVAD patients, we have begun prospectively to study this as well as other potential markers of ventricular recovery. The future of VADs may rest in part on techniques developed to promote and assess ventricular recovery, thus lessening the burden on the donor organ supply.

SELECTED REFERENCES

Farrar DJ, Hill JD. Univentricular and biventricular Thoratec VAD support as a bridge to transplantation. *Ann Thorac Surg* 1993;55:276–282.

Frazier OH. The development of an implantable, portable, electrically powered left ventricular assist device. *Semin Thorac Cardiovasc Surg* 1994;6:181–187.

Frazier OH, Macris MP, Radovancevic B, eds. *Support and replacement of the failing heart*. Philadelphia: Lippincott–Raven Publishers, 1996.

Frazier OH, Rose EA, Macmanus Q, et al. Multicenter evaluation of the HeartMate 1000 IP left ventricular assist device. *Ann Thorac Surg* 1992; 53:1080–1088.

Frazier OH, Rose EA, McCarthy P, et al. Improved mortality and rehabilitation of transplant candidates treated with a long-term implantable left ventricular assist system. *Ann Surg* 1995;222:327–338.

Goldstein DJ, Seldomridge JA, Chen JM, et al. Use of aprotinin in LVAD recipients reduces blood loss, blood use, and perioperative mortality. *Ann Thorac Surg* 1995;59:1063–1068.

McBride LR. Bridging to cardiac transplantation with external ventricular assist devices. *Semin Thorac Cardiovasc Surg* 1994;6:169–173.

McCarthy PM, Sabik JF. Implantable circulatory support devices as a bridge to heart transplantation. *Semin Thorac Cardiovasc Surg* 1994;6:174–180.

Minami K, Posival H, El-Bynayosy A, et al. Mechanical ventricular support using pulsatile Abiomed BVS 5000 and centrifugal Biomedicus-pump in postcardiotomy shock. *Int J Artif Organs* 1994;17:492–498.

Oz MC, Argenziano M, Catanese KA, et al. Bridge experience with long-term implantable left ventricular assist devices: are they an alternative to transplantation? *Circulation* 1997;95:1844–1852.

Oz MC, Goldstein DJ, Pepino P, et al. Screening scale predicts patients successfully receiving long-term implantable left ventricular assist devices. *Circulation* 1995;92:[Suppl II]169–173.

Rose EA, Goldstein DJ. Wearable long-term mechanical support for patients with end-stage heart disease: a tenable goal. *Ann Thorac Surg* 1996;61:399–402.

Rose EA, Levin HR, Oz MC, et al. Artificial circulatory support with textured interior surfaces: a counter-intuitive approach to minimize thromboembolism. *Circulation* 1994;90:[Suppl II]87–91.

Vetter HO, Kaulbach HG, Schmitz C, et al. Experience with the Novacor left ventricular assist system as a bridge to cardiac transplantation, including the new wearable system. *J Thorac Cardiovasc Surg* 1995; 109:74–80.

Votapka TV, Pennington DG. Circulatory assist devices in congestive heart failure. *Cardiol Clin* 1994;12:143–154.

Management of End-Stage Heart Disease, edited by Eric A. Rose and Lynne Warner Stevenson. Lippincott–Raven Publishers, Philadelphia ©1998.

CHAPTER 17

Total Artificial Heart

Robert T. V. Kung

The final decade of the 20th century may prove to be the turning point in the quest to develop a total artificial heart (TAH) adequate for clinical use. Already during this decade, the first temporary artificial heart, the BVS 5000 (Abiomed, Inc., Danvers, MA), was introduced clinically after the Federal Food and Drug Administration (FDA) approved the device for use as postcardiotomy support in 1992. Two years later, the FDA approved use of the Heart-Mate left ventricular assist device (LVAD; Thermo Cardiosystems, Woburn, MA) as a bridge to transplantation. Trials are being conducted to demonstrate the safety of long-term support with the LVAD. The culmination in the development of mechanical circulatory support devices, however, will be the day the first fully implantable TAH is introduced clinically.

The extended journey began in 1964, when the National Heart Institute established the artificial heart program. As early as 1969, an artificial heart was implanted by Cooley to keep a patient alive until a donor heart could be found and transplanted. The original goal of the program was to develop a fully implantable artificial heart. Soon, however, problems with compatibility of blood materials, availability of power sources, and the risk of infectious complications caused the program to shift its attention toward the development of an LVAD. Although development of an implantable LVAD faced obstacles similar to those with the TAH, they seemed easier to overcome. Support for the LVAD program continued through the 1980s, laying the foundation for the ventricular and biventricular assist devices now in clinical use.

Although the National Heart and Lung Institute, later renamed the National Heart, Lung and Blood Institute (NHLBI), focused on the LVAD, artificial heart research continued at the University of Utah. In the early 1980s, a pneumatically actuated heart was developed by a team led by Kolff and Jarvik. Despite significant infection and thromboembolic problems, valuable lessons were learned

from these implantations. The blood pump needed to be improved and more reliable heart valves needed to be developed. Most important, however, we learned that the success of the TAH depends on the quality of life that it affords to its recipient. Thus, a fully implantable TAH must be developed if the TAH is ever to become a viable treatment for patients with end-stage heart failure.

Toward the later part of the 1980s, the NHLBI initiated a program for the development of the untethered, fully implantable TAH. This program nurtured the current generation of TAH systems. Its development teams are Abiomed/Texas Heart Institute and Penn State/3M Sarns. Each group is completing feasibility testing of their respective system in preparation for the formal preclinical reliability testing that will begin in 1998.

Much of the clinical experience with the LVAD and the TAH has been gained primarily in the bridge-to-transplantation population, where the limited donor heart supply restricts the use of these devices to 2,000 cases per year. Long-term assist devices will realize their full potential only when such devices are used to support their recipients for the duration of their lives. A randomized trial (REMATCH; Randomized Evaluation of Mechanical Assistance for the Treatment of Congestive Heart Failure) was begun to compare the effectiveness of the LVAD versus medical therapy in patients with New York Heart Association (NYHA) Class IV congestive heart failure (CHF) who are not eligible for transplantation (age 65–72 years). Similar trials for the TAH will most likely begin around the turn of the century.

ROLE OF THE LEFT VENTRICULAR ASSIST DEVICE AND THE TOTAL ARTIFICIAL HEART

As the implantable LVAD and the TAH begin to fulfill their original purpose as long-term devices, it has become increasingly important to identify the patient populations who will most benefit from these devices. Previous estimates of the target population, most notably the Olmstead

Abiomed, Inc., Danvers, Massachusetts 01923

County study, have considered the potential number of subjects for cardiac replacement, either by transplantation or by the TAH. The study was conducted to determine the need for the TAH. Based on the Olmstead County statistics between 1979 and 1983 for heart failure (more specifically, severe depression of left ventricular function, and exclusions due to sudden death and co-morbidities), 14% of patients who died of heart failure were considered candidates for cardiac replacement. The age group considered was between 15 to 69 years. The study concluded that approximately 16,500 people in the United States could benefit from cardiac replacement annually. If age constraints are not considered, the number could rise to approximately 80,000.

Studies of patients supported with the LVAD have shown good results; however, the LVAD may not be effective in patients with (a) acute myocardial infarction, especially those with apical infarcts; (b) chronic obstructive pulmonary disease, in whom right heart support is required to overcome the high pulmonary resistance; (c) aortic valve or mitral valve implants, in whom absence of valve motion would lead to clot formation and potential for strokes; (d) intractable arrhythmia, resulting in compromised right heart function; (e) significant aortic valve insufficiency, Grade III to IV; (f) left ventricular thrombus; (g) endocarditis, leading to infection of the device; and (h) rejection of a transplanted heart. Most of these patients may be saved by implantation of the TAH.

The *1991 Morbidity and Mortality Statistics* published by the NHLBI in 1994 allows us to assess further the number of cardiac deaths that could be averted by the implantable LVAD or TAH. Table 1 lists the major diagnostic categories and the associated number of cardiac deaths in each category. The diagnostic category is based on the ICD-9 code relating death to hospital admission diagnosis. The categories are not necessarily the cause of death, but may be a major underlying factor contributing to eventual pump failure and death. For example, hypertension by itself does not result in cardiac death; however,

hypertension may be a contributor to CHF and subsequent death. Coronary heart disease remains the primary cause of death. The heart failure group consists of patients whose primary diagnosis is CHF. Most transplant recipients fall into the heart failure and cardiomyopathy categories. Thus, up to 63,000 patients per year may benefit from cardiac replacement—yet only 2,300 patients received transplantations in 1991.

In estimating how many patients could benefit from mechanical assistance, exclusion factors (such as sudden death) must be accounted for. Figure 1 shows a distribution of patients into various categories leading to death. Of the 721,000 cardiac deaths in 1991, 67.3% were due to coronary heart disease, 5.7% to arrhythmia, and most of the remaining 27% to CHF. In the coronary heart disease group, approximately 46% of deaths were attributable to sudden death. The remaining 54% probably died from progressive hemodynamic deterioration.

The remaining diagnostic groups were assumed to have the same rate of sudden death as patients with CHF. Such an assumption is valid because the proportion of patients experiencing sudden cardiac death is approximately 56% of total deaths as a result of first-time indications of coronary heart disease with no prior history of such disease. In general, sudden death comprises one half of all cardiac deaths, and is nearly independent of the type of cardiac disease, with the exception of arrhythmia.

Table 2 summarizes the deaths due to disease categories that could benefit from mechanical assistance. The total number of 418,000 subjects would be reduced by 50% if the co-morbidity rate given by Kottke were used, resulting in a potential patient population of 209,000. By imposing an age limit of 75 years, a further reduction of 50% would result, yielding a potential patient population of 105,000 who could benefit from mechanical support. This estimate is consistent with that given by Funk. The preferred device for each diagnostic indication is also listed.

The purpose of our analysis was not to project total numbers of patients suitable for mechanical assistance, but rather to determine the relative applicability of the TAH versus the LVAD. Although the TAH may be used in all of these patient categories, the LVAD may not. Most patients who die as a result of acute myocardial infarction could not be helped by the LVAD. Patients with myocarditis, if they are at all candidates for cardiac replacement, would need a TAH because the infected heart must be removed. Because the nidus for infection remains, the use of an LVAD in such a patient would lead to device infection. Patients with pulmonary embolism invariably have pulmonary hypertension, a condition that requires a TAH instead of an LVAD. Patients resuscitated from cardiac arrest would most likely require a TAH because of global damage to their hearts, a condition for which LVAD would not provide adequate support. The congestive heart failure patient group is the current target population for trans-

TABLE 1. *Cardiac deaths by categories*

Diagnostic category	No. of deaths
Coronary heart disease	485,000
Acute myocardial infarction (54.1%)	
Chronic ischemic (45.9%)	
Pulmonary embolism	12,000
Carditis (valvular, endocarditis,	96,000
myocarditis, pericarditis)	
Arrhythmias	41,000
Congestive heart failure	87,000
Heart failure (44.8%)	
Cardiomyopathy (27.6%)	
Hypertension (27.6%)	
Total	721,000

721,000 CARDIAC DEATHS
(1991)

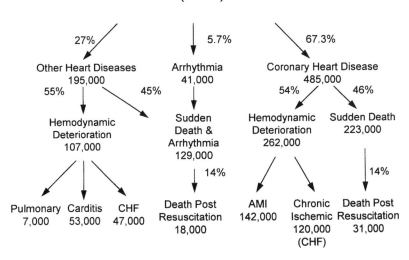

FIG. 1. Distribution of cardiac patients into various categories leading to death, based on 1991 mortality data.

plantation; their enlarged hearts, permit good filling of the device, make them ideal for LVAD implantation.

Of the cardiac deaths that could be averted by use of mechanical support, a TAH would be more appropriate in 60%, whereas the remaining 40% could be supported with either an LVAD or the TAH. Disregarding the problems inherent in relying solely on the TAH (without the native heart for back-up), the TAH could be used effectively in patients with both right and left ventricular failure, whereas the LVAD cannot be used in patients in whom right heart support is essential.

TOTAL ARTIFICIAL HEART DEVELOPMENT AND STATUS

The development of an implantable TAH requires combining the art of medicine with the science of engineer-

ing. The device must be anatomically compatible, physiologically responsive, hemodynamically effective, hematologically nonactivating, and operationally reliable, while providing the recipient with a good quality of life. In brief, the device must be safe, reliable, effective, and permit the recipient to live without restrictions in lifestyle. Thus, the TAH of the future will be free of percutaneous tethers, wires, and tubes.

The status of systems in development has been reviewed by Pierce et al., and this will not be repeated here. Each of the systems is designed to deliver up to 8 L/minute of cardiac output at physiologic pressures, and operate for a minimum of 20 minutes from its rechargeable internal power source and a minimum of 8 hours from its external source.

The Abiomed system, however, will be described here. This TAH is a product of collaboration between Abiomed and the Texas Heart Institute. Distinct design features of

TABLE 2. *Potential mechanical circulatory support patient population*

Diagnostic indications	No. of deaths[a][b]	Number of MCS candidates	Percentage	Preferred device
Acute myocardial infarction	142,000	36,000	34.0%	TAH
Chronic ischemic	120,000	30,000	28.7%	LVAD, TAH
Carditis	53,000	13,000	12.7%	TAH
Pulmonary	7,000	2,000	1.7%	TAH
Postresuscitation	49,000	12,000	11.7%	TAH
Congestive heart failure	47,000	12,000	11.2%	LVAD, TAH
Total	418,000	105,000[c]		

MCS, mechanical circulatory support; LVAD, left ventricular assist device; TAH, total artificial heart.
[a]Co-morbidity could reduce the applicable numbers by 50%.
[b]An age limit of 75 years would further reduce the applicable population by 50%.
[c]All numbers are rounded off to thousands.

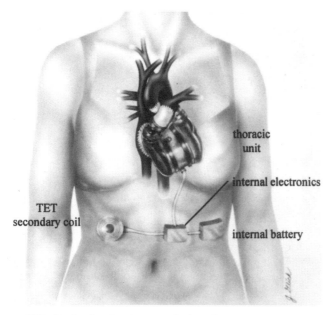

FIG. 2. Anatomic placement of system components.

the Penn State/3M Sarns system are elucidated as appropriate.

Our design philosophy has been to engineer a device with configurational flexibility. A hydraulic fluid drive mechanism without direct mechanical contact actuation of the blood bladders meets this criterion. In addition, to improve reliability and lower the cost of manufacturing,

component dimensions are designed not to require high tolerances. Our energy converter, blood pump, and valve designs adhere to these guidelines. Our goal is to design a device whose implantation does not cost more than the cost for transplantation in a United Network for Organ Sharing Status II patient ($129,000).

The anatomic placement of system components is illustrated in Figure 2. The thoracic unit, consisting of the energy converter and two blood pumps, approximates the shape and volume of the natural heart and is implanted in the pericardial volume vacated by the excised natural heart. The internal battery pack, internal electronics, and transcutaneous energy transmission coil are placed abdominally as shown in Figure 2.

The blood pumps (85-mL total volume; 70-mL stroke volume; 82% ejection fraction) are seamless, with no steps from proximal to the inflow valve to the outflow graft, distal to the outflow valve. Valve connector junctions have been implicated as initiation sites for thromboemboli. The seamless design eliminates such nidi for embolus generation. The inflow cuff has a quick-connecting mechanism that impedes pannus ingrowth. This is achieved by the use of a properly dimensioned protrusion of the inlet conduit into the cuff. Blood motion around the outer wall of the conduit prevents tissue growth along the outer wall of the protrusion. Figure 3 shows no tissue ingrowth into the protruding inflow after the device was implanted for 3.5 months in a calf. A quick-connecting mechanism allows convenient joining

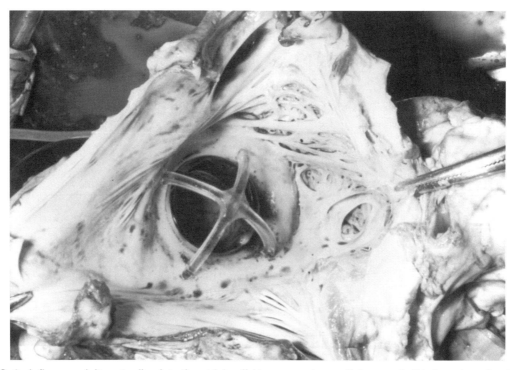

FIG. 3. Inflow conduit protruding into the atrial cuff. No pannus ingrowth is seen in this long-term implant. An inflow cage in the shape of a cross, which is not in contact with the inflow conduit, serves to avoid atrial tissue blockage of total artificial heart inflow. This structure is not in contact with the inflow conduit.

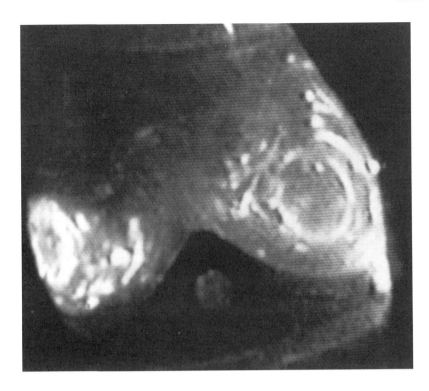

FIG. 4. Light scattering off of suspended particles in fluid illustrates vortical flow in the valve sinus.

of the outflow conduit and the graft. Internal blood pump surfaces, including the integral trileaflet valves, are fabricated from a nontoxic, nonmutagenic polyetherurethane, Angioflex (ABIOMED, Danvers, MA), which has the required durability and flexing cycle life. Valves have been cycled in excess of one billion beats, an equivalent of more than 20 years of real-time service at physiologic pressure differences of 90 mm Hg. These valves are designed with sinuses that maintain vortical blood motion even during valve closure to avoid stagnation and deposition. Such vortical motion is illustrated in a time-exposure photograph of light scattering off of suspended particles in a flowing fluid (Figure 4). The light streaks follow vortical streamlines. Figure 5 shows a TAH valve explanted after 56 days to be free of deposition. The pumps incorporate a free diaphragm for coupling to the energy system. A major point of distinction between the two systems under development is the valves used in the systems. In contrast to the integrally fabricated polyetherurethane valve used by our group, Penn State/3M Sarns uses Bjork-Shiley Delrin disc valves (Shiley, Irvine, CA).

The electrohydraulic energy system drives the blood pump membrane using a hydraulic fluid (methyl silicone) operating at physiologic pressures. As a result of fluid coupling, the membrane motion during filling and ejection normally follows the least resistant path with minimum strain. The hydraulic fluid and blood are immiscible, with negligible fluid transfer (3×10^{-2} mL/year) across the membranes. The energy converter includes a unidirectional (3,000–9,000 rpm) centrifugal

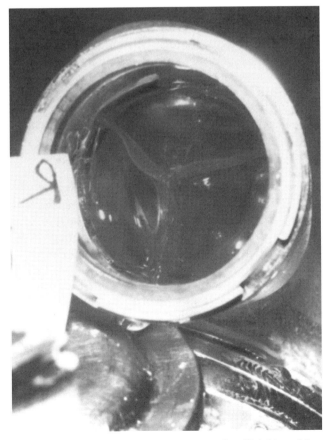

FIG. 5. Explanted trileaflet valve in a total artificial heart free of deposition.

pump driven by a brushless direct-current motor. Flow reversal is accomplished by a two-position, rotary porting valve. The pump motor impeller and the porting valve are the primary moving parts of the energy converter. The motor sits immersed in the hydraulic fluid that fills the energy system housing. This ensures that temperatures are uniform throughout the system. Waste heat is transferred to the blood across the pump diaphragms with a minimal increase in the blood temperature (<0.2°C) and from the housing to contacting body fluids and surfaces (temperature increase <4°C). The choice of a unidirectional, continuous-rotation pump is based on bearing life considerations. An added benefit is that a more efficient centrifugal pump can be used. For the flow regime consistent with physiologic interest, the centrifugal pump has twice the efficiency of an axial flow pump. In contrast to the fluid-driven blood pump membranes used in our system, direct pusher-plate actuation of the blood membrane or sac is used in the Penn State/3M Sarns system.

Electronic control circuits are miniaturized and consist of a microcontroller, electrically erasable programmable, read only memory (EEPROM), random access memory analog sensing circuits, analog-to-digital converter, control logic, and power field effect transistors (FETs) for driving the rotary valve limited-angle torque motor and the centrifugal pump motor.

The internal battery uses 11 nickel-cadmium 0.9 A·hour cells that can provide 45-minute operation under normal physiologic conditions with a life of 2,000 cycles. A 1.35-·hour, 14.4-V lithium-ion system has been evaluated. Weighing approximately 200 g, the lithium-ion package can provide 45 minutes of operation at a reduced cycle life; however, it has the advantage of having a large reserve capacity (additional 45 minutes). The battery pack, shaped to fit between the subcostal and iliac region extraperitoneally, is amenable to surgical replacement without shutting down the system.

A transcutaneous energy transmission/telemetry system (TET/TS) allows power to be transferred without skin penetration (efficiency 75%). Bidirectional internal and external communication is achieved through radio frequency transmission (19,200-baud data rate).

The internal system efficiency is 14% from battery power to blood power at nominal flows of 5 L/minute and aortic afterloads of 100 mm Hg. This efficiency level is competitive with that of the natural heart. The metabolic needs of the heart are about five times what it can generate in flow power. Although the system's cardiac output is designed to be 8 L/minute, maximum output exceeds 10 L/minute, an output sufficient for highly demanding activities.

In the TAH, pumping is achieved by alternately driving the left and the right pumps. Because the pumps are hydraulically coupled, the system ejects blood alternately from the left and the right blood chambers, accompanied by alternate filling of the right and the left blood chambers, respectively.

It is well established, however, that left–right cardiac output differences exist. A difference of approximately 5% is attributable to the bronchial branch flow. In permanent systems, this flow difference compensation has to be considered in conjunction with the system compliance and control.

A third hydraulic chamber (~15 mL in volume) is incorporated on the proximal (atrial) side of the left pump inflow valve with its own flexible diaphragm in contact with blood at the inflow. This chamber serves as a fluid reservoir to maintain the natural imbalance between the left- and right-side flows (the left can be as much as 15% higher than the right), changing the right hydraulic chamber fluid volume during a beat in response to the left atrial pressure without actively pumping blood. This hydraulic shunt chamber diverts fluid from the right hydraulic chamber, reducing its stroke volume. The amount of shunting is proportional to the left atrial pressure. High left atrial pressure leads to high shunting or lower right-sided stroke volume and output, and vice versa. This mechanism is capable of maintaining balanced left and right atrial pressure. This is validated in the atrial pressures from a series of studies in calves, shown in Figure 6. Typically, the left and right atrial pressures are within 5 mm Hg of each other. The filling pressures are high because the cardiac output required by the calf readily outstrips actual device output.

In contrast to this technique, the Penn State/3M Sarns system uses gas compliance for managing flow differ-

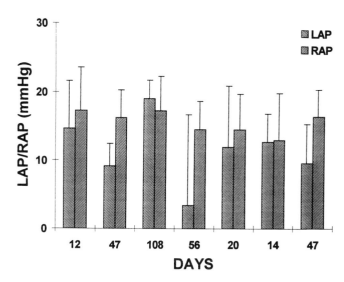

FIG. 6. Balanced left and right atrial filling pressures in a series of long-term implants. Atrial pressures were measured from atrial cuff lines.

ence. Periodic gas refilling through a subdermal port is required to maintain proper compliance.

The inputs for control are provided by two pressure sensors, one in each hydraulic chamber. The hydraulic pressures are used to determine the outputs: left and right motor speeds (rate of filling/ejection) and beat rate. The motor speeds are adjusted to maintain maximum ejection, based on the systolic hydraulic pressure at the end of diaphragm movement on each side. The beat rate increases and decreases according to the right-side filling pressure, resulting in a Starling-like response. The left-side filling pressure is not used for control purposes. The strategy is independent of outflow impedances. The TAH reacts (both in stroke volume and beat rate) to changes in the available fill volume, and adjusts the motor speeds to accommodate afterload changes.

The device as currently configured fits into more than 90% of men and more than 70% of women in the United States. A smaller model with a maximum flow of 6 to 7 L/minutes instead of the 10 L/minutes of our current system is needed to accommodate people too small to use the current TAH.

The Phase I goal has been to demonstrate 2-month *in vivo* and 3-month *in vitro* operation. We have achieved 2-month survivals with the implanted thoracic unit and the electronics, internal battery, and the TET/TS in calves. *In vitro* operation has exceeded 3 months. Studies are ongoing and continuing. The system is ready to begin preclinical reliability testing.

THE PATH TO CLINICAL TRIAL

As part of our preparation for the introduction of the TAH into clinical trial, we have addressed many of its pertinent user-related features. Foremost among these issues are the shape of the TET and the ergonomics of the external wearable power pack. The circular TET performs very well, although power transfer is somewhat sensitive to the alignment between the internal and external coils. Hence, the secondary coil must be implanted in the subcutaneous tissue layer, a region of low vascularity that is prone to irritation and potential skin erosion. To overcome these limitations and permit implantation of the secondary coil in the fascial layer, a broader-area coil will reduce the sensitivity to lateral alignment mismatches and increase the tolerance to the larger gap between the secondary and the primary coil. Figure 7 shows a set of flexible, oval-shaped TET coils designed for better implant fit in the waist region.

The external batteries consist of modules of lithium-ion batteries, with a 2-hour pack (1 lb.) and a number of 4-hour packs (2 lbs.). The 2-hour pack can be carried in a pocket or connected to a charger when sedentary, whereas the 4-hour packs can be slipped into a belt pouch capable of carrying three packs. The external electronics

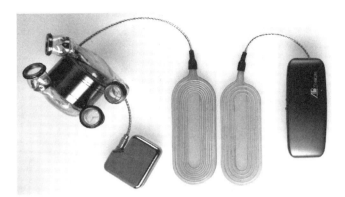

FIG. 7. Photograph showing models of the internal components (*left*) and the external components (*right*). The internal components shown are the heart, the internal battery (a similar internal electronics pack is not shown) and the internal secondary coil. The external components shown are the primary coil and the electronic control and battery pack.

are contained in the 2-hour package. This modular approach allows the recipient to participate in many physical activities, from office work to sports using a 2-hour pack, to extended outings using the three 4-hour packs. Figure 7 shows the system with its internal and external components (4-hour pack not shown).

The goal of the NHLBI program is to produce a system whose recipients have survival rates comparable with those of cardiac transplant recipients (a 1-year reliability of 80%, a 2-year reliability of 70%, and a 5-year reliability of 60%), but without the morbidity associated with immunosuppression. Sequential goals can be set for the development program. At present, the goal is to demonstrate an 80% reliability for a 2-year life in the NHLBI program. Such a test program would entail more than eight systems on bench test for 2 years, and eight animal studies, each demonstrating 3-month duration of implant. Great strides have been made toward developing the implantable TAH. The path toward its clinical application is clearly marked; during the 21st century, the TAH will become a clinical reality.

SELECTED REFERENCES

Cooley DA, Liotta D, Hallman GL, et al. Orthotopic cardiac prosthesis for two stages cardiac replacement. *Am J Cardiol* 1969;24:723–727.
Copeland JG, Smith RG, Cleavinger MC. Development and current status of the CardioWest C-70® total artificial heart. In: Lewis T, Graham TR, eds. *Mechanical circulatory support*. London: Edward Arnold, 1995:186–197.
Devries WC, Anderson JL, Joyce LD, et al. Clinical use of the total artificial heart. *N Engl J Med* 1984;310:273.
Frazier OH, Rose EA, McCarthy P, et al. Reduced mortality and rehabilitation of transplant candidates treated with a long-term implantable left ventricular assist system. *Ann Surg* 1995;222:327–336.
Gray LA, Champsaur GC. The BVS 5000 biventricular assist device: worldwide registry experience. *ASAIO J* 1994;40:M460–M464.
Guyton RA, Schonberger JP, Everts PA, et al. Postcardiotomy shock: clinical evaluation of the BVS 5000® biventricular support system. *Ann Thorac Surg* 1993;53:346–356.

Hosenpud JD, Novick RJ, Breen TJ, Keck B, Daily D. Registry of the International Society for Heart and Lung Transplantation: twelfth official report—1995. *J Heart Lung Transplant* 1995;14:805–815.

Kannel WB, Plehn JF, Cupples LA. Cardiac failure and sudden death in the Framingham Study. *Am Heart J* 1988;115:869–875.

Kannel WB, Thomas HE Jr. Sudden coronary death: the Framingham Study. *Ann NY Acad Sci* 1982;382:3–18.

Kung RTV, Yu LS, Ochs BD, et al. Progress in the development of the Abiomed total artificial heart. *ASAIO J* 1995;41:M245–M248.

Kung RTV, Yu LS, Ochs BD, et al. An atrial hydraulic shunt in a total artificial heart. *ASAIO J* 1993;39:M213–M217.

Lorell BH. *Mortality, incidence and prevalence of heart failure: current and projected clinical need for mechanical circulatory support.* Report of the Workshop on the Artificial Heart: Planning for Evolving Technologies. Bethesda, MD: National Heart, Lung, and Blood Institute, January, 1994.

Parnis SM, Yu LS, Ochs BD, et al. Chronic in vivo evaluation of an electrohydraulic total artificial heart. *ASAIO J* 1994;40:M489–M493.

Pierce WS, Sapirstein JS, Pae WE Jr. Total artificial heart: from bridge to transplantation to permanent use. *Ann Thorac Surg* 1996;61:342–346.

Simon SR, Powell CH, Bartozkis TC, Hock DH. A new system for classification of cardiac death as arrhythmic, ischemic, or due to myocardial pump failure. *Am J Cardiol* 1995;76:896–898.

Snyder AJ, Rosenberg G, Reibson J, et al. An electrically powered total artificial heart. *ASAIO J* 1992;38:M707–M712.

Yu LS, Finnegan M, Vaughan S, et al. A compact and noise free electrohydraulic total artificial heart. *ASAIO J* 1993;39:M386–M391.

Management of End-Stage Heart Disease, edited
by Eric A. Rose and Lynne Warner Stevenson.
Lippincott–Raven Publishers, Philadelphia ©1998.

CHAPTER 18

Axial Flow Pumps

O. Howard Frazier

Over the past 50 years, many surgical advances have been made in the treatment of end-stage heart disease. From the introduction of cardiopulmonary bypass (which allowed surgeons to perform heart valve and coronary artery bypass operations) to the advent of cyclosporine (which transformed cardiac transplantation into a viable option for patients with end-stage heart disease), treatments for end-stage heart failure have progressed significantly.

One of the major focuses of our research has been myocardial replacement therapy. At the moment, the preferred method of myocardial replacement therapy is cardiac transplantation. Unfortunately, transplantation has some limitations. First, the shortage of donor hearts restricts the number of patients who can receive this therapy. Second, patients who do undergo transplantation may experience accelerated atherosclerosis in their donor heart. Thus, alternative therapies for heart failure must be found.

For many years, cardiac surgeons have focused on mechanical circulatory support as a means of treating patients with end-stage heart failure. DeBakey and associates used the first left ventricular assist device in 1963. Cooley and Liotta then implanted the first total artificial heart in 1969. These accomplishments illustrated that mechanical devices could effectively support the circulation of patients with heart failure. Then, with the advent of cyclosporine came a renewed interest in transplantation and, consequently, a renewed interest in mechanical assist devices. Since then, assist devices have moved out of the research laboratory and into the clinical arena. Ventricular assist systems (VAS), including temporary external systems like the Thoratec (Thoratec Corporation, Berkeley, CA) and the BVS 5000 (Abiomed Cardiovas-

cular, Inc., Danvers, MA) and long-term implantable systems like the Novacor (Baxter Healthcare Corporation, Oakland, CA) and the HeartMate (Thermo Cardiosystems, Woburn, MA), are now regularly used to bridge patients to transplantation.

Unfortunately, not every patient who needs ventricular support can be treated with the current long-term VASs. For example, patients whose body surface area is less than 1.5 m^2 (many women and most children) cannot be treated with a HeartMate because it is too large to be implanted. In addition, the difficulty in designing a compliance chamber (an implantable chamber used for internal venting of the pump) has prevented such pulsatile devices from becoming fully implantable.

To address such problems, engineers and physicians are collaborating to develop a new generation of assist devices: the axial flow pumps. These pumps are small enough to be implanted in children and powerful enough to support the circulation of an adult man. Currently, a short-term axial flow pump, the Hemopump (Medtronic, Inc., Grand Rapids, MI), is undergoing clinical testing with good results. In addition, there are ongoing animal studies of several long-term axial flow devices, including the Baylor/NASA pump (Baylor College of Medicine, Houston, TX), the Nimbus Axipump (Nimbus, Inc., Rancho Cordova, CA), and the Transicoil VAS (Transicoil, Inc., Valley Forge, PA), which incorporates the Jarvik 2000 blood pump. A discussion of each of these devices is presented in this chapter.

SHORT-TERM CIRCULATORY SUPPORT: THE HEMOPUMP

The Hemopump is an intraaortic axial flow pump used to provide short-term ventricular support to patients in cardiogenic shock (Figure 1). In contrast to the commonly used intraaortic balloon pump, the Hemopump unloads the ventricle directly. Thus, the device has the

Department of Surgery, University of Texas Medical School, Houston, Texas 77225-0345

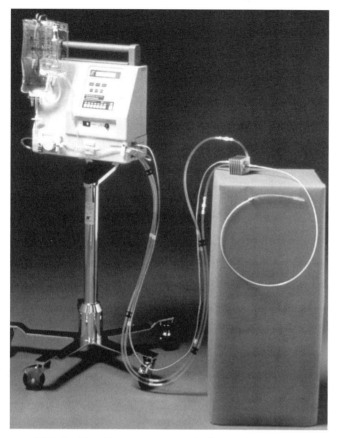

FIG. 1. The Hemopump ventricular assist system.

ability to reduce the end-diastolic or intraventricular cavitary pressure, an important factor in relieving ventricular wall stress and allowing ventricular function to improve. This device remains under research protocol in the United States; however, results thus far demonstrate that the Hemopump may be used effectively to treat patients in cardiogenic shock, including patients who are waiting for or who have undergone cardiac transplantation.

The Hemopump is particularly useful in patients with heart transplants undergoing acute rejection or donor heart failure. Implanting and removing a pulsatile left ventricular assist device (LVAS) like the HeartMate requires extensive surgery and increases the patient's risk of infection, which must be carefully avoided in the immunosuppressed transplantation patient. The catheter-mounted method of implanting and removing the Hemopump poses a much smaller risk of surgical complications and infection.

Description

The Hemopump consists of an axial flow pump enclosed within a silicone cannula, along with a drive cable and a purge fluid system. The pump has a diameter of 7 mm and is about the size of the cap on a small marking pen (Figure 2). The pump has a rotating speed of almost 25,000 revolutions per minute (rpm). When the pump rotates, blood is drawn from the ventricle and pumped into the thoracic aorta. The pump is capable of providing as much as 4.71 L/minute of flow despite its small size. Thus, the Hemopump can assume most of the work of the left ventricle, decreasing both left ventricular and pulmonary capillary wedge pressures.

Three different models of the Hemopump are available: 24-Fr femoral, sternotomy, and 14-Fr percutaneous. In each model, the pump is attached distally to an inflow cannula, which has a beveled, radiopaque tip designed to facilitate entry of the cannula across the aortic valve and into the left ventricular cavity. The cannula is positioned in the left ventricle; the pump rests in the ascending aorta (Figure 3).

The drive cable is enclosed in a polymeric sheath. Also enclosed in the sheath is the purge fluid system. This system maintains blood seal integrity and lubricates the pump and drive assembly. The fluid (40% dextrose in water) may help prevent the formation of thrombus.

The purge fluid system is controlled by an external roller pump located on the pump console. The pump console weighs approximately 25 lbs. and controls and powers the pump.

Animal Studies

The Texas Heart Institute initiated *in vivo* experimental studies of the Hemopump in 1986. We implanted several

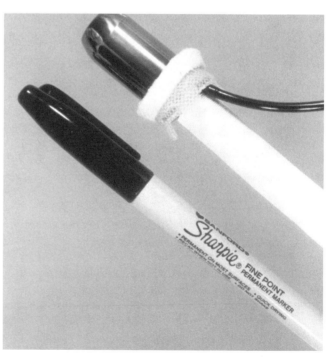

FIG. 2. The Hemopump is about the size of the cap on a small marking pen.

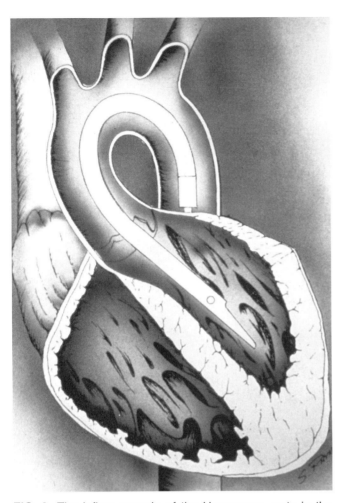

FIG. 3. The inflow cannula of the Hemopump rests in the ventricular cavity; the pump itself is located in the ascending aorta.

of these devices in calves. Initially, there was some fear that the high rpm generated by the pump would damage blood cells. After 14 days of pumping, however, we found that the Hemopump caused only minimal hemolysis. Thus, further experimental studies were begun. At The University of Texas—Houston Medical School, Smalling and associates examined the effect of Hemopump on dogs whose left anterior descending artery had been ligated. Results in this study were encouraging as well. They demonstrated that by reducing intraventricular pressures, the Hemopump could preserve the viability of the myocardium and allow recovery of the ventricle.

Clinical Studies

After the success of the animal trials, clinical trials were begun. The first pilot studies were performed at the Texas Heart Institute. The success of these trials led to a multicenter study, approved by the U.S. Food and Drug Administration, in which the Hemopump was used to support the circulation of patients in cardiogenic shock at 10 centers in the United States.

Selection Criteria

To be eligible for the clinical trial, patients had to have a cardiac index less than or equal to 2.0 L/minute/m², a systolic blood pressure less than 90 mm Hg, and a pulmonary capillary wedge pressure greater than 18 mm Hg. Patients had to have received maximum pharmacologic and volume therapy without recovery before being considered for support with the Hemopump. Patients were not eligible for the study if they had severe aortic valve stenosis or regurgitation, known dissecting aneurysms, known aortic wall disease, end-stage terminal illness, significant blood dyscrasia, or prosthetic aortic valves.

Insertion Techniques

Unlike an implantable, pulsatile LVAS, the Hemopump may be inserted with minimal surgical intervention. In most cases, the Hemopump is inserted through the femoral artery. The artery is incised, and a length of 12-mm woven Dacron is anastomosed to the arteriotomy site.

A thoracic approach may be used in patients with small femoral arteries (such as some women and children), in those with severe peripheral vascular disease, and in those who cannot be weaned from cardiopulmonary bypass and whose ascending aorta has already been exposed. A longitudinal ascending aortal arteriotomy may be performed, through which a 10-cm short cannula is inserted into the left ventricle.

With the aid of fluoroscopy, the cannula and pump are threaded through the artery and guided to the aorta; the inflow cannula is then passed across the aortic valve. The tip of the cannula is placed in the left ventricle so that it may draw blood from the ventricular cavity. The axial flow pump is located at the opposite end of the cannula, just beyond the subclavian take-off. When turned on, the pump pulls the blood from the ventricle and pushes it through the descending thoracic aorta.

Anticoagulation

To prevent the formation of thrombus, patients receive a 10,000-unit bolus of heparin before pump insertion. After insertion, patients receive a continuous heparin infusion beginning at 1,000 units per hour with a target partial thromboplastin time of 1.5 to 2 times the control value. Postsurgical patients, however, should not receive heparin until postoperative bleeding is controlled.

Results of a Clinical Trial

Survival

Fifteen patients (11 men, 4 women; mean age, 46 years, range 8.6–65.3 years) who participated in this trial were awaiting or had received a heart transplant. Two of these patients could not be treated with a Hemopump, one because of severe atherosclerosis of the iliofemoral system and the other because of the small size of the femoral artery. These two patients died early after treatment.

The other 13 patients underwent successful Hemopump insertion and were supported by the Hemopump for a mean 60.9 hours (range, 2.1–15.1 hours). Eight of these patients (61%) were weaned successfully from the device, 5 (38%) of whom survived to 30 days. The remaining 5 patients died during support or just after the Hemopump was removed.

The survival rate for patients after cardiogenic shock secondary to acute myocardial infarction is reported to be between 10% and 25%. The survival rate for these 15 patients was 38%, a significant improvement. Thus, Hemopump support could significantly improve the chances for survival after cardiogenic shock, especially for seriously ill patients with end-stage heart disease.

Complications

The hemodynamic status of these patients was monitored throughout the duration of Hemopump support. Although there had been some concern that the high rpm of the pump would cause damage to blood components, particularly the erythrocytes, the mean level of plasma free hemoglobin during support was less than 50 mg/dL. Thus, patients supported with a Hemopump seem to face about the same risk of severe hemolysis as do patients supported by an implantable LVAS.

There was also concern that the introduction of the catheter into the left ventricle would itself affect hemodynamic function. Despite the occurrence of dysrhythmias, however, cardiac output and mean arterial pressure remained stable in most patients, although a few required cardioversion therapy.

Fracture of the drive cable and ejection of the cannula did prove to be a problem in some patients. In addition, the intraventricular mural thrombus that can form after cardiogenic shock has led to thromboembolic complications in some patients. Although this is a very serious complication, it occurs infrequently (2.4% in one report). No thromboembolic complications have originated from the Hemopump itself.

Although the overall status of the patients was improved after support with the Hemopump, the ventricles of a few patients did not recover enough to be weaned from the device. In addition, some patients were not able to recover from end-organ failure. It appears that support by the Hemopump is most beneficial when the device is implanted early after cardiogenic shock occurs—before end-organ dysfunction becomes irreversible.

Other Considerations

There are many advantages in using the Hemopump instead of an LVAS or balloon pump to support patients with end-stage heart failure in cardiogenic shock. First, insertion of the Hemopump is no more invasive than insertion of an intraaortic balloon pump, and less invasive than implantation of an LVAS. The low level of invasiveness is particularly useful for heart transplant recipients because it spares them great risk of further surgical trauma or infection. The Hemopump also provides support without removal of heart tissue, which is required when implanting an LVAS. Finally, because of its small size, the Hemopump can be used to support the circulation in women and children.

There are limitations to the use of the Hemopump, however. Because patients supported with the device must remain in bed during support, the Hemopump is not suited for patients requiring long-term mechanical assistance. Many patients awaiting transplantation must wait for an extended period before an appropriate donor heart is found. In addition, patients with irreversible heart failure may require higher rates of flow than the Hemopump is able to provide. In such cases, implantation of a long-term LVAS (for example, the HeartMate) is appropriate. Such a device can effectively support the bridge-to-transplantation patient without requiring extended periods of immobility, and can even allow patients to await transplantation at home.

LONG-TERM CIRCULATORY SUPPORT

A number of axial flow pump systems intended for long-term support of the failing heart are under investigation.

Baylor/NASA Axial Flow Ventricular Assist Device

The Baylor/NASA ventricular assist device (VAD) is being developed jointly by Baylor College of Medicine and the National Aeronautics and Space Administration (NASA) Johnson Space Center (Houston, TX). It is intended as a long-term VAD that may be used to support a patient's circulation for more than 3 months. This device is 75 mm long, 25 mm in diameter, and has a mass of 53 g and a total displacement of 15 cm^3 (Figure 4A). Despite its small size, this pump should be able to provide a flow of 5 L/minute. As for hemolysis, *in vitro* testing has shown an acceptable level of 0.0029 ± 0.0009 g/100 L hemoglobin.

The pump components are made of polycarbonate and include an inducer/impeller, a flow straightener, and a diffuser (Figure 4B). The pump bearings consist of zirconia shafts and balls and sapphire and olive endstones. In addition to the pump, the VAD also has a 0.5-inch inflow cannula, a 51-Fr outflow cannula (Research Med-

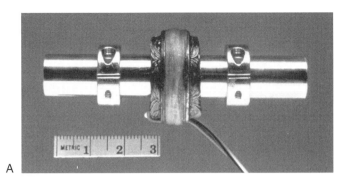

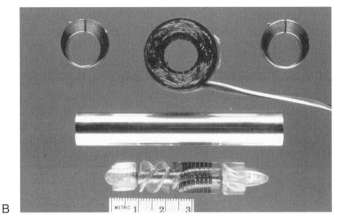

FIG. 4. The Baylor/NASA axial flow pump assembled **(A)** and disassembled **(B)**.

ical Inc., Salt Lake City, UT) and 0.5-inch Tygon tubing (Norton Performance Plastics Co., Akron, OH). The cannulae and tubing are made of polyvinylchloride and polycarbonate.

In Vivo *Trials: Phase I*

Thus far, only two calves have been implanted with the Baylor/NASA VAD. The goal of this trial was to maintain circulatory support for 2 or more days. The Baylor/NASA pump was attached to the back of the calf, with the inflow cannula entering the ventricle through an apical sewing ring and the outflow cannula exiting the ventricle through a vascular graft anastomosed to the thoracic descending aorta. Heparin was administered to the calves to maintain an activated clotting time of 250 seconds.

Eight pumps were implanted in the two calves for periods ranging from 18 to 203 hours. The first calf was implanted with seven different pumps and sacrificed on the 27th day. The second calf was implanted with one pump and sacrificed on the 12th day. Pumps were to be changed when significant complications or technical problems occurred. Four of the eight pumps operated successfully for 2 or more days (64, 87, 152, and 203 hours, respectively). In each pump study, the pump was removed because the formation of thrombus required that electri-

cal power to the pump be increased. In most cases, thrombus formed on the flow straightener and hub areas.

Modifications are now underway to rectify these problems, including the introduction of hub washout features and the repositioning of the internal pump parts. Because this was a Phase I study in which the goal for support was only 2 days, the materials were not antithrombogenic. Thus, components made of polycarbonate and polyvinylchloride in Phase I will consist of more biocompatible materials for the Phase II trial. The goal of the Phase II trial will be to support the calves for more than 2 weeks.

Nimbus Axipump

The Nimbus Axipump is another axial flow pump designed for long-term support of the circulation (Figure 5). It contains a static diffuser and an electromagnetically driven rotor. The device has a mass of 176 g and can produce up to 10 L/minute of flow. Although the first prototype of the Nimbus Axipump required a purge fluid system, the current prototype does not. The pump is connected transcutaneously to the drive console with an electrical drive line and purge line (Figure 6). The drive console regulates pump speed, which ranges between 6,000 and 13,000 rpm.

In Vivo *Studies*

The Nimbus Axipump was implanted in one sheep and two calves. The pump was inserted through a left thoracotomy. The outflow cannula was connected to a vascular graft, which was anastomosed to the thoracic descending aorta. The electrical drive cable and the purge line were attached to the drive console. A bolus of heparin was administered before the pump was turned on. When the animal's digestive system was again functioning normally, the heparin was replaced with warfarin, 5 mg/day.

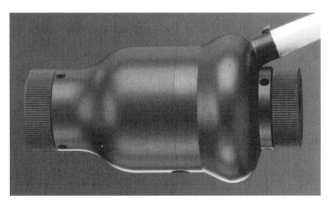

FIG. 5. The Nimbus Axipump. (Photograph used by permission of Nimbus, Inc., Rancho Cordova, CA.)

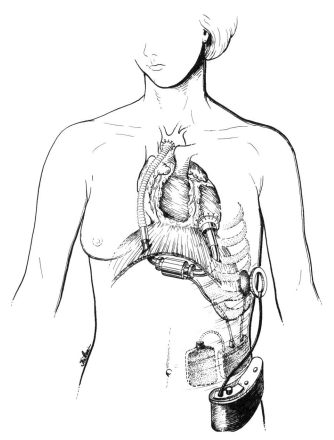

FIG. 6. Internal placement of the Nimbus Axipump. (Illustration used by permission of Nimbus, Inc., Rancho Cordova, CA.)

The sheep was supported by the Axipump for 28 days. On the 28th day, support was terminated because of a purge system failure. One of the two calves was supported for 57 days, the other for 52 days. One calf was euthanized because of low pump flow, the other to examine the pump and to determine whether end-organ damage had occurred.

In the sheep, thrombus was found in the wedge between the cannula tip and the ventricular wall at the coring site. In the calves, no thrombus was found around the cannula tip. Both calves, however, had small, multiple infarctions in both kidneys, and in both, the left lung had adhered to the heart and chest wall. In addition, a small area of atelectasis was found in each animal where the outflow graft and the left lung touched.

The pump was made of stainless steel and titanium. In the future, substances that are less thrombogenic will be used to coat the inner surface of the pump to avoid thrombus formation in the device.

Transicoil Ventricular Assist Device

The Transicoil VAS, which incorporates the Jarvik 2000 blood pump (Jarvik Research, Inc., New York, NY),

is an intraventricular assist device that may be used to bridge patients to transplantation and to provide long-term circulatory support for patients with end-stage heart disease. The Jarvik 2000 is small: it has a mass of 85 g and a displacement volume of 25 cm^3 (Figure 7). Despite its size, the pump is capable of providing over 12 L/minute of flow.

The only moving part in the pump is the rotor. The rotor contains a permanent magnet of a brushless direct-current motor, which regulates its power supply. The pump rotor is mounted on an axial flow impeller, which in turn is supported by ceramic, blood-immersed bearings. The pump impeller receives power from electromagnetic fields across the motor "air gap." The pump housing includes a 180-degree elliptical inflow cage and a 90-degree outflow elbow, which prevents the outflow graft from kinking. All blood-contacting surfaces are made of titanium.

In Vivo *Studies*

These studies have been designed to identify potential problems in device design and correct them before clinical trials begin. In a trial, the Jarvik 2000 was inserted into the left ventricles in seven calves.

To insert the device, a left lateral thoracotomy is performed at the fifth intercostal space, and a rib is removed. Heparin (1 mg/kg) is then administered to the calf, and a 16-mm, preclotted, low-porosity Dacron graft anastomosed to the descending thoracic aorta. A tapered, silicone-collared sewing ring is sutured to the left ventricular apex, in which a small cruciate incision is made. A conical obturator is inserted into the left ventricular cavity and used to apply back pressure to the apical endo-

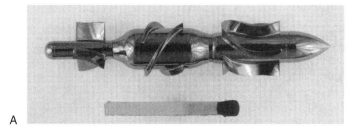

A

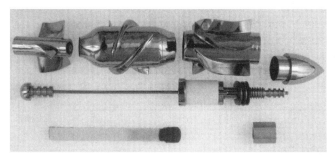

B

FIG. 7. The Jarvik 2000 (without the pump housing) shown assembled (A) and disassembled (B).

cardium. Using a cylindrical knife, the ventricular apex is cored, the obturator and knife removed, and the core plicated by hand. The pump is placed into the ventricle and a pursestring suture is drawn around the silicone collar. After air is removed from the graft, the pump can be activated.

Although these devices were designed to be completely implantable, electronics and batteries were not implanted during this study. Instead, the pump received power through a percutaneous drive line. The calves received 2.5 to 25 mg of warfarin, 400 mg of dipyridamole, and 1 g of aspirin daily.

In this study, the calves' circulation was supported by the Jarvik 2000 for an average of 107 days (range, 70–162 days). The continuous speed of the devices was 10,000 rpm, which produced an average flow of 5 to 6 L/minute. Blood urea nitrogen and serial serum creatinine levels remained normal. Plasma free hemoglobin levels were an average of 6.3 mg/dL (range, 4.3–11.4 mg/dL; normal, 1–4 mg/dL). The animals experienced only minimal hemolysis. The mean current remained steady throughout the study. Changes in current levels corresponded to changes in arterial pulse pressure, demonstrating that the Jarvik 2000 can produce pulsatile waveforms in circulation.

The calves were euthanized for various reasons, including a thrombus at the rotor–stator junction, infections, a broken electrical wire, and impeller blade–pump housing frictions. There was virtually no bearing wear in any pump, nor were there thromboemboli in the kidneys.

Future modifications to the Jarvik 2000 blood pump will include redesign of the rotor–stator junction. Testing of the entire Transicoil VAS will require the implantation of the battery and electronics system designed to run the Jarvik 2000. In addition, a new battery will be designed that is easier for the patient to use, as well as a new control system to meet the special needs of each patient.

CONCLUSIONS

Axial flow pumps may have an important role in the future of mechanical circulatory support. Unlike pulsatile pumps, these devices can be inserted or implanted relatively quickly. Furthermore, mechanical circulatory support systems that incorporate axial flow pumps do not require compliance chambers. In addition, they can be used in patients of all sizes, including small adults and children.

Clinical trials of the Hemopump have demonstrated its safety and efficacy in supporting the circulation of patients in cardiogenic shock. Animal studies of the long-term pumps (Baylor/NASA, Axipump, Jarvik 2000) have demonstrated their potential to provide safe and effective circulatory support. Further studies are needed to refine these devices before clinical trials can begin; however, if axial flow pumps fulfill their initial promise, they could ultimately prolong and improve the quality of the lives of thousands of patients with end-stage heart failure.

SELECTED REFERENCES

Butler KC, Maher TR, Borovetz HS, et al. Development of an axial flow blood pump LVAS. *ASAIO J* 1992;38:M296–M300.

Frazier OH, Macris MP. Clinical use of the Hemopump. In: Lewis T, Graham TR, eds. *Mechanical circulatory support*. London: Edward Arnold, 1995:146–152.

Frazier OH, Macris MP, Wampler RK, et al. Treatment of cardiac allograft failure by use of an intraaortic axial flow pump. *J Heart Transplant* 1990; 9:408–414.

Jarvik RK. System considerations favoring rotary artificial hearts with blood-immersed bearings. *Artif Organs* 1995;19:565–570.

Kaplon RJ, Oz MC, Kwiatkowski PA, et al. Miniature axial flow pump for ventricular assistance in children and small adults. *J Thorac Cardiovasc Surg* 1996;111:13–18.

Konishi H, Antaki JF, Boston JR, et al. Dynamic systemic vascular resistance in a sheep supported with a Nimbus Axipump. *ASAIO J* 1994;40: M299–M302.

Konishi H, Antaki JF, Litwak P, et al. Long-term animal survival with an implantable axial flow pump as a left ventricular assist device. *Artif Organs* 1996;20:124–127.

Macris MP, Myers TJ, Jarvik R, et al. In vivo evaluation of an intraventricular electric axial flow pump for left ventricular assistance. *ASAIO J* 1994;40:M719–M722.

Macris MP, Parnis SM, Frazier OH, et al. Development of an implantable ventricular assist system. *Ann Thorac Surg* 1997;63:367–370.

Mizuguchi K, Damm GA, Bozeman RJ, et al. Development of the Baylor/NASA axial flow ventricular assist device: in vitro performance and systemic hemolysis test results. *Artif Organs* 1994;18:32–43.

Parnis SM, Macris MP, Jarvik R, et al. Five-month survival in a calf supported with an intraventricular axial flow blood pump. *ASAIO J* 1995;41: M333–M336.

Poirier VL. The quest for a solution. We must continue. We must push forward. The 16th Hastings Lecture. *ASAIO Trans* 1993;36:856–863.

Rountree WD, Barbie RN, Neichin JN, Neichin ML. Johnson & Johnson Hemopump temporary cardiac assist system. In: Quaal SJ, ed. *Cardiac mechanical assist beyond balloon pumping*. St Louis: Mosby–Year Book, 1993:87–98.

Wampler RK, Frazier OH, Lansing AM, et al. Treatment of cardiogenic shock with the Hemopump left ventricular assist device. *Ann Thorac Surg* 1991;52:506–513.

Myocardial Enhancement Therapies

Management of End-Stage Heart Disease, edited by Eric A. Rose and Lynne Warner Stevenson. Lippincott–Raven Publishers, Philadelphia ©1998.

CHAPTER 19

Surgical Therapy for Heart Failure: Dynamic Cardiomyoplasty

George J. Magovern, Jr., Kathleen A. Simpson, James A. Magovern, and George J. Magovern, Sr.

Heart failure is initiated by a sustained loss of myocardial pumping power and subsequent decrease in systemic circulation. Medical therapy slows or masks the progression of symptoms arising from systemic compensatory mechanisms, without affecting the underlying cause of the disease. Cardiac transplantation is available only to a small percentage of patients with heart failure, and the efficacy of this procedure is further reduced by rejection, opportunistic infection, and posttransplantation coronary artery disease.

A long-term solution to the problem of heart failure depends on restoration of pumping power to the myocardium. Transfer of power through mechanical ventricular assistance or total heart replacement has been investigated since the late 1950s with some promise of future success. Stringent biomedical, economic, and quality-of-life requirements for development of a practical clinical device have delayed this worthwhile endeavor. New approaches to the problem should be studied as well.

SKELETAL MUSCLE POWER

Muscles are engines like the steam engine, an internal combustion engine, using energy stored in chemical fuel to generate mechanical movement.
Richard Dawkins in *The Selfish Gene*, used with permission from Oxford University Press

One of the most interesting fields in basic science and clinical research is the attempt to use intact skeletal muscle as a power source in cardiac assist. The fact that skele-

tal muscle is able to function at power levels analogous to those of the heart is well known, but skeletal muscle, unlike cardiac muscle, is fatigable and can sustain power output for only a short time.

Muscle function, in a simplified description, is controlled by nerve impulses that cause the release of acetylcholine and calcium ions, initiating muscle contraction. The force of skeletal muscle contraction depends on how many active motor units are recruited simultaneously.

In contrast, in the heart, a single impulse spreads throughout the myocardial syncytium, and all fibers contract as one, producing an "all-or-none" response. Skeletal muscle contraction can be made to simulate cardiac contraction by tetanization, during which muscle contractions are fused into a single, prolonged contraction by burst stimuli, creating an isometric phase of contraction similar to systole.

Skeletal muscle can be made to perform with increased fatigue resistance. This is possible because of a property skeletal muscle possesses known as muscle plasticity. Muscle plasticity allows skeletal muscle to respond to changes in neuromuscular activity with alteration in myofiber phenotype expression. Changes in neuromuscular activity can be artificially induced by low-frequency electrical stimulation, which affects genetic expression in Type II glycolytic, fast-twitch skeletal muscle. Type II fibers are converted to slow-contracting, oxidative Type I fibers with attributes similar to cardiac muscle, including much of its inherent resistance to fatigue. This transformation is typically accompanied by a 50% loss in power-generating capacity, but sufficient power remains to sustain work rates suitable for cardiac assist. Such transformation has been confirmed with histologic, morphologic, and functional testing in numerous animal and human studies, although the development of optimal

Department of Thoracic Surgery, Division of Cardiothoracic Surgery, Allegheny University Hospitals-Allegheny General, Pittsburgh, Pennsylvania 15212-4772 stimulation regimens for transformation remains under investigation.

SKELETAL MUSCLE FOR CARDIAC ASSIST

Multiple strategies have been used in the attempt to harness skeletal muscle power to augment cardiac output. The normal adult human heart supplies approximately 1 watt (W) of power in moving 5 L of blood against a 100-mm Hg afterload. Skeletal muscle ventricle techniques involve the construction of a contractile skeletal muscle pouch that is connected through a hydraulic system to the circulation. Skeletal muscle ventricles provide a maximum of about 0.2 W of power to the circulation, which is adequate for counterpulsation assist strategies based on a stroke volume of 40 to 50 mL.

Direct diastolic counterpulsation by circumferential wrap of a portion of the latissimus dorsi muscle (LDM) around the descending aorta trades a reduction in power for simplicity of application. Limited by the small volume of aortic blood displaced, maximum power output to the circulation is about 0.1 W. Laboratory studies have shown this technique to provide hemodynamic improvement similar to that of the intraaortic balloon pump.

Skeletal muscle ventricle and aortomyoplasty techniques operate at reduced levels of energy transfer because a wrapped configuration is less mechanically efficient than the normal *in situ* linear LDM contraction mode. Another approach to the use of skeletal muscle power is direct conversion of the muscle energy in linear LDM contraction to electrical or hydraulic power by means of a high-efficiency muscle energy collection device connected to the *in situ* LDM. This approach has three primary advantages: (a) decreased power loss, (b) less disruption to the LDM and thus a healthier muscle, and (c) availability of energy for a wide variety of mechanisms designed to exploit the energy output from the conversion device. Preliminary studies suggest that this strategy could supply approximately 1 W of power to a secondary mechanism. Development of prototype energy collection devices is in progress at our institution and at other laboratories.

In more advanced stages of heart failure, the myocardium needs to be stabilized and supported, as well as supplied with additional power to circulate blood. The use of electrically transformed and stimulated LDM to reinforce and augment the heart is termed "dynamic cardiomyoplasty."

Clinical and experimental studies of dynamic cardiomyoplasty have been ongoing since the mid-1980s. The historical origins of this concept as an outgrowth of early attempts to use unstimulated skeletal muscle to repair and reinforce ventricular defects is evident from the patient selection in early clinical trials of the procedure. Alain Carpentier used the technique in conjunction with resection of a large cardiac tumor in the world's first reported case, performed in Paris, in January, 1985. George J. Magovern performed cardiomyoplasty after

aneurysectomy in the first two cardiomyoplasty operations performed in the United States, in September, 1985, and February, 1986. The success of these initial procedures encouraged the use of the technique as an innovative surgical approach to therapy for heart failure. To date, over 500 procedures have been reported worldwide.

CLINICAL CARDIOMYOPLASTY: SURGICAL TECHNIQUE

Detailed descriptions of the procedure have previously been published (Figure 1). The LDM (usually the left LDM) is mobilized through a longitudinal flank incision extending from the axilla to a point proximal to the iliac crest. The LDM is released from its tendinous origin and insertion, preserving the neurovascular bundle. Chest wall-perforating vessels supplying the distal two thirds of the muscle are then woven into the axillary region of the

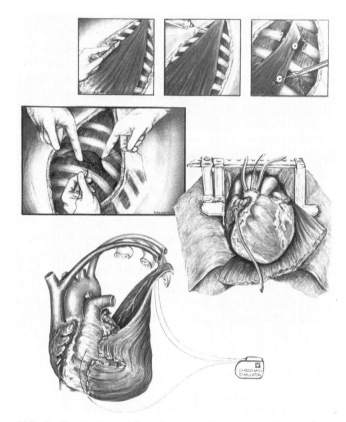

FIG. 1. Illustration of the steps involved in cardiomyoplasty surgery. The top panel shows mobilization of the latissimus dorsi muscle (LDM), injection of papaverine near the vascular pedicle to prevent vasospasm, and insertion of the muscle stimulation leads. The next panel demonstrates attachment of the tendon of the LDM to the bed of the resected rib, after first placing the muscle in the left hemithorax. The next drawing shows the left LDM inside the pericardial sac, before the muscle wrapping procedure. Pursestring sutures have been placed in the aorta and right atrium for cannulation in the event that cardiopulmonary bypass is needed. The bottom drawing shows the completed wrap, the muscle stimulator leads, the sensing lead on the right ventricle, and the cardiomyostimulator.

LDM for programmed stimulation of the muscle. One is placed adjacent to, but not in contact with the thoracodorsal nerve branches, and the second is placed 6 cm distal to the first. Transillumination of the muscle is used to aid in positioning the electrodes and to avoid injury to the neurovascular branches. The leads are temporarily attached to a pacemaker and stimulation thresholds and muscle contraction patterns are assessed.

A 5-cm section of the anterolateral second or third rib is removed and the muscle and its pedicle are translocated into the pleural space. The proximal humeral attachment of the muscle is fixed to the bed of the resected rib. Using a mid-sternotomy or left thoracotomy incision, the muscle is wrapped around the heart in one of several cuplike configurations to encompass primarily all of the left ventricle and most of the right ventricle (Figure 2). The geometric configuration of the wrap varies according to the size of the heart and the pathologic process. A posterior LDM wrap is often the choice used for global dysfunction and dilatation, whereas an anterior wrap may be better suited to regional dysfunction.

A sensing electrode is placed on the right ventricle and all leads are tunneled into a subrectus pocket in the abdominal wall and connected to a cardiomyostimulator. The most commonly used device has been the Medtronic SP1005/SP1005A cardiomyostimulator (Medtronic, Inc., Minneapolis, MN). This device senses the R-wave and stimulates the LDM to contract in synchrony with the heart. Echocardiography is used to fine-adjust the initiation of LDM contraction to the closing of the mitral valve. The Medtronic cardiomyostimulator is capable of delivering stimuli of variable duration, width, and voltage with a single- or multiple-impulse burst stimulus.

Right Latissimus Dorsi Cardiomyoplasty

In 1993, Furnary et al. analyzed the results of experimental studies on bilateral LDM cardiomyoplasty and documented significant ventricular augmentation from the right LDM alone. Further studies using the right LDM confirmed this finding, and the procedure was subsequently performed in at least one series of patients.

Mobilization and translocation of the right LDM is performed in a manner similar to that of the left LDM. Muscle wrap of the heart is done through a mid-sternotomy incision. The muscle is wrapped anteriorly, to avoid compression of the right atrium and inferior vena cava. The muscle does not encircle the heart in a cuplike configuration, but crosses the ventricles and is attached to the posterior pericardium to form a sort of muscular "sling." The procedure is then completed as described previously for left LDM cardiomyoplasty.

Concurrent Coronary Artery Bypass

At our institution, no patient undergoing cardiomyoplasty had evidence of significant ischemia on preoperative thallium scan. However, when a lesion of greater than 90% is identified in a proximal coronary artery, it is our practice to perform precautionary bypass grafting to prevent acute closure of the vessel in the perioperative period.

SKELETAL MUSCLE TRANSFORMATION AFTER CARDIOMYOPLASTY

A 6-week muscle-training program is begun after a 2-week recovery period. Twenty-four–hour stimulation is begun at the start of week 3 and continues for 6 weeks. Pulse frequency is gradually increased from 2 to 30 Hz during this period. At a constant pulse-train (burst) duration of 185 milliseconds, this schedule produces an

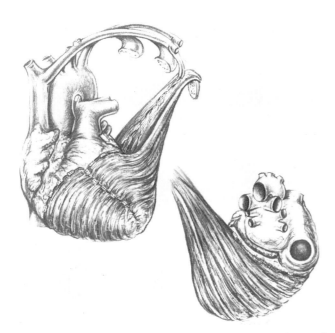

FIG. 2. View of a completed left latissimus dorsi muscle (LDM) cardiomyoplasty wrap, as shown from the anterior perspective (*top left*). View of a completed left LDM cardiomyoplasty wrap, as viewed from behind (*lower right*). The posterior aspect of the left ventricle is completely covered with skeletal muscle.

TABLE 1. *Stimulation schedule for latissimus dorsi muscle training*

Postoperative week	Frequency (H$_2$; pulses/sec)	Pulses/burst[a]
1, 2	No stimulation (recovery period)	
3, 4	2	1
5, 6	10	2
7, 8	15	3
9	20	4
10	25	5
11	30	6

[a]Burst duration is set at 185 msec throughout the training period. Pulse amplitude is set at twice the surgical threshold. Synchronization ratio is 2:1.

increase of one pulse per burst for each week of training, with the final burst containing six pulses. The synchronization ratio is set at 2 : 1 throughout this period (one LDM contraction occurs at every other cardiac cycle; Table 1).

PATIENT EVALUATION

At our institution, patients with heart failure are evaluated by a multidisciplinary heart failure group. Appropriate patients are referred for surgical options, including heart transplantation, coronary bypass, and cardiomyoplasty.

The standard evaluation protocol includes right and left heart catheterization with coronary angiography, echocardiographic assessment of valvular disease and ventricular function, and radionuclide multigated acquisition scan determination of left ventricular volume and right and left ventricular ejection fraction (LVEF). A myocardial viability study is used to identify reversible myocardial ischemia, and Holter monitoring is used to screen for significant arrhythmias.

Patients who appear to be likely candidates for transplantation undergo noninvasive assessment for peripheral vascular disease and carotid disease along with a complete psychosocial evaluation. Potential cardiomyoplasty patients complete metabolic exercise testing to evaluate myocardial oxygen consumption. A computed tomographic scan of the chest is performed to estimate the cardiothoracic ratio and the size of the LDM.

PATIENT SELECTION

Patients with reversible myocardial ischemia and operable coronary artery disease are offered coronary artery bypass, even in the absence of anginal symptoms. All remaining patients who qualify for heart transplantation are offered this option. Patients who do not qualify for coronary artery bypass or cardiac transplantation, or who choose not to be listed for transplantation, are considered for cardiomyoplasty.

Patients who are rejected for cardiac transplantation because of poor cardiopulmonary status are rarely acceptable for cardiomyoplasty. Cardiomyoplasty surgery is currently limited to those patients with evidence of sufficient cardiac reserve to withstand a major surgical procedure and the subsequent muscle training period. Cardiomyoplasty may, however, be a viable alternative for those patients denied transplantation because of age or psychosocial considerations.

In this country, cardiomyoplasty is performed under the guidelines of U.S. Food and Drug Administration (FDA) sponsored studies of the Medtronic cardiomyostimulator. The procedure may be offered to patients aged 18 to 80 years with New York Heart Association (NYHA) Class III

TABLE 2. *Selection criteria for dynamic cardiomyoplasty*

Inclusion
18–80 yr of age
NYHA Class III heart failure
Left ventricular ejection fraction 0.2–0.4
Available for postoperative follow-up study
Exclusion
Severe left heart failure (NYHA Class IV)
Significant right heart failure
Hypertrophic cardiomyopathy
Significant arrhythmia refractory to medical therapy
Irreversible pulmonary dysfunction (peripheral vascular resistance >3 Wood Units)
Renal or hepatic failure
Neuromuscular disease
Previous sternotomy

NYHA, New York Heart Association.

heart failure. LVEF must be less than 0.4 and greater than 0.2, and the patient cannot be dependent on intraaortic balloon pulsation or inotropic support (Table 2).

Patients with neuromuscular disease, renal or hepatic failure, or irreversible pulmonary dysfunction are excluded from surgery. Based on analysis of the initial clinical results in the United States, patients with biventricular failure (right ventricular ejection fraction < 0.4) or significant ventricular or atrial arrhythmia are unlikely to benefit from the procedure. Patients with previous cardiac operations are excluded because of the potential increased risks associated with resternotomy and anticipated complications with successful performance of the cardiac wrap.

RESULTS OF CLINICAL STUDIES

Allegheny General Hospital, 1985 to 1988

Five patients with ischemic cardiomyopathy underwent left LDM cardiomyoplasty. Standard dual-chamber pacemakers were used to stimulate the LDM in these first American clinical studies. Four patients were in NYHA Class IV and one patient was in NYHA Class III before surgery. Mean LVEF for the group was 0.29. All patients had concurrent cardiac surgical procedures—aneurysectomy or aneurysm repair in three patients and coronary artery bypass in two patients.

Three patients died of ventricular arrhythmia. These deaths occurred at 2, 28, and 28 months after surgery. Two patients are still alive more than 10 years after cardiomyoplasty. Pacemaker removal was necessary in one of these two patients 5 years after implant because of refractory infection. With the exception of the patient who died 2 months after surgery, all patients in this group demonstrated improvement in functional class (Figure 3). This subjective measure was not consistently matched by changes in hemodynamic parameters.

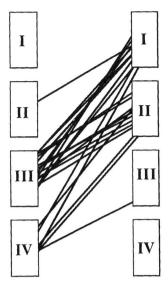

FIG. 3. Change in New York Heart Association Functional Class for patients who survived at least 6 months after cardiomyoplasty surgery.

Allegheny General Hospital, 1988 to 1991

This study was performed under an FDA Phase I protocol evaluating the safety and efficacy of the Medtronic SP1005 burst cardiomyostimulator. All patients were required to be in an advanced stage of heart failure for inclusion in this study. Ten patients were accepted for surgery—six with ischemic cardiomyopathy and four with idiopathic cardiomyopathy. Mean preoperative LVEF was 0.22. Concurrent surgery (coronary artery bypass) was performed in three patients.

There were four operative deaths in this group (three from cardiac failure, one from ventricular arrhythmia). Two patients died less than 6 months after operation (one from cardiac failure, one from ventricular arrhythmia). The remaining patients survived an average of 28 months (range, 7–49 months). All are now dead. Cause of death in the long-term survivors was cardiac failure in two patients and ventricular arrhythmia in two patients.

Left ventricular ejection fraction in the four long-term survivors increased to 0.31 after surgery ($p < 0.05$), and all of these patients improved by at least one NYHA functional class. Positive hemodynamic results failed to be sustained beyond 12 to 18 months postsurgery.

United States Combined Phase II Study, 1991 to 1993

Evaluation of the Medtronic burst stimulator (modified and designated as model SP1005A for this phase) was continued under an expanded FDA Phase II protocol involving 57 patients at 7 centers[1] in North and South America. Data analysis from the Phase I study was used to adjust selection criteria for Phase II. Thirty-seven patients (65%) had idiopathic cardiomyopathy, 19 patients had ischemic cardiomyopathy, and 1 patient had Chagas' disease. Fifty-two patients were in NYHA Class III before surgery; the remaining patients were in NYHA Class II (two patients) or NYHA Class IV (three patients). Mean preoperative LVEF was 0.22. Concurrent cardiac surgery was performed in four patients.

There were seven operative deaths (12%). Nineteen patients (33%) died between 1 and 21 months after surgery. Postdischarge deaths were largely due to arrhythmia (12/19, 63%). The remaining postdischarge deaths were due to cardiac failure in two patients and noncardiac causes in five patients.

Significant improvement in NYHA Class was seen in the 32 patients who survived at least 6 months after surgery. Before operation, 31 of these patients were in NYHA Class III, and 1 was in NYHA Class IV. At 6 months, 9 patients were in NYHA Class I, 16 patients were in NYHA Class II, and 7 patients were in NYHA Class III ($p < 0.001$). This pattern was repeated in the 12-month survivors.

Patients surviving at least 12 months after surgery had significant increases in LVEF (0.25 to 0.30, $p < 0.05$) and left ventricular stroke work index (26.1 to to 34.3 g m/m^2, $p < 0.05$). Improvement in ventricular wall motion, as measured by a segmental wall motion score, was also demonstrated in these patients ($p < 0.05$).

Allegheny General Hospital Phase II Subgroup, 1991 to 1993

Nineteen patients were studied under Phase II guidelines at our institution. Eight patients had idiopathic cardiomyopathy and 11 patients had ischemic cardiomyopathy. All patients were in NYHA Class III at the time of surgery. Mean preoperative LVEF was 0.26 in this group. Concurrent surgery (coronary artery bypass) was performed in two patients.

Perioperative myocardial infarction led to one operative death in this group; all other patients survived to discharge. Four deaths occurred less than 6 months after surgery, all due to arrhythmia. There were nine deaths between 9 and 43 months after surgery. Cause of death in these patients was arrhythmia in four patients and cardiac failure in five patients. Five patients are alive at 44 to 62 months postsurgery.

---

[1]Data from one center in Montreal, Canada, and one center in São Paulo, Brazil, were combined with data from the FDA study because these centers followed a protocol identical to that of the FDA Phase II study.

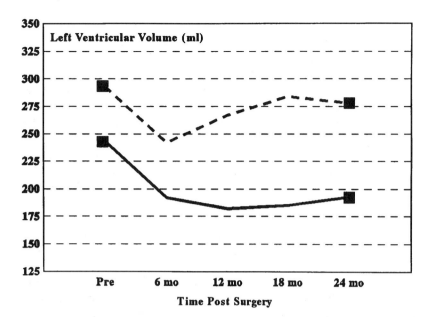

FIG. 4. Left ventricular volume determination (by multigated acquisition scan) in seven patients from the Allegheny General Hospital Phase II subgroup who survived at least 24 months after cardiomyoplasty surgery. Solid line represents the five patients with stabilization or decrease in left ventricular volume compared with preoperative baseline. Dashed line represents left ventricular volume data from all seven patients. (Two 24-month survivors are not included in this analysis because they did not have volume measurements performed at the 24-month time period.)

All patients who survived greater than 6 months had improvement in functional class, with a mean NYHA Class of 1.7.

Sixteen patients in this subgroup had cardiomyoplasty using the right LDM. These patients demonstrated impressive early increases in LVEF and reductions in left ventricular volume. At 6 weeks after surgery, LVEF had risen from 0.26 to 0.33 ($p < 0.03$). Left ventricular volume decreased concurrently with the increase in LVEF, although the decrease did not become statistically significant until 6 months after surgery (305 to 249 mL, $p < 0.01$). After the 6-month follow-up period, LVEF and left ventricular volume tended to return to baseline levels.

Stabilization of left ventricular volume at or below baseline levels was seen in five of the nine 2-year survivors in the Allegheny General Phase II subgroup (four patients with right LDM wrap and one patient with left LDM wrap; Figure 4).

CARDIOMYOPLASTY: MECHANISMS OF ACTION

Left Ventricular Systolic Augmentation

The cardiomyoplasty procedure was originally developed as a means of providing direct systolic assist through synchronous contraction of a myocardial LDM wrap. Experimental animal studies using diverse protocols have demonstrated evidence for systolic improvement after cardiomyoplasty. Cho et al. performed pressure–volume analysis of systolic function in the normal canine heart with trained LDM cardiomyoplasty. An increase in contractility was noted, but cardiac output was not affected because of a concomitant decrease in end-diastolic volume. In a model of heart failure induced by rapid ventricular pacing, Lee et al. found an increased

cardiac output, increased systolic shortening, and decreased left ventricular end-diastolic pressure. Cheng et al. demonstrated positive effects on both diastolic and systolic function in a canine model of doxorubicin-induced heart failure. In this study using both a chronic heart failure model and transformed LDM cardiomyoplasty, a comparison of stimulated versus unstimulated cardiac cycles revealed increases in peak ventricular filling rate, peak ventricular emptying rate, decreased left ventricular end-diastolic pressure, and increased LVEF.

Millner et al. reported on a comprehensive animal study that compared the hemodynamic effects of transformed LDM wrap, unstimulated LDM wrap, and unwrapped myocardium in three groups of sheep with chronic heart failure induced by coronary artery ligation. Hemodynamic function curves were recorded as the animals responded to increasing fluid challenge. Compared with animals with an unconditioned LDM wrap, stimulated cardiomyoplasty produced improvements in the function curves for left ventricular end-diastolic pressure, pulmonary capillary wedge pressure, and cardiac output. Similar improvement was noted when curves from the stimulated LDM group were compared with those for the group without cardiomyoplasty.

Impressive results have been achieved in laboratory trials with right LDM cardiomyoplasty. Significant hemodynamic improvement was first documented for the load-dependent parameters of aortic flow, aortic pressure, and left ventricular pressure. Further studies confirmed consistent, significant improvement in the load-independent parameter of preload recruitable stroke work, a sensitive measure of changes in contractility. In these studies, the stroke work was greater in cardiac cycles with LDM contraction than in those without LDM contraction (preload recruitable stroke work of 81 g·cm/cm³ with LDM contraction, vs. 64 g·cm/cm³ without LDM contraction). No effects on diastolic function were observed in these trials. It was hypothesized that the right LDM wrap was more advantageously oriented to assist systolic ejection because the right LDM contraction should compress the left ventricle in a direction parallel to the net vector of outflow through the aortic valve.

Evidence of systolic augmentation in clinical cardiomyoplasty trials has been inconsistent. Two of the four survivors from our first, small clinical series demonstrated improvement in LVEF with stimulated, as opposed to nonstimulated, LDM, and significant increases in LVEF were seen in the long-term survivors of the Phase I trial. Moreira and colleagues reported improved LVEF in a small series of patients operated on before 1990. The results of the Phase II combined trial included documentation of statistically significant effects on LVEF and left ventricular stroke work index. Early results with the right LDM cardiomyoplasty patient group at Allegheny General Hospital showed larger increases in LVEF. As in all clinical cardiomyoplasty trials, effects on systolic function were seen frequently, but not consistently, and the positive results were rarely sustained in later follow-up. These findings are important, however, in that they confirm that the procedure is capable of affecting systolic function.

Effects on Left Ventricular Morphology

Despite evidence of modest effects on postoperative hemodynamic function, clinical trial reports on cardiomyoplasty have consistently documented improvement in functional status as measured by the NYHA Class scale. This subjective finding was confirmed during the Phase II clinical trial, with significant positive results on a quality-of-life survey completed by patients before and every 6 months after surgery.

Additional mechanisms of action have been explored to help account for some of these findings. Studies using two different experimental models of heart failure, rapid ventricular pacing and coronary ligation, have documented a reduction in left ventricular dilatation with LDM wrapping of the failed heart. Similar effects were seen in patients during follow-up studies reported by Magovern and Carpentier. Cardiomyoplasty has thus been shown to delay or arrest the progressive ventricular dilatation that normally occurs in heart failure.

It has been suggested that the LDM can exert a "girdling" effect on the failing ventricle. Application of the LDM may increase the effective myocardial wall thickness, producing a reduction in wall stress. In a clinical investigation, Kass and associates evaluated hemodynamics in three cardiomyoplasty patients with the cardiomyostimulator turned off. Studies were performed at 6 and 12 months after surgery. Using conductance catheter techniques, the investigators documented improvement in left ventricular end-diastolic pressure, LVEF, right atrial

pressure, and a leftward shift in the left ventricular systolic pressure–volume relation. These effects were not changed by resumption of myostimulation and LDM contraction. The most reasonable explanation of these effects is that cardiomyoplasty can help to reverse the effects of chronic ventricular remodeling normally seen in heart failure. This process may be an important component of the long-term effects of cardiomyoplasty and may be responsible for some of the positive systolic effects noted in long-term survivors. Such a process would also represent the first therapeutic option for heart failure that targets the underlying cause of the disease.

FUTURE DIRECTIONS

Clinical and laboratory investigations of cardiomyoplasty have served to reveal the complexity involved with the application of this conceptually simple therapeutic approach to reduced cardiac output. These results are not consistent enough to suggest more extensive use of the procedure in the heart failure population at this time, especially considering that the procedure is most likely to produce benefits when performed in less seriously ill patients. Several key challenges have been defined by these studies, and practical solutions have been proposed.

Arrhythmia is the primary cause of death for cardiomyoplasty patients after hospital discharge, a finding that is not surprising in a population of patients with NYHA Class III to IV heart failure. Currently, options are limited for the cardiomyoplasty patient who fails medical management for arrhythmia. Implantation of an implantable cardioverter–defibrillator (AICD) is not recommended in these patients because little is known about possible interactions between the cardiomyostimulator and an AICD. A cardiomyostimulator incorporating AICD functions would be an ideal solution; however, development of strategies for the use of existing AICD devices in cardiomyoplasty patients can be expected to reduce mortality substantially.

Deterioration in hemodynamics and functional status has been noted in many patients who survive longer than 1 year after surgery. This observation has been confirmed in a study of the long-term effects of cardiomyoplasty in spontaneous canine cardiomyopathy. Postmortem examination of the LDM in cardiomyoplasty patients has revealed marked fibrosis, especially in the distal third of the muscle. Long-term stimulation of the LDM may not be feasible with the LDM training and maintenance protocol now in use. Transformation of fiber type in the wrapped LDM has been targeted to maximal fatigue resistance. With long-term stimulation, this goal appears to be met, with production of a muscle composed of primarily Type I fibers. Unfortunately, this fatigue resistance is conferred only with a concomitant loss in power. The goal of current studies has been to develop a stimulation protocol that produces a balanced muscle fiber mix, expressing both fatigue resistance and power.

Long-term use of burst stimulation patterns has also been shown to promote fibrosis in the LDM. Several clinical centers, including Allegheny General Hospital, have experimented with daily "rest" periods for the LDM. We have noted concurrent hemodynamic (LVEF) and functional improvement in some of our patients when this strategy is used, but the evidence is anecdotal.

In a clinical trial beginning in 1998, the cardiomyoplasty operation will be changed to a two-stage procedure to incorporate an adaptive "vascular delay" period for the mobilized LDM. During the stage one operation, the LDM is dissected from the chest wall, dividing the perforators and leaving the neurovascular bundle intact. The subcutaneous surface of the muscle is not dissected at this time, to retard the development of muscle edema. Mobilization with resection of the perforators, translocation, and cardiac wrap are performed during stage two, about 10 days later. This procedure has been routinely used in the laboratory to allow the LDM to produce new vascular patterns before translocation, especially in the distal LDM.

One explanation for patient-to-patient inconsistency in clinical results may be suboptimal synchronization between the cardiac cycle and LDM contraction. Schreuder and colleagues performed hemodynamic analysis in nine cardiomyoplasty patients in a range of synchronization delay periods. At optimal synchronization, a mean increase in cardiac output of 8% was demonstrated in stimulated compared with unstimulated cardiac cycles. Two of our patients have exhibited symptoms consistent with diastolic compromise. Analysis of echocardiographic studies in these patients appeared to show LDM contraction continuing into the diastolic phase of the subsequent cardiac cycle at the normal 2 : 1 stimulation schedule. Meticulous synchronization of LDM contraction to systolic ejection appears to be important for hemodynamic improvement. The new Medtronic Transform cardiomyostimulator, to be used in clinical trials beginning in 1996, features enhanced programmer control of LDM stimulation parameters. Studies with this device may help to resolve this issue.

One aspect of this procedure that has received little attention is the preoperative status of the LDM. Chronic heart failure has been shown to have deleterious effects on skeletal muscle metabolism. Howell et al. studied the effects on skeletal muscle of 6 weeks of heart failure induced by rapid ventricular pacing in an animal model. In the LDM, altered muscle blood flow, reduced contractile function, and abnormal metabolism were documented. Effects on force generation appeared to be more profound in the diaphragm, a slow-twitch, relatively fatigue-resistant muscle that is metabolically and histologically similar to the electrically transformed LDM. Thus, it appears that heart failure may affect the efficacy of the LDM first by reducing the capacity of the LDM to adapt to mobilization and translocation, and second by

decreasing the ability of muscle fibers to respond to long-term electrical stimulation.

Preoperative exercise regimens as well as transcutaneous electrical stimulation programs have been suggested as prophylactic interventions for the debilitated LDM, but no controlled trials have been reported. Fritzsche and associates described a series of animal studies in which an anabolic steroid was infused directly into the LDM during the training period. They report an acceleration in transformation to slow-twitch fiber patterns and an increase in force capacity in the steroid-treated LDM. Interpretation of these results has been controversial, but the idea of pharmacologic manipulation of the functional status of the LDM is an attractive concept.

SUMMARY

Heart failure is engendered by the loss of sufficient power to circulate blood. A long-term solution to this problem must include the restoration of effective pumping capacity to the myocardium. Use of the power generated by skeletal muscle is an appealing concept in theory, and many practical approaches for accomplishment of this task are under investigation. Cardiomyoplasty is the only such strategy that has been tested in the clinic. It remains one of the most viable experimental options for surgical treatment of heart failure because it appears to be capable of supporting and stabilizing the dysfunctional heart as well as supplying additional energy for pumping.

Results from clinical trials are too inconsistent to recommend more widespread use of cardiomyoplasty in the heart failure population at this time. However, sound laboratory investigations have demonstrated the potential of this technique, and realistic solutions have been proposed for the problems that have been encountered. A refined strategy for clinical application of cardiomyoplasty based on a more sophisticated understanding of the physiology and function of the LDM–myocardial complex is the goal of these efforts.

SELECTED REFERENCES

Acker MA, Hammond RL, Mannion JD, et al. Skeletal muscle as the potential power source for a cardiovascular pump: assessment in vivo. *Science* 1987;236:324–327.

Carpentier A, Chachques JC, Grandjean PA, et al. Dynamic cardiomyoplasty: a seven year clinical experience. *J Thorac Cardiovasc Surg* 1993;106:42–52.

Cheng W, Justicz AG, Soberman MS, et al. Effects of dynamic cardiomyoplasty on indices of left ventricular systolic and diastolic function in a canine model of chronic heart failure. *J Thorac Cardiovasc Surg* 1992;103:1207–1213.

Cho PW, Levin HR, Curtis WE, et al. Pressure–volume analysis of changes in chronic cardiomyoplasty. *Ann Thorac Surg* 1993;56:38–45.

Fritzsche D, Krakor R, Asmussen G, et al. Anabolic steroids (metenolone) improve muscle performance and hemodynamic characteristics in cardiomyoplasty. *Ann Thorac Surg* 1995;59:961–970.

Furnary AP, Magovern JA, Christlieb IY, et al. Component analysis of bilateral anterior cardiomyoplasty. *Ann Thorac Surg* 1993;55:72–77.

Howell, A, Maarek J-M, Fournier M, et al. Congestive heart failure: differential adaptation of the diaphragm and latissimus dorsi. *J Appl Physiol* 1995;79:389–397.

Kass DA, Baughman KL, Pak PH, et al. Reverse remodeling from cardiomyoplasty in human heart failure: external constraint versus active assist. *Circulation* 1995;91:2314–2318.

Lazzara RR, Trumble DR, Magovern JA. Dynamic descending thoracic aortomyoplasty: comparison with intraaortic balloon pump in a model of heart failure. *Ann Thorac Surg* 1994;366:366–370.

Lee KF, Dignan RJ, Parmer JM, et al. Effects of dynamic cardiomyoplasty on left ventricular performance and myocardial mechanics in dilated cardiomyopathy. *J Thorac Cardiovasc Surg* 1991;102:124–131.

Magovern JA, Magovern GJ Sr. Cardiomyoplasty. In LR Kaiser, IL Kron, TL Spray, editors: *Mastery of cardiothoracic surgery.* Boston: Little, Brown and Company, 1996:574–582.

Magovern JA, Magovern GJ, Maher TD, et al. Operation for congestive heart failure: transplantation, coronary artery bypass, and cardiomyoplasty. *Ann Thorac Surg* 1993;56:418–425.

Magovern GJ, Simpson KA. Clinical cardiomyoplasty: review of the ten-year United States experience. *Ann Thorac Surg* 1996;61:413–419.

Millner RWJ, Burrows M, Pearson I, Pepper JR. Dynamic cardiomyoplasty in chronic left ventricular failure: an experimental model. *Ann Thorac Surg* 1993;55:493–501.

Moreira LFP, Stolf NAG, Jatene AD. Benefits of cardiomyoplasty for dilated cardiomyopathy. *Semin Thorac Cardiovasc Surg* 1991;3:140–144.

Orton C. *Controversies in skeletal muscle assist* [Panel discussion]. Presented at the 42nd Annual Conference of the American Society for Artificial Internal Organs, Washington, DC, May 2–4, 1996.

Park SE, Cmolik BL, Lazzara RR, Trumble DR. Right latissimus dorsi cardiomyoplasty augments left ventricular systolic performance. *Ann Thorac Surg* 1993;56:1290–1294.

Schreuder JJ, van der Veen FH, van der Velde ET, et al. Beat-to-beat analysis of left ventricular pressure–volume relation and stroke volume by conductance catheter and aortic model flow in cardiomyoplasty patients. *Circulation* 1995;91:2010–2017.

Tobin G, Gu J-M, Tobin A-E. *Latissimus dorsi flap loss in cardiomyoplasty: anatomic basis and prevention by delay*. Presented at the World Symposium on Cardiomyoplasty, Biomechanical and Artificial Heart, Paris, France, May 24–26, 1993.

Trumble DR, LaFramboise WF, Duan C, Magovern JA. Functional properties of conditioned skeletal muscle: implications for muscle-powered cardiac assist. *Am J Physiol* 1997;273:C588–C597.

Management of End-Stage Heart Disease, edited by Eric A. Rose and Lynne Warner Stevenson. Lippincott–Raven Publishers, Philadelphia ©1998.

CHAPTER 20

Myocyte Transplantation

Clifford H. Van Meter, Jr.

The marked discrepancy between the number of patients with end-stage heart disease and the number of organs available for orthotopic transplantation has given rise to a plethora of clinical and laboratory research to develop and evaluate alternative strategies. Within the realm of myocardial enhancement, therapies have developed in the fields of cellular transplantation and genetic manipulation. In contradistinction to the use of new knowledge in molecular biology and genetic manipulation to lessen or prevent injury, this effort attempts to use these emerging technologies to repair or rebuild damaged myocardium.

Adult heart muscle has no capacity to regenerate after injury to the myocardium and therefore, once a significant amount of cardiac mass is damaged, the patient is prone to development of intractable heart failure that may be responsive only to cardiac transplantation. The unique characteristics of the mammalian cardiac muscle cell are the key to unlocking its potential for regeneration and at the same time provides the very obstacles that block the road to success in cardiac cellular transplantation. Complete understanding of the mechanisms that control the myocyte cell cycle could allow us to design manipulations or procedures that might initiate a more complete repair or regeneration of adult myocardium after injury. These strategies could involve transplantation of pluripotent myocytes into damaged heart muscle that could replicate and regenerate to a degree that functional muscle would result. Likewise, these cells could induce a reversion of cardiac cells in the hibernating transition zone to the biochemical state in which they existed during early fetal growth, when they still had the capability simultaneously to differentiate and proliferate.

Unlike skeletal muscle, cardiac muscle cell differentiation is unique in that it occurs early in fetal life in the dividing cell. It is believed that the reason for this is that the heart is one of the first organs to form during development and, as such, gains function while it is still growing by cell division. Inasmuch as cardiac cells continue to divide as they differentiate, it has been postulated that they may have two separate developmental programs for terminal differentiation. Parallel research is attempting to identify the genes that control myocyte differentiation as well as the myocyte cell cycle. The unlocking of this code might obviate the need for cellular transplantation by permitting an alteration of the biochemical environment and allowing viable but nonfunctional cells to regenerate.

In the rat, for example, it is known that at approximately days 17 to 20 of postnatal development, hyperplastic growth ceases for the life of the animal. The increase in muscle mass of the heart from that time on is due exclusively to hypertrophy of preexisting cells. It has been estimated that this hypertrophy may result in a more than tenfold increase in volume to form the adult myocyte. Why this mode of hypertrophy is a functional one resulting in the mature healthy adult myocyte, and later modes of hypertrophy are dysfunctional ones resulting in the cardiomyopathic heart, is one of the questions that remains to be answered in this complex and poorly understood phenomenon.

The use of skeletal muscle to augment the failing heart can take the form of cardiomyoplasty, aortic wraps as a counterpulsation device, or as a skeletal muscle ventricle in series with the patient's heart. Skeletal muscle myoblast implantation has also been used as a form of biologic augmentation. Experiments have been conducted into the skeletal muscle's ability to regenerate after injury. The presence of satellite cells capable of dividing and growing allows this muscle to repair itself. Satellite cells have been implanted in patients with neuromuscular disease in the hope of regenerating muscle function. Satellite cells have also been injected into the hearts of both mice and swine. These cells grow in this

Division of Cardiothoracic Surgery and Transplantation, Ochsner Foundation Hospital, New Orleans, Louisiana 70121 living matrix, but studies thus far do not confirm the presence of gap junctions. In addition, there is an inflammatory response of some degree associated with this implantation. This raises the question of whether this model of cellular transplantation will become maximally functional by accomplishing electrical coupling between transplanted cells and cardiac muscle cells and facilitating the cell-to-cell interactions that are necessary for coordinated function.

More recent areas of investigation have focused on the use of fetal muscle cells that may still have the ability to divide. Such cells are harvested and placed into the recipient adult myocardium. Early experiments in this area have focused on the use of syngeneic mouse cardiomyocytes. Subsequent genetic modification of cells so that they are more apt to grow after injection has also been reported.

This chapter discusses a series of experiments beginning with genetically modified cell lines and including neonatal, fetal, and adult myocytes. These cells were obtained from *in vitro* co-culture or cell harvest and used in a series of small animal experiments and ultimately in adult swine. We trace the progress from co-culture experiments to syngeneic and xenogeneic injection in rodents, followed by fetal and neonatal myocyte injections in rodents, to the current model of large animal xenogeneic transplants.

Once successful viability of transplanted myocytes has been confirmed, evaluation of electrical activity and function must be evaluated. I present our initial results in these areas of investigation, and finally discuss our hopes for future studies and potential clinical applications.

CO-CULTURE EXPERIMENTS

Initial experiments using day-old neonatal rat ventricular cardiomyocytes were conducted. The cells were isolated by the protocols of Claycomb and Palazzo and modified after Claycomb and Lanson. This technique, as previously described, involves harvesting of hearts from anesthetized rats with subsequent attachment to a Frederick's condenser and retrograde perfusion with *Joklik's* medium, followed by a collagenase preparation. Once softened, the hearts can be minced and subjected to subtle fresh collagenase digestion to allow the collection of washed, pooled cells. Once plated, these cells grow to confluence. The effort to develop a cell system that could be used to study cardiac muscle cell cycles advanced significantly when it was reported that the large T-antigen of the SV40 virus, under control of the atrial natriuretic factor promoter, induced large tumors composed of dividing myocytes in the right atria of transgenic mice. A tumor line (AT-1) was subsequently developed from these mice that was shown to actively synthesize DNA and divide in culture. After plating, the AT-1 tumor cells formed a synchronously contracting monolayer. Dramatically, as the cells divided, they would pull away from adjacent myocytes, cease beating, and progress through mitosis; subsequently, the daughter cells would resume beating shortly after division. These collective studies demonstrate that highly differentiated adult cardiac myocytes from both the ventricle and the atrium can be stimulated to divide without the loss of their highly differentiated state. These cardiomyocytes exhibit all the morphologic characteristics associated with

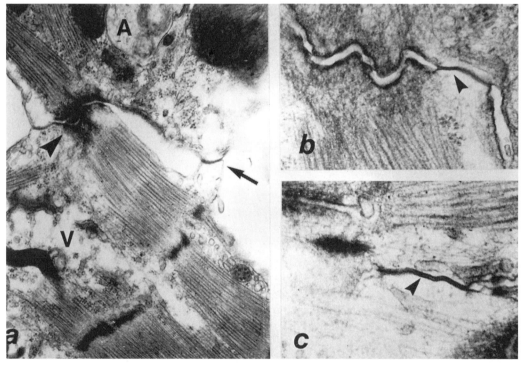

FIG. 1. Co-culture of adult rat ventricular cardiomyocytes (*V*) with AT-1 cells (*A*). Arrows indicate gap junctions (transmission electron microscope [EM] magnification 9000×).

adult cardiac myocytes. Co-cultured adult rat ventricular cardiomyocytes with neonatal rat cardiomyocytes or AT-1 cells were noted to form gap junctions (Figure 1). This was confirmed by immunohistologic chemical staining for the connexin protein, pan-cadherin. This *in vitro* work confirmed the assumption that by using either genetically altered or undifferentiated cells, xenogeneic cell transplantation was feasible.

SYNGENEIC AND XENOGENEIC INJECTIONS IN RODENTS

The second phase of experiments focused on transplantation of the the AT-1 cell by direct injection into the adult rat ventricle. The AT-1 cells were prepared as previously described, and this time were injected into syngeneic mice and immunosuppressed rats. Transplantation was accomplished by direct injection into the left ventricular wall, and cyclosporine A was administered by a gavage feeding. Histologic analysis indicated that in both models, the AT-1 cells formed nascent intercalated disks with each other and with host myocytes. Contractile proteins and atrial granules were also present (Figure 2).

The demonstration that these genetically altered AT-1 tumor cells would grow and form apparent gap junctions with host myocytes led to a subsequent series of experiments using myocytes with the potential to differentiate into adult cells.

FETAL AND NEONATAL MYOCYTE INJECTIONS

Fetal and neonatal mouse and rat cardiomyocytes were isolated by established protocols. In this process, cells are prepared by a series of saline rinses and subsequent trypsin and collagenase digestions. After final rinsing and pooling, the cells were injected into the adult rat and again were found to grow in the host myocardium and form rudimentary intercalated disks. Microscopy of the cells at this point indicated a more neonatal morphology (Figure 3). The experiments did, however, suggest that it would be possible to use neonatal allogeneic or even xenogeneic cells potentially to repair damaged host myocardium. An additional encouraging finding of these experiments was a noted increase in angiogenesis at the area of cell injection (Figure 4). This neovascularization indicated that the repair process could potentially augment the vascular supply not only to the transplanted cell, but to other areas of the ischemic host.

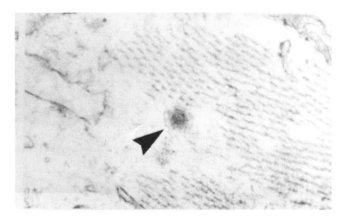

FIG. 3. Neonatal rat myocyte injected into adult rat ventricle. Note disordered contractile proteins to upper right of arrow (EM magnification 9000×).

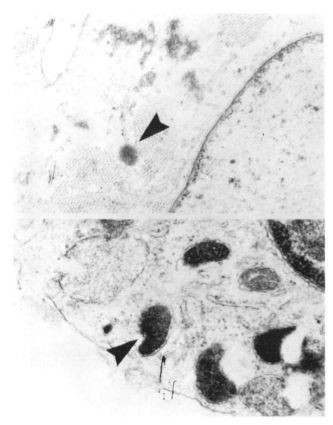

FIG. 2. AT-1 cell transplanted into adult rat ventricle. Arrow indicates atrial granule (EM magnification 9000×).

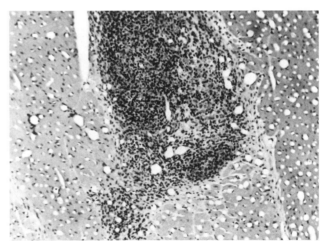

FIG. 4. Injected fetal rat myocytes in adult rat. Note marked angiogenesis in the area of cell injection (hematoxylin and eosin, magnification 400×).

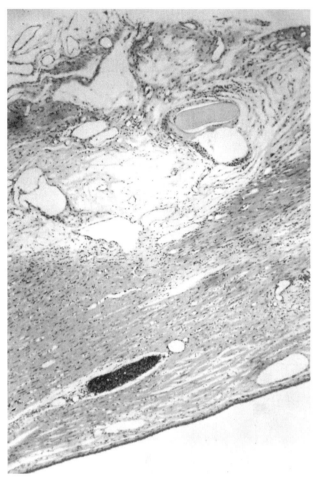

FIG. 5. Proline suture marking site of injection in adult pig myocardium (hematoxylin and eosin, magnification 400×).

LARGE ANIMAL XENOGENEIC TRANSPLANTATION

A series of experiments was then undertaken to determine if adult swine would accept these cells and cell lines. The swine model was chosen because of the similarity of the swine's coronary anatomy to that of humans and the consequent ease of creating percutaneous infarctions in these animals. Adult Yorkshire swine were anesthetized with ketamine and pentobarbital, intubated, and ventilated with isoflurane by a pressure-controlled ventilator. Long-term, subcutaneous-infusion catheter venous access was accomplished. Bretylium and diltiazem were given by infusion to prevent dysrhythmia. Under aseptic surgical technique, a median sternotomy was performed and a pericardial well created. Isolated cardiomyocytes in Joklik's medium were directly injected into the myocardium with a 26-gauge needle using a tuberculin syringe. Approximately 1 × 10 cardiomyoblasts were transplanted with each injection, in a volume of approximately 100 μL. Additional control injections were performed using 100 μL of Joklik's medium alone. Injection sites were marked with a 7-0 Prolene suture into the myocardium in the area of injection (Figure 5). The sternotomy was closed and the pericardial and thoracic spaces evacuated of residual air.

Animals were started on an immunosuppressive protocol consisting of oral cyclosporine to maintain levels of 150 to 300 ng/dL by TDX (Abbott Laboratories, Abbott Park, IL) assay. The animals were also given prednisone at a dose of 0.3 mg/kg/day. Creatinine kinase (CK) and CKMB isoenzyme fractions were obtained within 24

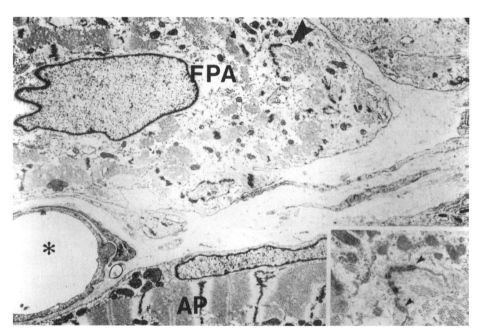

FIG. 6. Fetal pig atrial myocytes (*FPA*) injected into adult pig ventricle (*AP*). Asterisk identifies new vessel aligned with endothelial cell (EM magnification 9000×).

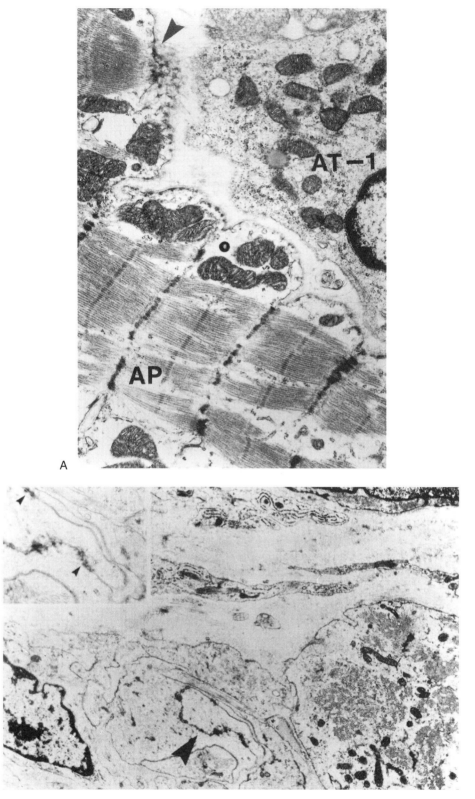

FIG. 7. A: AT-1 cells (AT-1) in adult pig ventricle (*AP*) (EM magnification 9000×). **B:** Arrows indicate nascent gap junction (magnification 100×) (EM magnification 33,300×).

hours of injection. There were no significant increases in CK or CKMB levels, indicating no myocardial death from the cellular implantation. No animals had significant illness, and all survived to subsequent harvest. Two had postoperative fevers related to local inflammation at the area of the venous access, and responded to antibiotic therapy.

At the end of 1 month, the animals were again anesthetized and under sterile conditions the chest was opened through a median sternotomy. Dissection was undertaken to free adhesions and the animals were heparinized. The great vessels were isolated and the beating heart excised. Selective cannulation of the left and right coronary arteries was accomplished and flushing with saline was followed by infusion of a buffered 4% paraformaldehyde–1% glutaralehyde fixative for 40 minutes. The excised hearts were then fixed an additional 7 days in 4% glutaraldehyde–0.1 molar sodium cacodylate. The injection sites were then identified and 1 cm² areas around these sites excised and rinsed for an additional week in 0.1 molar sodium cacodylate buffer with frequent changes. The blocks were further sectioned and prepared appropriately for light and electron microscopy.

Neonatal rat myocytes, AT-1 cells, neonatal porcine myocytes, and fetal human atrial and ventricular myocytes were implanted into the adult pig ventricle. In all of these experiments, cells were identified in the transplanted region. There appeared to be no gross encapsulation or significant inflammatory cell response that would indicate significant rejection of the allogeneic or xenogeneic transplanted cells. In addition, in all injection sites there was a demonstrated marked increase in neovascularization that was thought to be a result of cellular transplantation (Figure 6). Sham injections of Joklik's medium containing no cells did not result in this degree of neovascularization.

Using electron microscopy, nascent junctional contacts between host ventricular cardiomyocytes and transplanted AT-1 cells have been identified (Figure 7), again suggesting that in the large animal, these transplanted cells may also significantly add to the overall contractile mass of damaged host myocardium.

CELLULAR TRANSPLANTATION INTO DAMAGED MYOCARDIUM

Infarcts were performed in adult Yorkshire swine after anesthesia with ketamine and phenobarbital under isoflurane anesthesia delivered by pressure ventilation. The femoral artery was identified and cannulated with an introducer sheath and coronary angiography performed with Renografin (E. R. Squibb, Inc., Princeton, NJ). A 5-Fr H1 embolization catheter was then placed and maneuvered down the left anterior descending artery or one of the obtuse marginal coronary arteries. A copper embolization coil (Cook Co.) was then placed using a 0.035 guidewire for deployment. Myocardial infarction was confirmed electrocardiographically by the presence of marked ST segment evaluation. Occlusion was confirmed by repeat coronary angiography. High doses of bretylium and diltiazem were administered to prevent fibrillation, and standby DC cardioversion was prepared in case of arrhythmias. With this model, approximately 60% to 70% of the animals survived a myocardial infarction and went on to recover for 1 month.

At the end of that time, the animals were prepared in a fashion similar to that previously described, with a median sternotomy. The zone of myocardial infarction was easily identified by direct visualization. The infarct zone at that time was confirmed through the use of a Doppler thickening probe placed on the surface of the myocardium, which measured myocardial thickening in the region of interest (Figure 8). These ultrasonic microcrystal probes generate the measurable curves in normal myocardium, and demonstrated myocardial thinning in the region of infarction (Figure 9). These probes were left in place, sutured to the cardiac surface with 7-0 Prolene sutures. AT-1 cells and neonatal pig myocytes were then implanted in the area of infarction and at the border zone between infarcted tissue and normal myocardium. The sternotomy was closed, and the animals were maintained on an immunosuppressive regimen as previously described for a month.

The animals were again anesthetized per protocol; however, this time repeat readings were taken before sacrifice with the Doppler thickening probe in the area of interest to determine if there was physiologic improvement in myocardial function. Preliminary data indicate that there needs be some improvement in the function of the myocardium, and studies are ongoing to delineate the overall myocardial thickening and electrical activity of

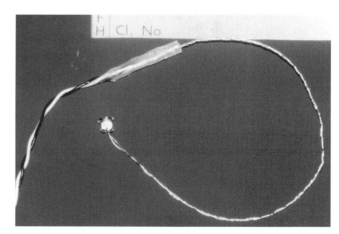

FIG. 8. Microcrystal Doppler thickening probe.

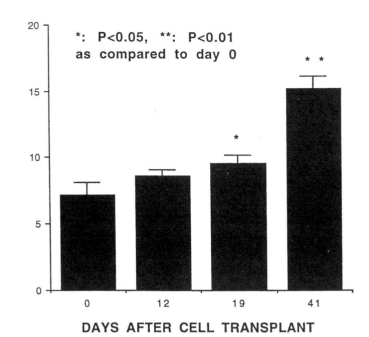

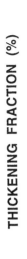

FIG. 9. Ultrasonic probe-generated data demonstrating increasing thickening fraction in region of infarct after cellular transplantation.

the cells in the region of interest by measurement of monophasic action potentials.

The micrographs in Figure 10 depict the neonatal pig cells transplanted into an infarct zone. The transplanted cells can be seen growing in the center of a zone of infarction with no normal myocardium adjacent. Even in the area of infarction, these cells are able to grow and induce neovascularization, which would be necessary for the overall improvement in function required in a recipient with ischemic cardiomyopathy.

GROWTH FACTOR-ENHANCED CELLULAR TRANSPLANTATION

The use of myoblast transplantation has generated much interest in the repair of damaged myocardium. With the presence of neovascularization in the area of transplanted cells, the question to be explored is whether the direct injection of certain chemokines responsible for angiogenesis would improve collateral flow in patients who had ischemic cardiomyopathy. The direct injection

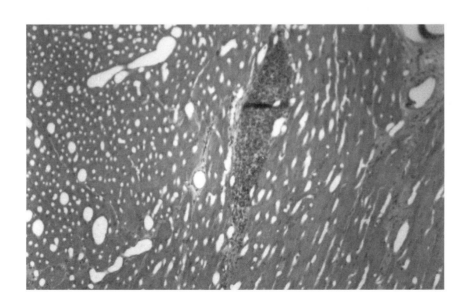

FIG. 10. Neonatal pig cardiomyocytes injected into adult pig infarct (hematoxylin and eosin, magnification 400×).

of vascular endothelial growth factor (VEGF), basic fibroblast growth factor (FGF), and sham injections was carried out in an effort to induce neovascularization in both normal and infarcted tissue in the adult swine. The injection process was similar to that used in myoblast transplantation, and the VEGF and FGF were injected both as liquid compounds and bound to heparin-bonded agarose microcarrier beads.

In preliminary studies, there was an increase in vascularity in the basic FGF- and VEGF-injected sites that was most evident with the injection of the heparin-bonded beads alone. This series of ongoing experiments poses the clinical question of whether the direct injection of these compounds would increase neovascularization in both damaged and normal cardiac tissue, with the potential end-point of improved blood flow throughout the myocardium. This type of therapy would be akin to trans-myocardial laser revascularization in terms of neovascularization, but would potentially be accomplished at a lower cost. It might be possible to do this procedure percutaneously by intracoronary injection of growth factors at the time of coronary angiography.

Although the clinical possibilities are exciting, the basic line of research is just beginning, and the methodology with regard to dosing and carriers is still being developed.

FUTURE STUDIES OF MYOCYTE TRANSPLANTATION AND POTENTIAL CLINICAL APPLICATIONS

Tremendous strides have been made in the field of myocyte transplantation since the initial development of tumor cell lines and successful *in vitro* co-culturing. Results of these initial experiments are encouraging in that they indicate the possibility of repairing certain hearts with either allogeneic or xenogeneic transplanted cells. Direct transplantation of neonatal or genetically altered cardiomyocytes could result in three mechanisms of action for repair of a failing myocardium. First, an actual increase in viable myocytes could be induced in adequate mass to achieve functional repair. Whether these cells differentiate and manifest adult contractile proteins remains to be seen; without any impediment to the ability to differentiate, and retention of the capability to replicate, it is presumed that these cells will be able to multiply and produce adequate amounts of adult contractile protein. Second, the profound angiogenesis noted at the areas of transplantation implies that these cells can be used to induce repair of damaged myocardium by their ability to induce neovascularization. This appears to occur even in zones of infarction (Figure 11), and may play as important a role in myocardial repair as the contractile function of the cells themselves. Finally, it is conceivable, but less probable, that the presence of these cells that retain the ability to divide and differentiate may alter the chemical and hormonal milieu of the dilated model of heart failure such that cells may dedifferentiate and again realize their capacity for self-repair.

This field of study may provide valuable knowledge about and insight into areas parallel to myocyte transplantation with equal or greater potential for clinical application. Increased understanding of the mechanisms that control the myocyte cell cycle and terminal differentiation may allow future investigators to design manipulations that initiate repair or regeneration of failed myocardium. In addition, considerable insight into the field of xenogeneic transplantation is gained on the cellular level. It is possible that the amount of rejection present in these transplanted xenogeneic cells is significantly less than that seen in whole-organ xenographs because of a lack of cell surface markers in isolated neonatal myocytes. The use of pure myocytes with no endothelial

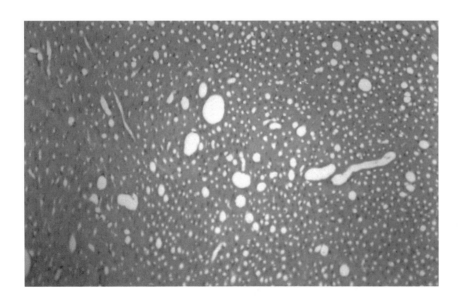

FIG. 11. Infarcted adult pig myocardium remote from area of myocyte transplantation. Note marked neovascularization (hematoxylin and eosin, magnification 300×).

cells in the transplantation model may explain why the recognition of the major histocompatibility complex antigens seem to be less strong than in the whole organ.

Clearly, we have barely begun to realize the possible clinical and research benefits of cardiomyocyte transplantation. Although it has the potential to act as a patch to repair a damaged heart, further investigation of this technique will offer a wide array of knowledge that, when applied, can potentially decrease the need for solid organ transplantation and ultimately expand our knowledge of transplantation as a whole.

SELECTED REFERENCES

Claycomb WC. Biochemical aspects of cardiac muscle differentiation, DNA synthesis and nuclear cytoplasmic deoxyribonucleic acid polymeric activity. *J Biol Chem* 1975;250:3229–3235.

Claycomb WC. Control of cardiac muscle cell division. *Trends in Cardiovascular Medicine* 1992;2:231–236.

Claycomb WC, Lanson NA Jr. Isolation and culture of the terminally differentiated adult cardiac muscle cell. *In Vitro* 1984;20:647–651.

Claycomb WC, Palazzo MC. Culture of the terminally differentiated adult cardiac muscle cell: a light and scanning electron microscope study. *Dev Biol* 1980;161:249–265.

DelCarpio JB, Barbee RW, Perry BD, Claycomb WC. Cardiomyocyte transfer into the mammalian heart: cardiac growth and regeneration. *Ann NY Acad Sci* 1995;752:267–285.

Delcarpio JB, Lanson NA Jr, Claycomb WC. Morphological characteristics of cardiomyocytes isolated from a transplantable cardiac tumor derived from transgeneic mouse (AT-1 cells). *Circ Res* 1991;69: 1591–1600.

Field LJ. Atrial natriuretic factor-SV40 T-antigen transgenes produced tumors and cardiac arrhythmias in mice. *Science* 239:1029–1033.

Kao RL, McGovern JA, Tong JY, McGovern GJ. Muscle regeneration of injured myocardium. *J Cell Biochem* 1991;45[Suppl 15C]:73(abstr).

Kiortsis V, Koussoulakus S, Wallace H, ed. *Recent trends in regeneration research*. New York: Plenum Press, 1989.

Koh GY, Klug MG, Soonpaa MH, Field LJ. Long-term survival of C2 C12 myoblast grafts in part. *J Clin Invest* 1993;92:1548–1554.

Mauro A. Satellite cell of skeletal muscle fibers. *Journal of Biophysical and Biochemical Cytology* 1961;9:493–497.

Rumyantsev PP, ed. *Growth and hyperplasia of cardiac muscle cells*. New York: Academic Press, 1991.

Smart F, Claycomb W, DelCarpio J, Van Meter C. Cultured cardiomyocytes. In: Cooper DK, Miller LW, Patterson GW, eds. *Transplantation and replacement of thoracic organs*. London: Kluwer Academic, 1992; 785–795.

Soonpaa MH, Koh GY, Klug MG, Field LJ. Formation of nascent intercalated disks between grafted fetal cardiomyocytes and host myocardium. *Science* 1994;264:98–101.

Zibaitis A, Greentree D, Ma F, et al. Myocardial regeneration with satellite cell implantation. *Transplant Proc* 1994;26:3294.

Management of End-Stage Heart Disease, edited by Eric A. Rose and Lynne Warner Stevenson. Lippincott–Raven Publishers, Philadelphia ©1998.

CHAPTER 21

Ventriculectomy

Patrick M. McCarthy, Vigneshwar Kasirajan, Randall C. Starling, Nicholas G. Smedira, and James B. Young

The media have focused a great deal of attention on the Batista procedure (partial left ventriculectomy, or left ventricular volume reduction surgery). Although there are fundamental reasons to think that this operation holds promise for some patients with end-stage cardiomyopathy, more research and follow-up are needed before the true role of this procedure becomes clear. In addition, the operation is so new that most reports are anecdotal, and manuscripts are in preparation or not yet published by peer-reviewed journals. Therefore, in this chapter we briefly outline what we think are the important points of the rationale for the Batista procedure, our early clinical experience, and what we anticipate for future investigations.

RATIONALE FOR THE BATISTA PROCEDURE

The concept of reducing heart size to improve cardiac function is not new. Even before coronary bypass surgery, the beneficial effects of ventricular aneurysmectomy on left ventricular end-diastolic pressure and clinical symptoms had been reported. More recently, medical therapies, such as angiotensin-converting enzyme (ACE) inhibitors or carvedilol, have shown that pharmacologic effectiveness correlates with decreased left ventricular end-diastolic volume and improved left ventricular ejection fraction. The novel concept introduced by Randas Batista was to remove left ventricular muscle, not scar, and thereby decrease wall tension (by a reduction in radius) according to the law of LaPlace. Batista reasoned that he was returning the heart to a more normal mass-to-diameter ratio and that it would therefore function as a more efficient pump. Furthermore, computer-generated models confirm the beneficial effect of reduction in left ventricular diameter on left ventricular function.

We believe that an important part of the operation that acts synergistically with reduction of left ventricular volume is repair of the associated mitral valve lesion found in patients with dilated cardiomyopathy. Reports indicate that even patients with severe left ventricular dysfunction and 4+ mitral regurgitation show clinical improvement after mitral valve repair. As part of his operation, Batista would sew the anterior and posterior mitral valve leaflets together (Alfieri repair) to reduce mitral regurgitation (Figure 1).

What is missing from the rationale behind the Batista procedure has been animal experiments. Unfortunately, most existing animal models do not simulate the expected chronic outcome after the Batista procedure. However, several centers are developing models to test the procedure.

We recognized that, at present, we are on the learning curve regarding patient selection, surgical techniques, and perioperative care. Our initial indications for surgery were patients that met the following criteria: (a) a left ventricular end-diastolic diameter of at least 7 cm on at least one recent echocardiogram, (b) New York Heart Association (NYHA) Class III to IV heart failure despite optimal medical therapy, and (c) confirmed heart transplantation candidacy. The latter was chosen to make the operation as safe as possible for patients during our earliest applications. We reasoned that patients who did not improve after the Batista procedure could be relisted for heart transplantation, and patients who failed after surgery could receive an implantable left ventricular assist device (LVAD) as a bridge to transplantation. A series of baseline, intraoperative, and postoperative studies were then designed for patients undergoing the procedure. This report briefly outlines the earliest experience at the Cleveland Clinic Foundation.

Departments of Thoracic and Cardiovascular Surgery, Cleveland Clinic Foundation, Cleveland, Ohio 44195

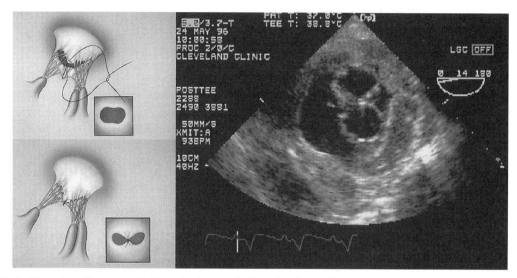

FIG. 1. To reduce the central jet of mitral regurgitation, the free edges of the anterior and posterior mitral leaflets are sewn together to create a double-orifice mitral valve. Also, a Cosgrove-Edwards ring was used for posterior annuloplasty. (Reproduced with permission from McCarthy PM, Starling RC, Wong J, et al. Early results with partial left ventriculectomy. *J Thorac Cardiovasc Surg* 1997;114:755–765.)

PARTIAL LEFT VENTRICULECTOMY WITH MITRAL VALVE REPAIR

Patient Population

Between May 1996 and August 1997, 57 patients were chosen out of thousands of potential referrals for the Batista procedure. Fifty-four patients (95%) were deemed candidates for heart transplantation. Three patients were not deemed suitable candidates for transplantation because of elevated age or significant co-morbidities. All patients were thought to have idiopathic dilated cardiomyopathy, and one patient had familial cardiomyopathy. Of the patients referred for the Batista procedure meeting our inclusion criteria, most were rejected because they were "too well" (including some patients already listed for transplantation elsewhere), and for these patients, continued or increased medical therapy was recommended. Therefore, the patient population reflects advanced heart failure despite optimal medical therapy. Most patients were in NYHA Class IV (61.4%) at the time of surgery. Others were in Class III (36.8%), but had had previous hospitalizations, and had previously displayed Class IV symptoms. One patient was on implantable LVAD support, but the device was infected and the patient showed signs of cardiac recovery. At the time of surgery, 40% of the patients were hospitalized and were receiving at least one inotrope; three patients were also on intraaortic balloon pumps. Baseline hemodynamic studies (despite a high incidence of inotropic support) documented cardiac failure with a mean cardiac index of 2.1 ± 0.6 L/minute/m², pulmonary artery pressures of 51 ± 12, 36 ± 8, and 27 ± 8 mm Hg (systolic, mean, and diastolic, respectively), and a pulmonary capillary wedge pressure of 24 ± 8 mm Hg. Peak oxygen consumption was 10.6 ± 4 mL/kg/minute. By echocardiographic examination, forward left ventricular ejection fraction averaged $13.5\% \pm 6\%$, left ventricular end-diastolic diameter averaged 8.1 ± 1 cm, and mitral regurgitation was 2.8 (range, 0–4+).

Surgical Approach

The surgical technique evolved from our earliest surgeries, which were very similar to those used by Batista in Brazil (mitral valve repair using the Alfieri technique only, and left ventricular resection on a beating heart). Because of reports of postoperative exsanguinating hemorrhage through the suture line, all patients had closure of the ventriculotomy with strips of felt (Figure 2). As the

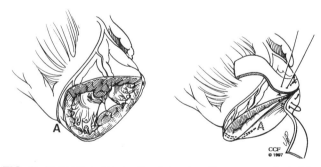

FIG. 2. In most patients, the lateral wall was resected. After reinforced closure, the left anterior descending at the apex (*point A*) was wrapped around the new apex. (Reproduced with permission from McCarthy PM, Starling RC, Wong J, et al. Early results with partial left ventriculectomy. *J Thorac Cardiovasc Surg* 1997;114 [*in press*].)

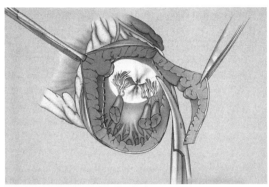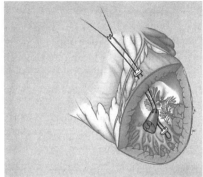

FIG. 3. To remove more left ventricular wall and further reduce left ventricular size, one or both papillary muscles were transected and the head of the papillary muscle was resuspended. (Reproduced with permission from McCarthy PM, Starling RC, Wong J, et al. Early results with partial left ventriculectomy. *J Thorac Cardiovasc Surg* 1997;114:755–765.)

experience progressed, more complex mitral valve repairs were added, including a posterior annuloplasty using a Cosgrove-Edwards ring in 95% of patients. Moreover, in a significant proportion of patients (53%), resection of one or both papillary muscles to allow further ventricular resection with resuspension of the resected papillary muscle heads through the ventriculotomy was undertaken (Figure 3). Medical therapy of heart failure was resumed after surgery (digoxin, diuretics, maximum tolerated ACE inhibitors), and warfarin was added because of the risk of left atrial or ventricular thrombus. Amiodarone (200 mg/day) maintenance was administered because of reports of sudden death in the Brazil experience.

Results

There were two in-hospital mortalities, one from multiorgan failure and one from pneumonia. Ten patients (17.5%) required early LVAD insertion because of marginal cardiac function. Of these, one patient had recovery of cardiac function and was later weaned from LVAD support. Five patients were transplanted, and two are well on LVAD support. Excluding LVAD patients, the mean intensive care unit length of stay was 3 days, and mean hospital length of stay was 12 days. Hospital charges were significantly less than for patients undergoing transplantation, including patients who failed.

Patients were reactivated for transplantation if they clinically deteriorated and did not improve despite adjustments in medical therapy. The actuarial survival rate 1 year after surgery was 82.1%, and freedom from relisting for transplantation, death, or need for LVAD was 58% (mean follow-up, 9 months). Three patients died of sudden cardiac death, three of recurrent heart failure, and one after transplantation. This 1-year survival rate is similar to that for a cohort of patients undergoing transplantation at the Cleveland Clinic for dilated cardiomyopathy since 1990. Multivariate analysis of preoperative,

echocardiographic, and intraoperative variables showed age younger than 40 years to be the only significant risk factor for failure. However, younger patients were statistically different from those older than 40 years of age with regard to increased inotrope need, higher incidence of Class IV failure, and higher pulmonary artery pressure.

On follow-up, most patients were symptomatically improved (mean preoperative NYHA Class of 3.7; 2.2 at follow-up). Peak oxygen consumption significantly increased from 10.6 ± 4 to 15.4 ± 4.5 mL/kg/minute ($p < 0.001$). Perioperative changes in left ventricular volume were sustained, with 3-month left ventricular end-diastolic diameter reduced to 6.3 ± 0.9 cm ($p < 0.001$ vs. baseline) and improvement in forward ejection fraction from $13.6\% \pm 6\%$ to $23\% \pm 7.7\%$ ($p < 0.001$).

CONCLUSIONS AND FUTURE DIRECTIONS

The theoretic considerations previously outlined, coupled with the long-term survival of some patients undergoing the Batista procedure in the Brazil experience, warrant that this operation undergo further investigation. Another compelling argument in support of partial ventriculectomy is the need for new strategies for patients with end-stage cardiac failure. The number of donors is woefully inadequate for human heart transplantation, and other alternatives like permanent LVAD insertion and xenotransplantation are limited or unavailable.

It is not known whether the Batista procedure will become a practical alternative for patients with end-stage heart disease. Only further follow-up and rigorous scientific scrutiny will determine the role of this operation. It is our initial clinical impression that patient selection will be improved with the use of dobutamine echocardiography, cardiac magnetic resonance imaging, positron emission tomography scans, and a favorable clinical response to dobutamine. The occurrence of late sudden cardiac death in three of our patients has led us to initiate a trial of implantable cardioverter–defibrillator use in all patients after surgery (patients will be randomized to the use of amiodarone). Depending on the results of our initial experience, it may be that a randomized clinical trial will be needed for widespread acceptance of this procedure. The practical barriers to performing this clinical trial, however, are formidable, and include limited enrollment, lack of sponsoring agency or company, and variable surgical technique in a multicenter study.

Based on this early experience, observation of long-term survivors from Brazil, and early experience from other selected centers, we do think that the operation should continue to be investigated. Whether the Batista operation will play a role in the treatment of end-stage cardiomyopathy remains unanswered.

SELECTED REFERENCES

Bach DS, Bolling SF. Early improvement in congestive heart failure after correction of secondary mitral regurgitation in end-stage cardiomyopathy. *Am Heart J* 1995;129:1165–1170.

Batista RJV, Nery P, Bocchino L, et al. Partial left ventriculectomy to treat end-stage heart disease. *Ann Thorac Surg* 1997;64:634–638.

Batista RJV, Santos JLV, Takeshita N, et al. Partial left ventriculectomy to improve left ventricular function in end-stage heart disease. *J Card Surg* 1996;11:96–97.

Bocchi E, Moraes AV, Bacal F, Moreira LF, Stolf N. Clinical outcome after surgical remodeling of the left ventricle in candidates to heart transplantation with idiopathic dilated cardiomyopathy: short-term results. *Circulation* 94[Suppl 1]I:172(abstr).

Bolling SF, Deeb GM, Brunsting LA, Bach DS. Early outcome of mitral valve reconstruction in patients with end-stage cardiomyopathy. *J Thorac Cardiovasc Surg* 1995;109:676–683.

Cosgrove DM, Arcidi JM, Rodriguez L, et al. Initial experience with the Cosgrove-Edwards annuloplasty system. *Ann Thorac Surg* 1995;60:449–504.

Dickstein ML, Spotnitz HM, Rose EA, Burkhoff D. Heart reduction surgery: an analysis of the impact on cardiac function. *J Thorac Cardiovasc Surg* 1997;113:1032–1040.

Favaloro RG. Ventricular aneurysm: clinical experience. *Ann Thorac Surg* 1968;6:6627–6645.

Fucci C, Sandrelli L, Pardini A, et al. Improved results with mitral valve repair using new surgical techniques. *Eur J Cardiothorac Surg* 1995;9;621–627.

Hogness JR, Van Antwerp M, eds. *The artificial heart: prototypes, policies, and patients.* Washington, DC: National Academy Press, 1991:4.1–4.18.

James K, Starling R, Sapp S, et al. Economic comparison of two surgical therapies for heart failure: ventricular remodeling versus cardiac transplantation. *Circulation* 1997(abstr) [Suppl 1]I:368.

Konstam MDA, Rousseau MF, Kronenby MV, et al. Effects of the angiotensin converting enzyme inhibitor enalapin 7 on the long-term progression of ventricular dysfunction in patients with heart failure. *Circulation* 1992;86:431–438.

McCarthy JF, McCarthy PM, Starling RC, et al. Partial left ventriculectomy and mitral valve repair for end-stage congestive heart failure. *Eur J Cardiothorac Surg* 1998.

McCarthy PM, Starling RC, Wong J, et al. Early results with partial left ventriculectomy. *J Thorac Cardiovasc Surg* 1997;114:755–765.

Packer M, Bristow MR, Cohn JN, et al. The effect of carvedilol on morbidity and mortality in patients with chronic heart failure. *N Engl J Med* 1996;334:1349–1355.

The SOLVD Investigators. Effect of enalapril on mortality and the development of heart failure in asymptomatic patients with reduced left ventricle ejection fraction. *N Engl J Med* 1992;327:685–691.

Management of End-Stage Heart Disease, edited by Eric A. Rose and Lynne Warner Stevenson. Lippincott–Raven Publishers, Philadelphia ©1998.

AFTERWORD

Novel Cardiac Replacement Therapies

A Vision for the Future

Daniel J. Goldstein, Maria Rosa Costanzo, and Eric A. Rose

Despite advances in the understanding of the pathophysiologic mechanisms underlying congestive heart failure—from the molecular to the organ level—end-stage heart disease refractory to maximal medical therapy continues to claim the lives of approximately 40,000 patients every year in the United States. Although heart transplantation is an accepted therapy for end-stage heart disease, some serious obstacles preclude its widespread application. These include the critical shortage of donor hearts because of the inability of donor organ supply to meet the demands of the increasing number of potential heart transplantation candidates, and the high incidence of allograft coronary artery disease, which is the main limiting factor to long-term survival in heart transplant recipients. According to data from the United Network for Organ Sharing (UNOS), approximately one third of the patients awaiting solid organ transplantation die before a suitable donor organ becomes available. Angiographic allograft coronary artery disease occurs in approximately 50% of the recipients by 5 years after heart transplantation. These observations underscore the crucial need for alternatives to human heart replacement, despite the unquestionable ability of heart transplantation to improve the quality of life and lengthen the survival of patients with end-stage heart disease.

Currently, both biologic and mechanical alternatives to human heart replacement are being studied. The common denominator of these investigational approaches is the replacement or functional augmentation of the diseased native heart.

BIOLOGIC ALTERNATIVES

Concordant Xenotransplantation

Until relatively recently, the use of closely related primate donors (concordant xenotransplantation) was considered by many investigators to be the most promising alternative to human heart replacement. Unfortunately, the primates most suitable for this purpose—chimpanzees, gibbons, and orangutans—are all endangered species, and therefore the use of their organs for the transplantation of human recipients would quickly decimate the existing populations. Conversely, the use of nonendangered primates, such as baboons and cynomolgus monkeys, as organ donors is limited by blood type incompatibiliies and their small size, which make them unsuitable for adult human recipients.

Regulatory and ethical barriers, coupled with the concerns expressed by virologists that lethal infections, such as those caused by the human immunodeficiency or Ebola viruses, may be transmitted from primate donors to human recipients, have severely hindered scientific progress in this field. Because of these concerns, neither the U.S. Food and Drug Administration (FDA) nor the Centers for Disease Control and Prevention have been able to define their positions on concordant xenotransplantation.

Discordant Xenotransplantation

Discordant xenotransplantation (transplantation of human recipients with organs from nonprimate donors) is

D. J. Goldstein and E. A. Rose: Department of Surgery, Columbia-Presbyterian Medical Center, New York, New York 10032

M. R. Costanzo: Department of Medicine, Rush-Presbyterian-St. Luke's Medical Center, Chicago, Illinois 60612 currently the subject of intense investigation. However, our understanding of discordant xenotransplantation is still insufficient to justify the use of this approach in clinical trials.

Pigs have been studied as potential donors of discordant xenoorgans for several important reasons. These include pigs' ABO blood type compatibility with the human species, and the virtually unlimited supply of these animals. In addition, because approximately 90 million pigs are killed every year by the food industry, the ethical issues regarding the use of pigs as organ donors have not been the subject of the bitter controversy that surrounds the retrieval of organs from primate donors. Many other attributes increase the likelihood for the successful transplantation of pig organs into human recipients. A useful feature of pigs is the wide range of sizes of these animals to accommodate the diverse physiologic and geometric needs of human recipients. Of even greater importance for the successful clinical application of discordant xenotransplantation has been the creation of transgenic pigs that express the genes coding for human thrombomodulin, CD59, and inhibitors of complement activity and thrombosis. The pivotal significance of these scientific advances is underscored by the knowledge that activation of the complement cascade by human natural antibodies directed against pig glycoprotein antigens and the resulting widespread thrombosis are the principal mechanisms mediating destruction of the xenoorgan.

Indeed, research in the field of xenotransplantation has primarily focused on overcoming hyperacute rejection. More recent experimental evidence, however, has shown that the rejection barrier to successful discordant xenotransplantation is far more complex than previously anticipated. In this regard, experiments conducted by Michler and colleagues in a pig-to-baboon xenotransplantation model have shown that the rejection mediated by natural killer cells, noncomplement-dependent antibody-induced cytotoxicity, and direct neutrophil responses is an immune mechanism that can still destroy xenoorgans after they have survived hyperacute rejection. These findings clearly indicate that a much greater understanding of acute and chronic xenoorgan rejection is crucial before discordant xenotransplantation can become a clinical reality.

Fetal Myoblast Transplantation

Another current focus of intense investigation in the area of human heart replacement is the substitution of damaged myocardial tissue with allogeneic or xenogeneic fetal or neonatal myoblasts (analogous to the efforts that have been directed toward the transplantation of fetal brain cells for the treatment of Parkinson's disease). *In vitro* and *in vivo* experiments have shown that cellular engraftment is achievable, that gap junctions and intercalated disks are formed between transplanted neonatal cells and host myocytes, and that extensive neovascular-ization of normal and damaged myocardium occurs. Furthermore, when xenogeneic cells are transplanted, rejection is less severe than that occurring against a whole xenoorgan because of the absence of xenoantigens on the surface of neonatal myocytes. Additional efforts in the area of myoblast transplantation are focused on measurement of the electrical activity and contractile function of the engrafted cells. Despite considerable progress in this area, two critically important questions awaiting conclusive answers pertain to the magnitude and duration of the augmentation of contractile function attributable to the transplanted cells.

SURGICAL AND MECHANICAL ALTERNATIVES

High-Risk Conventional Cardiovascular Surgery

Until the aforementioned alternatives to human heart replacement become clinically applicable, every effort should be made to identify and treat reversible causes of heart failure, such as ischemia, valvular disease, and arrhythmias. Indeed, high-risk surgical revascularization, by recruiting hibernating myocardium and protecting the remaining normal myocardium, has been shown to produce significant hemodynamic and functional improvement in many patients with ischemia-induced left ventricular dysfunction. Growing experience also indicates that valve replacement or repair can significantly benefit patients in whom left ventricular dysfunction is worsened by mitral regurgitation due to ischemic heart disease or dilated cardiomyopathy. Because approximately 50% of patients with advanced heart failure die unexpectedly, and a high proportion of sudden death is caused by cardiac dysrhythmias, the detection and treatment of these life-threatening events has the potential of significantly improving survival of patients with end-stage heart disease. In patients with malignant ventricular tachyarrhythmias complicating a ventricular aneurysm, cardiac transplantation can be deferred or avoided if the life-threatening arrhythmias can be controlled with aneurysmectomy or ablation of the arrhythmic foci, in combination with high-risk revascularization. The results presented in this book by our surgical colleagues suggest that these high-risk, conventional surgeries will be used with increasing frequency in an attempt to forestall the progression of cardiomyopathy and relieve the pressure on the scant supply of donor organs.

Dynamic Cardiomyoplasty

Some investigators have proposed to provide accessory contractile function for the failing myocardium by using transformed skeletal muscle. This approach requires the mobilization of the latissimus dorsi muscle, which is subsequently wrapped around both ventricles. The muscle is then connected to a pacer–stimulator that makes it possible for the muscle to contract in synchrony with the heart. The action of the pacer–stimulator transforms the skeletal muscle over a period of 6 to 8 weeks into a fatigue-resistant, spontaneously contracting muscle. Although the pacing algorithms and geometric configuration of the wrap have been significantly improved, the role of cardiomyoplasty in the treatment of patients with advanced heart failure has not yet been defined. Results of clinical trials conducted in more than 300 patients have shown that in patients with New York Heart Association (NYHA) Class IV heart failure, dynamic cardiomyoplasty is associated with mortality rates as high as 23% in the early perioperative period and an additional 20% in the short to medium term. Although survival has been reported to be much better in patients with NYHA Class III heart failure, it remains unclear why these patients, who in general improve with optimal medical therapy, should be subjected to such an extensive surgery. The effects of dynamic cardiomyoplasty on exercise tolerance and quality of life were studied in nonrandomized trials, and therefore remain unproven. In addition, there have been reports in long-term survivors that the hemodynamic and functional improvements are not sustained because of fibrosis occurring in the transformed skeletal muscle. These observations underscore the need for further investigation before dynamic cardiomyoplasty can become an acceptable type of biologic circulatory support.

MECHANICAL ALTERNATIVES

External Blood Pumps

The successful use of external blood pumps has been limited by serious complications, such as hemorrhage, thromboembolism, and infection, that ultimately result in multiple organ failure.

Because of these life-threatening complications, the use of these devices should be limited to short-term circulatory support in patients who cannot be weaned from cardiopulmonary bypass after high-risk cardiovascular surgery. In addition, because patients supported with external blood pumps are bedridden, these pumps cannot be used as long-term mechanical bridges to heart transplantation.

Implantable Blood Pumps

The development of implantable left ventricular assist devices (LVADs) undoubtedly represents the most significant advance in the field of mechanical circulatory support. The development of *fully implantable* LVADs has been the focus of intense investigation. However, many remaining obstacles have precluded their clinical application. These include inadequate device reliability, the development of a compliance chamber, the need for reop-

eration in the event of device failure, and the requirement for life-long anticoagulation. Therefore, although fully implantable systems are obviously more desirable, critically important technical refinements are needed before these devices can be tested in long-term clinical trials. The current clinically applicable alternative to fully implantable mechanical circulatory support devices are the "wearable" LVADs, of which the Heartmate (Thermo Cardiosystems, Woburn, MA) and Novacor (Baxter Healthcare Corporation, Novacor Division, Oakland, CA) LVADs are examples. Although still tethered to external power sources, patients supported with these devices can enjoy unrestricted ambulation and independence because of technical advances that have significantly reduced the size of the control and power units.

The experience gained in patients requiring LVADs as a bridge to transplantation has confirmed that these devices are effective for short- and medium-term support of the circulation, and has imparted valuable lessons regarding the use of the LVADs as a permanent alternative to, rather than a temporary substitute for heart transplantation. It has become apparent, for example, that hemodynamic stability can be successfully achieved with left ventricular support alone in more than 90% of the patients, even in the presence of significant right ventricular dysfunction. In this setting, the achievement of adequate circulatory support is contingent on effective replacement of the left heart and treatment of pulmonary vascular hypertension. To achieve these goals, it is critical that blood loss and transfusion of blood products be minimized by the use of meticulous hemostatic techniques and blood-sparing agents such as aprotinin. The LVAD investigators now widely recognize that the transfusion of blood products, prompted by intraoperative bleeding, worsens pulmonary vascular hypertension, which in turn leads to refractory right heart failure and death. Another valuable lesson learned from the use of LVADs as bridges to transplantation is that the use of porcine inflow and outflow valves and of textured blood-contacting surfaces is associated with a risk of thromboembolic events lower than that observed with the use of mechanical valves and of smooth blood-contacting surfaces. Textured blood-contacting surfaces are less thrombogenic because they become covered by a tenacious thrombus that evolves into a stable pseudointimal layer. Because of the decreased risk of thromboembolic events, most patients undergoing the implantation of LVADs with textured blood-contacting surfaces do not require long-term anticoagulation with warfarin and receive only antiplatelet agents, such as aspirin. Observations made in LVAD recipients indicate that at in least 33% of these patients, infections develop originating from the exit site of the transcutaneous connections. Rigorous daily wound care and prompt initiation of the appropriate antimicrobial therapy are critical measures to prevent these infections from becoming life threatening.

The length of the experience with the use of LVADs as bridges to transplantation is approximately 10 years. This considerable experience has enabled the definition of patient selection criteria, refinement of device operation, and characterization of patient adaptation to the devices. The use of the wearable LVADs is associated with attenuation of the myocardial histologic abnormalities produced by chronic heart failure, decreased neurohormonal activation, improvements in end-organ function, and enhancement of quality of life. The latter is attributable to the ability of LVAD recipients to enjoy unrestricted ambulation, participate in physical rehabilitation programs, and eventually be discharged from the hospital. The clinical improvement that can be achieved with the wearable LVADs, the acceptable complication rates, and the critical donor organ shortage justify the evaluation of wearable LVADs as a permanent alternative rather than as mere "bridges" to heart transplantation in patients with heart failure refractory to optimal medical therapy.

The efficacy and safety of LVADs has persuaded the FDA to grant an investigational device exemption to compare wearable LVADs with maximal medical therapy in patients with advanced heart failure in a randomized, clinical trial called Randomized Evaluation of Mechanical Assistance for the Treatment of Congestive Heart Failure (REMATCH). The study population will consist of patients with NYHA Class IV heart failure who remain highly symptomatic despite maximal tolerated medical therapy, including intermittent or continuous intravenous inotropic support. In addition, patients can be enrolled in the REMATCH trial only if they are *not* suitable candidates for heart transplantation. The rationale for the exclusion of these patients from the study is that crossovers to heart transplantation would confound the results of the trial.

The primary hypothesis of the REMATCH trial is that the 2-year survival rate of the patients randomized to undergo implantation of wearable LVADs will be 25% greater than that of patients assigned to continue maximal medical therapy. Exercise tolerance, quality of life, and cost effectiveness of the wearable LVADs are some of the important variables that will be assessed in the REMATCH trial. If the LVADs are found to be superior to medical therapy in terms of functional improvement and costs, the role of mechanical circulatory assistance as an accepted treatment of advanced heart failure will be firmly established.

MANAGEMENT OF END-STAGE HEART DISEASE: CURRENT AND FUTURE OPTIONS

The magnitude of the impact the previously discussed technologies will have on the treatment of the growing population of patients with end-stage heart failure is not known.

Current Options

The therapeutic options for patients with end-stage heart failure remain limited (Figure 1). Patients with chronic end-stage heart failure are commonly treated with a pharmacologic regimen that includes digoxin, diuretics, and angiotensin-converting enzyme (ACE) inhibitors. Since the late 1980s, the respective roles of these drugs have undergone profound changes. The ACE inhibitors have become the mainstay of heart failure therapy. The results of large, multicenter, randomized trials have unequivocally shown the benefits of ACE inhibitors in terms of survival, functional capacity, and hospitalization in all patients with chronic left ventricular dysfunction, regardless of etiology and severity of symptoms. Current recommendations include the use of ACE inhibitors at the doses shown to produce benefits in the large clinical trials, and the indefinite use of ACE inhibitors in patients with *symptomatic* left ventricular dysfunction. Unfortunately, only approximately 50% of patients with heart failure are receiving ACE inhibitors, and vigorous efforts to educate the medical community are needed to translate the recommendations that have emerged from the trials into clinical practice. Trials have also shown the effectiveness of angiotensin II receptor antagonists. Because angiotensin II antagonists block the effects of the renin–angiotensin–aldosterone system at the tissue level, these drugs can be used in patients who experience intolerable adverse effects related to ACE inhibitor-induced inhibition of bradykinin breakdown. The role of digoxin has been reevaluated in two withdrawal studies and in a large survival trial called the DIG (Digitalis Investigator Group) trial. The results of these studies suggest that withdrawal of digoxin is associated with more frequent episodes of decompensation in patients with symptomatic heart failure. Digoxin, however, does not appear to have an appreciable effect on survival. Thus, although digoxin is no longer considered as the first-line drug for the treatment of left ventricular dysfunction, its use is recommended in patients with advanced, symptomatic heart failure. The use of diuretics is recommended for patients with symptomatic volume overload. In patients without this condition, diuretics, by reducing the effective blood volume, produce further neurohormonal activation and therefore may hasten rather than delay the progression of heart failure. If heart failure symptoms persist despite the use of digoxin, diuretics, and ACE inhibitors, direct arterial vasodilators, such as hydralazine and nitrates, can be added to the therapeutic regimen. The discovery that myocardial receptors are downregulated during heart failure, and that beta blockade results in receptor upregulation, has led to the study of the effects of beta blockers in patients with heart failure. The Metoprolol in Dilated Cardiomyopathy (MDC) trial has shown that this selective blocker of beta$_1$ receptors reduced the combined end-point of death and

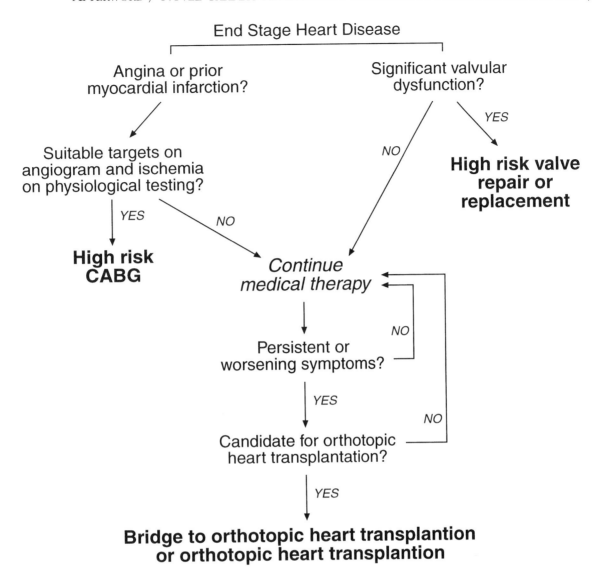

FIG. 1. Current options in the management of end-stage heart disease.

need for heart transplantation in patients with nonischemic, dilated cardiomyopathy. More recently, the nonselective beta blocker carvedilol has been shown to improve symptoms, functional capacity, and survival and to decrease hospitalization rates in patients with mild to moderate heart failure. A larger study is needed to determine if carvedilol produces similar benefits in patients with severe, NYHA Class IV heart failure. Some issues regarding the use of beta blockers in patients with heart failure need further definition. These include the identification of patients who can derive the greatest benefit from beta blockade, and the optimal doses of these drugs.

Technical surgical refinements, improved methods of myocardial preservation, and optimization of perioperative care have enhanced the odds that patients with ischemic or valvular heart disease complicated by heart failure might derive significant clinical benefits from high-risk revascularization or valvular repair or replacement. In appropriately selected patients, the hemodynamic and functional improvement achievable with conventional cardiovascular surgery is such that heart transplantation can be deferred of even avoided. A successful surgical outcome depends critically on the identification of enough viable myocardium and the preoperative optimization of the hemodynamic condition.

Because of the availability of the aforementioned therapeutic strategies, *only* patients requiring repeated hospitalizations for decompensation of heart failure refractory to medical or surgical therapy should be evaluated as potential candidates for heart transplantation. Candidates who deteriorate before a suitable donor heart becomes available can be offered the option of implantation of a wearable LVAD. Recipients of LVADs are automatically listed for urgent heart transplantation and maintain this priority status even when they become clinically stable. The possibility that stable LVAD patients be listed for heart transplantation at a lower priority status is being seriously considered by UNOS. This change would prevent the use of LVADs from affecting the order in which donor hearts are allocated.

Since the early 1980s, heart transplantation has progressed from a rarely performed experimental procedure to a widely accepted therapy for end-stage heart disease. The success of heart transplantation is no longer controversial. Unfortunately, very few therapeutic options are available to several subgroups of patients with end-stage heart disease. These include patients who have absolute contraindications to heart transplantation, recipients of heart transplantation in whom accelerated allograft coronary artery disease develops, and victims of acute hemodynamic collapse. The patients currently lacking effective therapeutic options may become the principal beneficiaries of the mechanical circulatory support devices under development.

Future Directions

Future Role of Cardiac Transplantation

Heart transplantation will likely remain a viable therapeutic option for patients with end-stage heart disease, despite the severe limitations imposed by third-party payors on the reimbursement of expensive therapies. However, the widening discrepancy between the number of patients with end-stage heart failure and that of donor hearts has resulted in a progressive prolongation of the waiting times. Thus, an increasing number of waiting patients deteriorate to the point of requiring continuous intravenous inotropic support before a suitable donor heart becomes available. The consequence of this disturbing trend is that the already scarce donor hearts are being allocated with decreasing frequency to ambulatory patients.

If, however, the use of mechanical circulatory support devices becomes more prevalent, patients with advanced heart failure will likely be in a situation similar to that of patients with end-stage renal disease. Patients with heart failure that progresses to end-stage disease will have the option of undergoing the implantation of an LVAD, with the understanding that mechanical circulatory support may be continued indefinitely. The subset of recipients of long-term mechanical assistance who are deemed suitable candidates for heart transplantation will undergo the procedure in the event that a donor heart becomes available.

The increased use of mechanical assistance in patients with end-stage heart failure may improve heart transplan-

tation outcome and reduce health care costs. The hemodynamic and clinical benefits produced by mechanical assistance convert high-risk, terminally ill patients into stable heart transplantation candidates. Because these patients can subsequently return to their homes, the costs resulting from repeated hospitalizations of critically ill patients in the intensive care unit will be dramatically reduced.

After heart transplantation, mechanical assistance may be used to rescue patients whose allograft fails either acutely or chronically because of coronary artery disease. In the setting of allograft coronary artery disease, mechanical assistance can be used either as a bridge to a second heart transplantation or as a permanent alternative to human heart replacement.

Acute Cardiogenic Shock

Some subsets of patients with severe heart failure are not appropriate candidates for the implantation of wearable LVADs. These include patients with cardiogenic shock, patient with chronic heart failure that acutely decompensates despite the administration of intravenous inotropic agents, patients who cannot be weaned from cardiopulmonary bypass, or heart transplant recipients with early or late allograft failure.

The intraaortic balloon pump (IABP), which is the most commonly used type of short-term mechanical circulatory support, can successfully rescue patients with cardiogenic shock occurring in the setting of an acute myocardial infarction. The IABP, however, has had limited success in the treatment of acute heart failure due to nonischemic heart diseases, such as acute myocarditis. The limitations of the IABP and the ineffectiveness of LVADs in patients with cardiogenic shock have spurred the increased use of short-term circulatory support devices at some centers. The use of short-term mechanical assistance is also appropriate when the possibility exists that cardiac function might normalize. In addition, devices for short-term support of the circulation may be life saving in patients who require transfer to centers equipped for the implantation of LVADs.

In the first decade of the 21st century, the indications for the use of short-term circulatory support devices are likely to be expanded by the development of modified compression pumps surrounding the heart, of a refined Abiomed BVS 5000 external pulsatile assist device (Abiomed Cardiovascular, Inc., Danvers, MA), and of new centrifugal pumps.

The widespread clinical implementation of the total artificial heart lags several years behind that of implantable LVADs. It is predicted that continued governmental support will enable clinical testing of the total artificial heart within the first decade of the 21st century. Potential candidates for the implantation of the total artificial heart include patients with prohibitive contraindications to heart transplantation, and recipients with allograft coronary artery disease not eligible for a second transplant.

An important observation emerging from these considerations is that there is no single device capable of rescuing all patients with severe heart failure. The optimal environment for implantation of mechanical circulatory support devices is at specialized cardiac care centers that have available a multidisciplinary team with expertise in the areas of mechanical assistance, heart transplantation, and investigational therapies for heart failure.

SUMMARY

A therapeutic approach that can arrest the progression of heart failure has not yet been identified. Similarly, a single treatment strategy that can benefit all patients with heart failure does not exist. In fact, the most valuable lesson imparted by the large clinical trials conducted since the late 1980s in patients with heart failure is that therapy for heart failure produces the greatest benefits when it is highly individualized. The expectation for the near future is that the range of therapeutic approaches will grow to include heart transplantation, mechanical and biologic assistance, and novel pharmacologic strategies. Mechanical assistance and new drugs may never entirely replace heart transplantation, but they may become more widely used options to improve the quality of life and the survival of patients who would otherwise die while waiting for a suitable donor heart, or those with co-morbidities that preclude heart transplantation. The future of patients with heart failure, therefore, is made brighter by the growing choices available for the treatment of this syndrome.

SELECTED REFERENCES

Argenziano M, Oz MC, Rose EA. The continuing evolution of mechanical ventricular assistance. *Curr Probl Surg* 1997;34:317–388.

Baker DW, Jones R, Hodges J, et al. Management of heart failure: III. the role of myocardial revascularization in the treatment of patients with moderate or severe left ventricular systolic dysfunction. *JAMA* 1994;272: 1528–1534.

CONSENSUS Trial Study Group. Effects of enalapril on mortality in severe congestive heart failure. *N Engl J Med* 1987;316:1429–1435.

Hoopes CW, Platt JF. Molecular strategies for clinical xenotransplantation in cardiothoracic surgery. *Semin Thorac Cardiovasc Surg* 1996;8: 156–174.

Magee JC, Platt JL. Xenograft rejection: molecular mechanisms and therapeutic implications. *Therapeutic Immunology* 1994;1:45–58.

Michler RE, Shah AS, Itescu S, et al. The influence of concordant xenografts on the humoral and cell-mediated immune responses to subsequent allografts in primates. *J Thorac Cardiovasc Surg* 1996;112: 1002–1009.

Mickleborough LL, Maruyama H, Takagi Y, et al. Results of revascularization in patients with severe left ventricular dysfunction. *Circulation* 1995;92[Suppl II]:73–79.

O'Connell JB, Bourge RC, Constanzo-Nordin MR, et al. Cardiac transplantation: recipient selection, donor procurement, and medical follow-up. *Circulation* 1992;86:1061–1079.

Shaw AS, Itescu S, O'Hair DP, et al. Importance of cell-mediated immune responses in rejection of concordant heart xenografts in primates. *Transplant Proc* 1996;28:775–776.

Starzl TE. Clinical xenotransplantation. *Xenotransplant* 1994;1:3–7.

Van Meter CH Jr, Claycomb WC, Delcarpio JB, et al. Myoblast transplantation in the porcine model: a potential technique for myocardial repair. *J Thorac Cardiovasc Surg* 1995;110:1442–1448.

Subject Index

263

hierarchy of, 144t
incidence of, 129
epidemiology of, 13
etiologies of, 129
exercise capacity in, 113–127
future health care for, 10–11
health care costs of, 3–6, 9
international, 5–6
hemodynamic parameters of, 136–137
hemodynamics of, 73–74
hospitalization for, 9
incidence and prevalence of, 53
by age and sex, 3, 4f
increasing, 3
ischemic
high-risk revascularization for, 149–150
transplantation for, 150
left ventricular dilatation in, 135
low serum sodium in, 135–136
management of, 22
managing persistent severe symptoms after
initial therapy for, 132f
mortality rates for, 25
new treatment strategies for, 9–10
number of hospital discharges with, 3
NYHA Class III, 136f
NYHA Class IV
actuarial survival in, 136f
evaluation for surgery, 138–139
symptoms of, 135
NYHA classifications of and exercise
capacity, 113–114
office-based treatment for, 9
optimal medical therapy for, 130–133
assessment after, 137–139
assessment before, 134–137
outpatient therapies for, 131t
positive inotropic agents for, 53–70
randomized, controlled, multicenter survival
trials in, 42–43t
readmission rates for, 3–5
reduction of elevated filling pressures of,
130–131
refractory
ACE inhibitors for, 40
hospitalization for, 48
severe
approach to, 39–52
clinic visit frequency for, 47
flexible diuretics in, 46–47
hospitalization for, 47–48
syndrome of, 53
treatment of
end-points for evaluation of, 25–35
evolution of, 73–88
history of, 73–74
surgical, 129–145, 231–238
ventricular rate and regularity control in, 110t
Heart Failure Functional Status Inventory,
34–35
The Heart (Hurst), 73
Heart transplantation. See also
Allotransplantation; Xenotransplantation
appropriateness of, 45
bridge to, 204–205
candidate evaluation for, 177–178
cost-benefit ratio of, 8
costs of, 182–183
compared with overall medical cost of
heart failure, 8
phases of, 8–9
postoperative, 9
preoperative, 9
demand for, 13–14

estimates of, 15–19
met, 14t, 18f
total, 14t, 18f, 19
unmet, 14t, 19f
diagnoses possibly indicating, 15t
donor criteria for, 178
downshifting risks of, 140
evaluation of candidates for, 137–139
future role of, 183, 260
graft atherosclerosis in, 181–182
historic perspective on, 177
immunosuppression and antibiotic
prophylaxis in, 178
improving outcomes and changing therapies
for, 144f
indications for, 145f
lymphoproliferative disorders after, 182
need for
total, 14t, 16f
unmet, 14t, 16, 17f
unrecognized, 14t, 16, 17f
need-demand-supply relationship for, 22f
outlook for candidates for, 140–143
peak oxygen consumption as selection
criterion for, 120–122
pediatric, indications for, 15t
projecting future of, 22–23
rejection of, 179–181
selection criteria for, 13
supply for
estimates of, 19–22
potential vs. actual, 14–15
survival rates for, 179–182
with and without, 141f
unrecognized need-met and unmet demand
relationship for, 21f
waiting list for, 17f
reported deaths on, 18f
HeartMate LVAD, 202–203, 221
surgical considerations of, 206–207
Hemodialysis, 50
Hemodynamically active drugs, 74
Hemodynamics
controlling derangement of, 50–52
in evaluation of advanced heart failure,
136–137
managing deterioration of, 144
monitoring of
invasive, 51
for severe heart failure patient, 49
six-month mortality related to, 49f
with treatment for heart failure, 28–30
Hemopump, 221–222
animal studies of, 222–223
anticoagulation with, 223
clinical studies of, 223
clinical trial results of, 223–224
complications of, 224
description of, 222
insertion techniques for, 223
selection criteria for, 223
Heparinization
during LVAD implantation, 210
in VAD implantation, 206–207
Hepatitis, 192
Herpesviruses, 192
Hexamethonium, 73
Hospitalization
with ACE inhibitors, 25–26
for advanced heart failure, 47–48
costs of, 9
with digoxin for heart failure, 27
rates of for heart failure by age, 40f
reduction of with ACE inhibitors, 6–7

with treatment for heart failure, 27–28
Human immunodeficiency virus (HIV),
191–192
Hydralazine
with ACE inhibitors, 131
for advanced heart failure, 39, 131t
for chronic heart failure, 130
clinical trials for, 42t
cost-effectiveness of, 7–8
functional capacity with, 31
for heart failure, 75t
in hemodynamic management, 51
Hydralazine-isosorbide dinitrate, 28
Hydralazine-nitrate, 30
Hyperkalemia, 50
Hypermagnesemia, 92
Hyperthyroidism, 46
Hypokalemia, arrhythmias with, 92
Hypomagnesemia, arrhythmias with, 92
Hypotension, symptomatic, 48
Hypothyroidism, 46

I
IABP. See Intraaortic balloon pump
Ibopamine
for advanced heart failure, 131t
for congestive heart failure, 62
Ibutilide
in heart failure, 93t
intravenous, 95
ICDs. See Implantable cardioverter-defibrillator
Immunoglobulin, in xenograft rejection, 187
Immunology
in xenografts, 190–191
xenotransplantation and, 186–191
Immunosuppression
for heart transplantation, 178
survival and after heart allotransplantation,
180f
in xenogeneic myocyte transplantation,
244–246
Implantable blood pumps, 257–258
Implantable cardioverter-defibrillator
in advanced heart failure treatment, 40
after cardiomyoplasty, 237
after ventriculectomy, 253–254
for arrhythmias in heart failure, 95–96
cost-effectiveness of, 9
for syncope, 102
for ventricular ectopic activity, 102–103
for ventricular fibrillation survivor, 101
for ventricular tachycardia, 98–99
Implantable devices. See also Blood pumps;
Left ventricular assist devices;
Ventricular assist devices
automatic, 131t, 143–144
long-term, 201–203
pulsatile
removal of, 207
surgical considerations of, 206–207
Infectious disease, 191–192
Influenza vaccines, prophylactic, 178
Inotropic agents. See also specific agents
acute decompensation with, 46
in advanced heart failure treatment, 40
chemical structures of, 59f
functional capacity with, 31
mechanisms of action of, 54–57
Class I, 57–64
Class II, 64–67
Class III, 68
Class IV, 68–70
positive
cardiac contraction and, 55–57